CANNABIS IS MEDICINE

*How Medical Cannabis and CBD Are Healing
Everything from Anxiety to Chronic Pain*

DR BONNI GOLDSTEIN

Copyright © 2020 Dr Bonni S. Goldstein

The right of Dr Bonni S. Goldstein to be identified as the Author of the Work has been asserted by her in accordance with the Copyright, Designs and Patents Act 1988.

First published in 2020 by Little, Brown Spark,
An imprint of Little, Brown and Company, a division of Hachette US Book Group, Inc.

First published in Great Britain in 2020 by HEADLINE HOME
an imprint of HEADLINE PUBLISHING GROUP

1

Apart from any use permitted under UK copyright law, this publication may only be reproduced, stored, or transmitted, in any form, or by any means, with prior permission in writing of the publishers or, in the case of reprographic production, in accordance with the terms of licences issued by the Copyright Licensing Agency.

Every effort has been made to fulfil requirements with regard to reproducing copyright material. The author and publisher will be glad to rectify any omissions at the earliest opportunity.

Cataloguing in Publication Data is available from the British Library

Trade paperback ISBN 978 1 4722 7662 9

Printed and bound in Great Britain by Clays Ltd, Elcograf S.p.A.

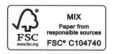

Headline's policy is to use papers that are natural, renewable and recyclable products and made from wood grown in well-managed forests and other controlled sources. The logging and manufacturing processes are expected to conform to the environmental regulations of the country of origin.

HEADLINE PUBLISHING GROUP
An Hachette UK Company
Carmelite House
50 Victoria Embankment
London EC4Y 0DZ

www.headline.co.uk
www.hachette.co.uk

For my family, who love and support me unconditionally.
And for my patients, who are the true pioneers
in the fight to use cannabis as medicine.

Contents

Author's Note: First, Do No Harm   ix

Introduction   3

How to Use This Book   5

PART I: The Science of Cannabis

Chapter 1:   The Cannabis Plant   9

Chapter 2:   The Endocannabinoid System   26

Chapter 3:   The Safety Profile of Cannabis   46

Chapter 4:   The Medicinal Effects of Phytocannabinoids: The Science Explained   58

Chapter 5:   How to Use Cannabis as Medicine   92

Chapter 6:   Medical Risks of Cannabis Use   136

PART II: Medical Symptoms and Conditions

Anxiety and Depression   155

Appetite Stimulation   161

Arthritis   164

Asthma   168

Attention Deficit Hyperactivity Disorder   169

Autism Spectrum Disorder   174

Contents

Autoimmune and Inflammatory Conditions ... 178

Cancer ... 183

Chronic Pain and Neuropathy ... 194

Diabetes ... 200

Epilepsy ... 203

Fibromyalgia ... 212

Gastrointestinal Disorders ... 216

Glaucoma ... 224

Infectious Diseases ... 226

Liver Disease and Hepatitis C ... 228

Migraine Headaches ... 231

Multiple Sclerosis ... 235

Neurodegenerative Disorders ... 238

Post-Traumatic Stress Disorder ... 249

Schizophrenia ... 253

Skin Disorders ... 256

Sleep Disorders ... 260

Spinal Cord Injury ... 264

Tourette Syndrome ... 267

Traumatic Brain Injury ... 270

Acknowledgments ... 275

Appendix A: The History of Cannabis ... 277

Appendix B: The Pharmacokinetics of Phytocannabinoids ... 285

Appendix C: Phytocannabinoids and Their Effects ... 289

Appendix D: Terpenoids and Their Effects ... 295

Notes ... 303

Index ... 345

Author's Note

First, Do No Harm

I don't recall exactly when I learned my mother had suffered from seizures. I think I was in high school when she finally talked to me about her medical history, and while there had always been intimations, I felt shocked to hear about it. When I look back on my childhood, I see clues, despite her keeping it a secret from just about everyone.

My mother didn't drive when I was a little girl growing up in Brooklyn. Because there was an abundance of public transportation, it didn't seem that strange, and most of my friends' mothers didn't drive either. When we moved to the suburbs in New Jersey, I noticed that my mother was the only one who didn't drive. We never talked about it, and eventually my mother did get her driver's license, but it was many years before I learned the real reason she didn't have one in the early part of my childhood.

At about the same time that I began dreaming about being a doctor, I became aware that my mother took medications every night. Two big prescription bottles sat in the upper cabinet next to the kitchen sink, and whenever I asked about them, she gave a vague answer. I remember getting a sense that this wasn't something she wanted to talk about, so I stopped asking. A few years later, when I was a teenager, I was standing next to her by the kitchen cabinet where the medicine bottles were kept and again asked her about her medications, completely unaware of the story she finally decided to share.

That day she told me that when my sister was two years old and I was just an infant, she had her first grand mal seizure in a Brooklyn playground, followed by two more seizures over the next few days. She eventually went to see a neurologist, and while she was in his office she had another seizure. She was hospitalized and immediately, she, my father, my grandmother, and my uncles were told that she might die. Diagnostic studies of the brain in the early 1960s were quite limited, and the doctors did not know what was causing the seizures. Started on phenytoin (Dilantin) and phenobarbital, she responded positively and was told to continue taking them for the rest of her life.

My grandmother, an uneducated and superstitious immigrant, was in complete denial that my mother had epilepsy. She was terrified and embarrassed at the same time. Because of this, my parents became tight-lipped about what had happened. It just was not discussed or shared with anyone.

I learned much later that even though the medications stopped her seizures, the side effects were difficult to tolerate. She became excessively hirsute and had significant lethargy and fatigue, making the care of two small children particularly challenging. She also had severe gingival hypertrophy, an overgrowth of gum tissue and a common side effect of phenytoin, which led to a lifetime of problems with her gums that still continue. I recall being in middle school and finding out that my mother had to have oral surgery for a terrible problem she was having with her gums. She stayed in bed for days with severe pain after the procedure. I can still see her there with ice on her swollen cheeks, black-and-blue, unable to talk or eat. Little did I know at the time that this was a result of her seizure medication.

After my sisters and I graduated from high school, my mother decided that she just couldn't tolerate the side effects of the medication any longer and that she was finished with it. She didn't consult her doctor or even gradually wean herself off the drugs but rather just stopped taking them. Fortunately, she experienced no repercussions from this arguably risky decision and remains seizure-free today. Meanwhile, I continued to pursue my medical degree and eventually became a doctor, working primarily in pediatric emergency medicine and urgent care. I loved my work, saving lives at the county hospital and teaching medical students and residents, but once I had my son, things changed. I had thought I could manage working nights and being with my son during the days, but after a few years, it grew more and more difficult, as I didn't feel truly present when home with my family. I was a very good pediatric ER doctor, but my frustrations from the exhaustion of night work and trying to be a caring physician in a broken system eventually wore me down.

After I took a leave of absence, a sick friend asked me about medical cannabis, putting it on my radar for the first time. Once I started reading the scientific literature, I grew incredulous that despite the discovery of the endocannabinoid system, the most widespread receptor system in the human brain, and my years of science-based education and medical training, I knew absolutely nothing about cannabis and how it works. Intrigued, I continued to read and study everything I could find about cannabis and soon decided to work part-time in a local medical cannabis clinic. I was surprised to find that the patients I met were just everyday people who went to work, had families, and had medical conditions that were not responding to conventional medications or traditional Western medical interventions. These were people who simply wanted a better quality of life.

I haven't looked back since.

Cannabis was not medically available or used as an anticonvulsant during the years my mother took antiseizure medications. In 1970, five years into her epilepsy diagnosis and treatment, the federal government classified cannabis as a Schedule I controlled substance with the passage of the Controlled Substances Act. Defined as a "drug or other substance that has a high potential for abuse, has no currently accepted medical use in treatment in the United States, and is lacking accepted safety for use of the drug or other substance under medical supervision," cannabis maintains its Schedule I classification to this day. This has virtually shut down all research on the multitude of compounds in cannabis that we now know have low risk for abuse, true and proven medical use, and an excellent safety profile, especially with medical supervision. Scientists had started significant cannabis research in the 1960s and were gaining knowledge of the phytocannabinoids, but this act by Congress completely closed the door on advancing cannabinoid science. After the discovery of the endo-cannabinoid system in the late 1980s, investigations in the field have exploded, especially in the last decade and mostly outside the US.

I am angry that my mother suffered, and continues to suffer, from the side effects of medications she took to alleviate her epilepsy. My mother's suffering was in part due to the propagation of false claims about canna-bis, claims based on ignorance and greed. The false claims persist, despite the fact that millions of patients who could be helped by cannabis con-tinue to suffer with medical conditions that are not responding to con-ventional treatments, and millions more grapple with intolerable side effects of those treatments. As a physician, I took an oath to "do no harm." After treating thousands of patients with medical cannabis, I can assert that the compounds in cannabis relieve unnecessary suffering with few or no adverse side effects.

I have witnessed sick and desperate patients have a complete turn-around in the quality of their lives. Cannabis medicine must be available as an option or alternative to current first-line treatments, especially if those treatments have harmful or potentially fatal side effects. If a phar-maceutical with the properties of cannabis were synthetically created and introduced today, the medical community would embrace it with open arms and tout it as a miracle drug.

It's been over fifty years since my mother developed epilepsy when I was a small child, and I get emotional thinking about her needless suffer-ing. Many physicians find their vocation from early experiences with ill relatives and friends. While I had little awareness of my mother's strug-gles with seizures and medications, I find that her life and experience have indeed informed mine. I wish medical cannabis had been available to my mother. I cannot undo what she endured. I can help others, though, by sharing the current knowledge about cannabis and cannabi-noid science. I have written this book so you and your loved ones, who may be suffering as my mother did, can move past the false propaganda that continues to this day and understand how **cannabis is medicine**.

CANNABIS
IS
MEDICINE

Introduction

Written by my patient Elise, as told to me in February of 2016, and whose story appears in chapter 5:

As a little girl, whenever I was alone—outside digging in the dirt or absentmindedly swinging on the swing set, splashing or playing in the bathtub—I would start humming a tune. I'd start softly and then grow bolder, add in little trills and jazzy riffs, each note a bit louder than the next. As I got older, I'd experiment with dropping my voice down to get to the lower notes and more dramatic effects. I had been exposed to singers like Judy Garland, Billie Holiday, Frank Sinatra, and Nat King Cole, and then to songwriter-artists like Joni Mitchell, Bob Dylan, and Carole King. I listened to James Taylor, Cat Stevens, and '60s Motown, and I recall at age twelve or thirteen thinking that Phoebe Snow was the ultimate in cool. Singing brought me freedom and joy, always, or at least until the pain started and I was diagnosed with rheumatoid arthritis. Over those years and the many that followed, in my late teens and early twenties, I didn't do that much singing, but on the occasions when I did, singing was one of the few things I could do to forget almost completely the way my body felt. During those moments, I tasted a little bit of freedom and was released from the pain and the loss of everything I used to be—all of my former life—even for a few minutes. I have noticed lately, though, that during the process of taking my cannabis medicine that I am humming again, albeit weakly with little breath or power. The humming grows stronger as I feel the medicine through my system, and I find myself adding jazzy riffs right and left, treating my voice like a slide trombone. I can go mournfully low and tragic like Billie and then trill upwards sweet and high like Ella. I imagine myself as sultry and sassy, as confident as Peggy Lee. It's as if cannabis has helped me to unlock the box in which I've kept my own personal songbird. This may be a small thing, but if anyone knows how it feels to be trapped in a constantly malfunctioning body, they would realize what an enormous gift it is to feel well, to feel strong and capable at something again for the first time in over a decade. I was locked in a prison of illness and pain, and cannabis unlocked the door for me to break free.

How to Use This Book

I have spent the last decade educating and explaining medical cannabis to patients, politicians, and medical professionals. In order to understand how cannabis can do all that it is advertised to do, you must first understand the plant itself. In the first part of this book, chapter 1 discusses the many different compounds that make up the cannabis plant. Chapter 2 explains our endocannabinoid system, its purpose, and how it interacts with the compounds found in cannabis. Diseases associated with an imbalance of the endocannabinoid system are also discussed. The safety of cannabis use is discussed in chapter 3. Chapter 4 delves deeply into the science of the various medicinal compounds found in the cannabis plant, reviewing the latest research of how and why they are effective. Chapter 5 gets into how to use cannabis as medicine, including how to read labels, ratios versus concentrations, and dosing. Special considerations for certain conditions and populations are discussed in chapter 6. Part II details a multitude of ailments in which cannabinoid medicine may play an important role.

Interspersed throughout the book are incredible stories of patients who have had success with using cannabis medicine. These patients were able to overcome medical conditions that were negatively affecting their quality of life, and they were all so eager to share their journey that led them to cannabis treatment. (Note that the names of some of the patients who shared their stories have been changed to protect their privacy.)

The appendixes include a time line of the history of cannabis as well as information on the pharmacokinetics of cannabis medicines, discussing the absorption, metabolism, and excretion of cannabinoids. Facts about the phytocannabinoids and terpenoids are listed in two charts that readers can use as references.

This book is not meant to give specific medical advice for your particular condition, as the use of cannabis medicine is not "one size fits all." Each person has their own goals of treatment and will respond uniquely to the many options within the cannabis medicine armamentarium. **The goal of this book is to help you understand if cannabis may be an option for you or your loved one.** The latest scientific information is presented in addition to my clinical experience with patients; however, research on cannabis is still severely restricted, leaving us with many unanswered questions. Please consult your physician before starting a cannabis regimen.

PART I

The Science of Cannabis

CHAPTER 1

The Cannabis Plant

In order to understand the medicinal value of the cannabis plant, you first need to learn about the many compounds found within it. The cannabis plant is dioecious (meaning it has male and female plants) and is made up of more than five hundred different chemical compounds.[1] When taking cannabis as medicine, you are by definition taking a mixture of many natural compounds that work together in balance with one another. In contrast, pharmaceutical medications routinely contain only one active compound.

The Latin name of the plant is *Cannabis sativa,* in the family called Cannabaceae. Other plants in this family are *Humulus* (hops) and *Celtis* (hackberries). These plants share an evolutionary origin but are quite different from one another. **The cannabis plant contains biologically active compounds called phytocannabinoids, terpenoids, and flavonoids.** These chemicals interact with the brain and body chemistry, causing certain effects. Hundreds of different cannabis varieties are grown all over the world, each containing varying amounts of the more than five hundred different compounds. Some varieties may have more or less of certain cannabinoids or terpenoids; it is these differences that cause the various medicinal effects. Contrary to popular vernacular, plants do not have "strains." We call the different varieties or types of cannabis "chemovars," which is short for "chemical varieties."

What Are Phytocannabinoids?

The term "cannabinoids" is very general and refers to a group of chemical compounds that are typically made up of twenty-one carbon atoms in a three-ring structure. The prefix "phyto" added to the word refers to the cannabinoids that are found exclusively in the cannabis plant. The two predominant and most studied phytocannabinoids are THC (delta-9-tetrahydrocannabinol) and CBD (cannabidiol). Approximately 140 phyto-cannabinoids have now been identified, and likely more will be discovered; however, only a few have been researched significantly.

Other phytocannabinoids found in the cannabis plant, often referred to as "minor" or "secondary" cannabinoids, include cannabinol (CBN), cannabigerol (CBG), cannabichromene (CBC), cannabicyclol (CBL), cannabivarin (CBV), cannabidivarin (CBDV), and tetrahydrocannabi-

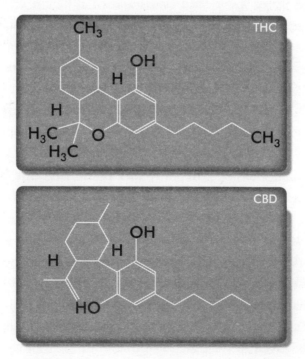

Molecular structures of THC and CBD.

varin (THCV). The medicinal effects of the most commonly used phyto-cannabinoids are reviewed in detail in chapter 4.

A Few Important Notes About Phytocannabinoids

- Phytocannabinoids were initially thought to be species-specific to the cannabis plant, which means they are not found in any other plant species. However, phytocannabinoids other than THC have been discovered in a few other plants, namely those from the genera *Echinacea, Helichrysum* (sunflowers), and *Radula* (liverworts).
- As mentioned, the term "cannabinoids" is very general, and it refers to a specific group of chemical compounds. Cannabinoids are found naturally in two places: plants and animals, including humans. "Phytocannabinoids" refers specifically to the cannabinoids that occur naturally in plants. "Endocannabinoids" refers specifically to the cannabinoids made by cells in humans and other animals. Cannabinoids can also be synthesized in a laboratory setting; these are referred to as "synthetic cannabinoids" and are primarily used in research.
- Do not get confused by the acronym "CBD." CBD stands for the phytocannabinoid "cannabidiol," not "cannabinoids." Many people incorrectly say "the CBDs," but CBD is not plural. THC is not referred to as "THCs" because it is one compound. CBD also is one compound.

How the Cannabis Plant Makes Phytocannabinoids

Phytocannabinoids are synthesized and concentrated in a viscous resin in an unfertilized female plant's glandular trichomes, which are tiny, sticky hairlike formations on the cannabis flowers.

When the cannabis plant synthesizes phytocannabinoids, geranyl diphosphate—the precursor to both phytocannabinoids and terpenoids—couples with olivetolic acid to produce cannabigerolic acid, which is then exposed to three enzymes: THCA synthase, which creates THCA; CBDA synthase, which creates CBDA; and CBCA synthase, which creates CBCA.

THCA and CBDA are the predominant phytocannabinoid compounds in the raw flowers of the cannabis plant and are the precursor

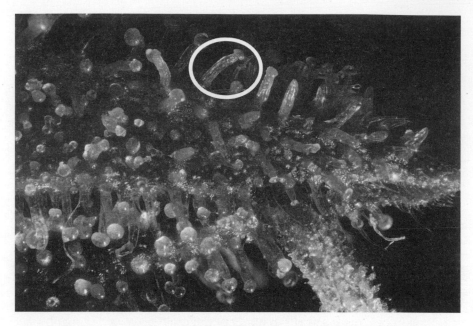

Trichome of female cannabis flower (circled).

compounds to THC and CBD, respectively. THCA and CBDA convert to THC and CBD, respectively, when they are exposed to heat. This chemical reaction is called "decarboxylation."

One way different types of cannabis plants are categorized is based on the genetically determined expression of the chemical composition of the phyto-cannabinoids, often called the "chemical phenotype," or "chemotype."

- *Type I:* High THC content and low CBD content; often called "drug-variety" (more than 0.3 percent THC by weight)
- *Type II:* Roughly equal THC and CBD content
- *Type III:* Dominant CBD; can be fiber-variety (less than 0.3 per-cent THC by weight) or drug-variety
- *Type IV:* Dominant CBG (cannabigerol) content
- *Type V:* No detectable phytocannabinoids

The majority of medicinal cannabis plants are genetically Type I and thus take the pathway that leads to THCA and ultimately THC. A small

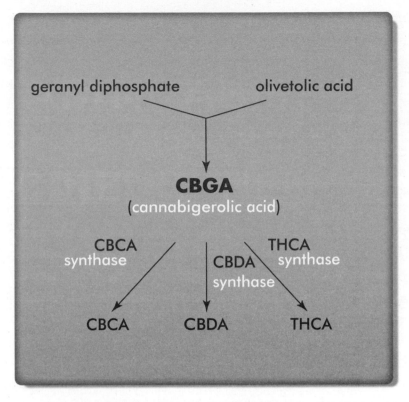

How the cannabis plant synthesizes phytocannabinoids.

number of plants are Type II, meaning they have genetics that will lead to a higher amount of CBDA; we call these plants CBD-rich chemovars. The genetic dominance for THC explains why most drug-variety plants are higher in THC potency and lower in CBD potency. The rampant cross-breeding of chemovars over the past few decades has also promoted higher THC content. The average THC content of cannabis confiscated by law enforcement in 1972 was 1 percent, increasing to 4 percent in the 1990s, to a national average of 17 percent as of 2017.[2] THC-rich cannabis flowers currently available in California dispensaries have THC content between 15 and 28 percent, with a corresponding CBD content of less than 1 percent. Concentrated forms of THC-rich cannabis (such as hashish) can be as high as 90 percent potency. The increase in THC content has led to a decrease in CBD content, and at one point it was thought that CBD-rich plants might no longer exist. However, the popularity and increased demand for CBD in the past decade has led to the stabilization of Type II plant genetics, leading in turn to the increased availability of CBD-dominant cannabis products.

Type I and Type II are what we call "medical marijuana" or "medical cannabis" and are available through state-regulated dispensaries. Type III is either medical cannabis with high CBD content or fiber-variety "hemp" products that have become very popular in recent years. The concern with hemp products is that they remain unregulated and the CBD content claimed on labels is frequently incorrect. (More on this to follow.)

The Entourage Effect

Of the 140 known phytocannabinoids, only a few have been thoroughly studied. Each of these phytocannabinoids, when isolated in a lab, has been shown to possess its own array of medicinal properties. However, when taken together as they occur naturally in the whole plant, they balance one another in a synergistic action first called "the entourage effect" by Israeli researcher Raphael Mechoulam, who was the first to isolate THC and CBD in the early 1960s. **The entourage effect means that the cannabinoids work better together than when isolated from one another. This synergy can enhance or modulate effects beneficially.**[3]

As an example of synergistic enhancement, both THC and CBD, when taken separately, have been found to provide pain relief, but studies show that CBD enhances pain relief when used in conjunction with THC, compared to THC used by itself.

As an example of opposing effects, CBD may decrease some of the intoxication, memory loss, and increased heart rate THC can induce.[4]

What Are Terpenoids?

Terpenoids—also called "terpenes"—are the essential oils that occur naturally and exist in all plants, including the cannabis plant. More than twenty thousand terpenes have been described, of which about two hundred occur in cannabis.[5] These oils give cannabis its odor, color, and flavor. They have evolved within the cannabis plant as a defense mechanism against insects, bacteria, fungi, and other plant predators. Terpenoids can be categorized by how many carbon units they contain: monoterpenes (10 carbons), sesquiterpenes (15 carbons), diterpenes (20 carbons), and triterpenes (30 carbons).

Some Important Facts About Terpenoids

- Terpenoids are genetically controlled.
- Production increases with light exposure.
- Production decreases as soil fertility decreases.
- The US Food and Drug Administration recognizes terpenoids as safe.
- Terpenoids vaporize near the same temperature as THC.
- Concentrating cannabis into hash or wax may reduce the terpene content and may cause medicinal effects to change.
- The terpenoid profile of any cannabis plant can be determined by laboratory analysis.

Terpenoids are known to be biologically active, just like phytocannabinoids, interacting with human cells, neurotransmitter receptors, and other parts of human physiology.[6] The unique combination of phytocannabinoids and terpenoids in a specific cannabis plant accounts for the varying effects felt when different types of cannabis plants are used. Most importantly, phytocannabinoids and terpenoids work synergistically to provide certain therapeutic effects. Terpenoids are also synergistic with each other, again enhancing their medicinal effects.

An example of a prominent cannabis terpenoid is limonene. It is a monoterpene found in lemon and other citrus fruits, and is the second most common terpenoid found in nature. Limonene has potent antidepressant and antianxiety activity as well as anticancer effects.[7] It also has been used successfully to decrease the symptoms of gastroesophageal reflux.[8]

Table 1 shows four of the most important terpenoids in the cannabis plant, including other plants where they are found, known medicinal effects, and aroma. (Please refer to the terpenoid chart in appendix D for a full list of the clinically important terpenoids.)

Table 1

Terpenoid	Also found in	Medicinal effects	Aroma
Limonene	Caraway seeds	Analgesic	Citrus
	Citrus rinds	Antianxiety	Orange
	Dill seeds	Anticancer	Spicy
	Juniper berries	Antidepressant	
	Peppermint	Anti-inflammatory	
	Rosemary	Antioxidant	
		Bronchodilator	
		GERD suppressant	
Beta-caryophyllene	Basil	Analgesic	Spicy
	Black pepper	Antibacterial	Woodsy
	Cinnamon	Anticancer	
	Cloves	Antifungal	
	Hops	Anti-inflammatory	
	Lavender	Anti-itching	
	Oregano	Antimalarial	
	Rosemary	Gastrointestinal relief	
		May reduce alcohol intake	
Alpha-pinene	Basil	Analgesic	Pine
	Dill	Anti-inflammatory	"Skunky"
	Eucalyptus	Bronchodilator	
	Parsley	Increases focus and alertness	
	Pine trees		
	Rosemary	Increases permeability of blood–brain barrier	
	Sage	Reduces THC-induced memory loss	
Linalool	Birch trees	Active against acne bacteria	Citrus
	Citrus	Analgesic	Floral
	Coriander	Antianxiety	Spicy
	Lavender	Antibacterial/antifungal	
	Rosewood	Anticonvulsant	
		Antidepressant	
		Anti-inflammatory	
		Antimalarial	

Terpenoid	Also found in	Medicinal effects	Aroma
Myrcene	Bay leaves	Analgesic	Clove
	Eucalyptus	Antianxiety	Earthy
	Hops	Antibacterial	Fruity
	Lemongrass	Anticancer	
	Mangoes	Antidepressant	
	Parsley	Anti-inflammatory	
	Wild thyme	Antioxidant	
		Muscle relaxant	
		Sedating/hypnotic	

The following are some examples of known synergies between phyto-cannabinoids and terpenoids for specific conditions. Patients often choose their products based on these synergies. Knowing the specific makeup of each product is necessary for patients to find what works best.

- *Pain relief:* THC+CBD + beta-myrcene + beta-caryophyllene
- *ADD/ADHD:* THC + beta-myrcene + beta-caryophyllene + pinene
- *Anxiety:* CBD + limonene + linalool
- *Depression:* THC+CBD+CBG + limonene
- *Insomnia:* THC + linalool + myrcene
- *Inflammation:* CBD+CBG + beta-caryophyllene

Cannabis plants can be tested for their terpenoid profiles as well as phytocannabinoid content. The terpenoid makeup of the plant is like a fingerprint for the chemovar. Different growers may be growing the same chemovars but calling them different names, or they may be calling chemovars the same names yet terpenoid testing reveals they are different. The terpenoid profile allows for detailed comparisons of chemovars and is very important to patients who find relief with one particular chemovar. If you know which terpenoids and terpenoid combinations are helpful for your condition, you can check terpenoid testing results to see if a certain product is likely to be effective.

What Are Flavonoids?

Flavonoids are compounds that give plants their pigmentation, filter ultraviolet rays, attract pollinators, and prevent plant disease. They exist in fruits, vegetables, and flowers. More than five thousand flavonoids occur in nature; approximately twenty are found in the cannabis plant. These compounds are classified as aromatic polycyclic phenols and are made up of 15 carbon atoms. The total content of flavonoids in a cannabis plant's flowers and leaves can reach 2 to 2.5 percent of its dry weight.

Flavonoids have been shown in laboratory studies to have anti-inflammatory and antioxidant properties.[9] They also have antifungal, antibacterial, antiviral, anticancer, and antiallergic activity. Several studies in humans report the following benefits of flavonoids:

- Flavonoids in green tea decreased the risk of gastric cancer in women.[10]
- An intake of flavonoids was protective against smoking-related cancers.[11]
- Dietary flavonoids (anthocyanins from berries and flavonols from green tea and cocoa) may lower the risk of type 2 diabetes and cardiovascular disease.[12]

Flavonoids are reported to be synergistic with both phytocannabinoids and terpenes, enhancing and modulating the medicinal effects. Prominent flavonoids found in the cannabis plant include:

Quercetin
- Potent antioxidant, antiviral, anticancer
- Also found in red wine, green tea, berries, onions

Apigenin
- Anti-inflammatory, antianxiety
- Also found in parsley, celery, chamomile tea, celeriac

Cannaflavins A and B
- Potent anti-inflammatory
- Unique to cannabis

Flavonoids contribute to the entourage effect, synergizing with phytocannabinoids and terpenoids to enhance medicinal benefits. For instance, in a rat model of neuropathic pain, a cannabis extract containing phytocannabinoids, terpenoids, and flavonoids was more effective at relieving pain than an extract with the same phytocannabinoids without the terpenoids and flavonoids.[13]

Sativa or Indica?

You may have noticed I have not mentioned the terms "sativa" and "indica" in the discussion of the plant. According to the correct scientific nomenclature, cannabis variety *sativa* refers to the fiber-type plant, so-called hemp, meaning the genetics of this particular plant promote the growth of fiber with very little THC production.[14] These fiber types also carry the gene that allows the plant to synthesize a small amount of CBD with very little or no THC. Cannabis variety *indica* scientifically refers to the drug-type plant, so-called marijuana, which carries the genetics to synthesize THC.

The current use of the terms "indica" and "sativa" completely ignores this scientifically correct nomenclature. These terms have been hijacked to indicate certain effects, namely that sativa chemovars are "uplifting and stimulating" and indica chemovars are "relaxing and sedating." These terms are not correct and oversimplify the complexity of the different chemovars, leading patients to try products that may not be effective.

Knowing the cannabinoid and terpenoid profile of a plant or product is a much better way to understand what its effects will be rather than knowing whether it is reported to be indica or sativa. For example, THC-rich chemovars with significant amounts of the terpenoid myrcene are quite sedating and are employed by many people to treat insomnia. Chemovars with higher amounts of limonene tend to have uplifting, antidepressant effects. Chemovars with higher amounts of linalool tend to have relaxing, antianxiety effects. Since cannabis plants are commonly crossbred and hybridized, it is difficult to know the cannabinoid and terpenoid profile without laboratory analysis. Fortunately, most states with cannabis regulations require laboratory analysis of products, allowing the patient to assess potential effects prior to use. If the terpenoid profile is not listed on a product, I recommend contacting the manufacturer and asking for the terpenoid profile reported on the lab analysis, called the Certificate of Analysis, or COA. In my experience, companies that are serious about their products share these results freely.

Interestingly, many patients who are inhaling flowers through vaporization learn to associate the smell of particular chemovars with their effects. One of my earliest patients was a young woman with severe depression. When we first met, she had already found success for her condition with cannabis, but she wanted to be part of California's legal system rather than buy cannabis on the underground market. When I asked her what chemovars helped her, she reported that she would smell the flowers and if they smelled citrusy or fruity, she knew they would be effective for her depression. She was smelling the terpenoid limonene.

The best way to determine the effects of a particular chemovar or product is to first evaluate the content of phytocannabinoids, calculate the ratio of CBD to THC if appropriate, and then look at the dominant terpenoids. This assessment will give significantly more information than the incorrect terms "sativa" and "indica."

Chemovar Names

Aside from their genetics, cannabis plants are living entities that respond to their environment. Growing conditions, harvesttime, and numerous other factors play an enormous role in the makeup of the final product. This is why the same chemovar grown in different places by different growers under different conditions can and likely will result in different phytocannabinoid and terpenoid content. For instance, a chemovar grown outdoors in Northern California is likely to have a different profile than the same chemovar grown in a greenhouse in Colorado. Patients who find a certain chemovar to be helpful must be aware that a similarly named chemovar may not have the same effects if it was grown under different cultivation conditions.

Hemp-Derived CBD

Among the five different types of cannabis, Type III fiber type, which is called "agricultural hemp" or "industrial hemp," has gained enormous popularity, as it is a "legal" source of CBD through the 2014 Farm Bill, which put hemp back on the map after eight decades of cannabis prohibition.

Many products made from hemp claim to contain CBD for medicinal purposes. Patients and caregivers continually report confusion when looking for CBD hemp products in stores and online, and rightly so. These products are completely unregulated and still should be considered "buyer beware." In 2015, the FDA tested a number of products claiming to contain CBD, and almost all of them lacked CBD or had amounts significantly lower than what was reported on the label. An additional problem with products made from hemp is possible contamination. This plant is a bioaccumulator, which means it accumulates toxic substances from the soil. If the soil is contaminated, for instance with metals, pesticides, gasoline, or solvents, these compounds can be pulled up into the plant. During the CBD extraction process, contaminants may be concentrated and may cause toxic side effects in the consumer. In fact, there are anecdotal reports of people becoming ill from so-called CBD products made from contaminated industrial hemp.

What is the difference between hemp and cannabis in terms of treating medical conditions? As Martin Lee from the organization Project CBD explains, the main difference between fiber-type and drug-type varieties is the content of resin, the sticky substance in the trichomes where the phytocannabinoids, terpenoids, and flavonoids are synthesized. High-resin plants contain a robust amount of these desired medicinal compounds. Hemp is low-resin and therefore typically quite low in phytocannabinoid content. Hemp is not an optimal source of CBD or other medicinal compounds. High-resin drug-type plants are much preferred as medicine when compared to low-resin hemp.[15]

But there is more to this story. The US government has inappropriately and narrowly defined industrial hemp as containing less than 0.3 percent THC by weight with no regard for the genetics of the plant. The vast majority of high-resin plants, including those that are CBD dominant, contain over 0.3 percent THC by weight and therefore are easy to identify as drug-variety cannabis. However, some cultivators are now growing high-resin CBD-dominant drug-type plants that are low enough in THC (under 0.3 percent THC by weight) that they meet the government's narrow definition of hemp. Although these plants are genetically drug-type cannabis and are high-resin, they can be sold online or outside a medical cannabis regulatory framework due to the low THC and are often mislabeled as hemp. I call these products "drug-type cannabis masquerading as hemp." Companies are incentivized to do this in order to have their sales not restricted to state-approved patients, to avoid the issue of federal illegality, and to avoid the cost and effort of complying with strict state cannabis product regulations.

How does one tell if a product is from a drug-type CBD-dominant plant or from a fiber-type hemp plant? The only reliable way to know is to check the Certificate of Analysis (COA), the report obtained from analytical testing. The COA should include cannabinoid and terpenoid content as well as the results of tests for mold, bacteria, pesticides, and residual solvents. All products sold in state-licensed cannabis dispensaries are required to have a COA available to patients and consumers. Whenever possible, products should be purchased at licensed dispensaries. If you are purchasing products online or from a non-dispensary retail store, ask for the COA. If they do not have a COA or refuse to share it, do not purchase the product. (Chapter 5 has more information about how to interpret a COA report.)

I encourage my patients to avoid products that come from fiber-variety hemp, as clinically I have found that drug-type cannabis is significantly more effective when treating most illnesses. However, as mentioned, there are quality products masquerading as hemp that are actually made from CBD-rich drug-variety plants with less than 0.3 percent THC. The COA of these products will show a diversity of cannabinoids and terpenoids, allowing patients to recognize that these are not true hemp.

———

Gavin's Story

Gavin was one of the first pediatric patients I treated with cannabis and I shared his story in my previous book, *Cannabis Revealed*. He has been on cannabinoid treatment for six years with incredible improvement in the quality of his life. Here is his original story with an update.

> *I sensed true desperation almost immediately when I met with four-year-old Gavin and his family. The despair was nearly palpable, even in Gavin's two grandmothers, who had accompanied the family to the office. Gavin himself appeared oblivious to his surroundings, made little eye contact, and was very hyperactive and distracted, moving around the office the entire time. He was a cute child, wearing a little fedora and glasses, but his face showed little emotion and we made no connection. "We need help so badly," the family said to me. "We can no longer live like this."*
>
> *Rebecca is a stay-at-home mother with a special-education degree whose first child, Gavin, was born six weeks early. While he had low*

muscle tone, something you'd expect from a preemie, he also didn't reach his early milestones, and at around age two Gavin's health and development began to fall apart. He was nearly two by the time he learned to walk, and at age three he was almost completely nonverbal. Ultimately diagnosed with complex partial seizures, cerebral palsy, and an unknown genetic anomaly, as well as cyclical vomiting and autism, Gavin was prescribed the anticonvulsant Keppra (levetiracetam) for his seizures. While the seizures stopped, Gavin's autistic behaviors increased, and within two months his meltdowns became uncontrollable. Rebecca and her husband had read online about "Keppra rage," a difficult side effect of this medication, and although they were happy that the seizures were controlled, the continuous and worsening behavioral issues became unacceptable. During this time, Rebecca saw the CNN documentary Weed and began to explore cannabis as a possible treatment. When she asked Gavin's neurologist about trying cannabis, he ignorantly told her, "The tar in the smoke will give him lung cancer." She was discouraged by this response but kept searching online for information and found support on Facebook. She eventually brought Gavin to my office in early 2014. With his behavior out of control, life with Gavin had become a daily struggle.

I started Gavin on CBD-rich cannabis oil, given by mouth. The effects were immediate. Within ten days, Gavin, previously nonverbal, began speaking. The change was so dramatic that Rebecca wanted to try weaning him off the Keppra to see if his seizures might also be controlled. She switched neurologists and found a supportive physician who helped her to wean Gavin off the Keppra over five months. When he was completely off the drug, an initial EEG showed some seizure activity, but Rebecca asked for three months to adjust the dosage of CBD before trying other pharmaceuticals. The subsequent forty-eight-hour EEG showed no seizure activity, and Gavin hasn't needed any further antiepileptic medications.

Although the use of CBD-rich oil for a number of months resulted in seizure freedom, improved verbal ability, and improved behavior, Gavin continued to have some unwanted behaviors related to his autism. It was at this point that we added THC-rich oil twice a day to the CBD. As we'd hoped, his behavior improved significantly.

Rebecca still marvels at the dramatic turnaround in Gavin due to cannabis medicine. In addition to seizure control, Gavin's incredible improvements in speech and autistic behaviors thrill her the most. Although everyone who knew Gavin saw that he was quite intelligent (even the speech pathologist had given him an iPad with communication apps because they knew of his capabilities), he previously had no real language or any imaginary play. One afternoon soon after Gavin began taking CBD oil, Rebecca was in her bedroom folding laundry. She looked up to see Gavin walking in with the laundry basket. He placed it on the floor, stepped into it, and declared, "Look, Mom! I'm an astronaut!"

Gavin has had no adverse side effects from cannabis use. He has not experienced any intoxicating effects. He is able to make connections with peers, and he transitions from activity to activity throughout the day with ease. He is happy and thriving, and reports from school are outstanding. Gavin's story moves me as both a physician and a mother. Although not every patient experiences this level of improvement, Gavin is an example of why cannabis treatment must be an available option for all children with challenging medical conditions. His quality of life has been improved so significantly that he is able to participate in his life fully as all children deserve.

Update: *Gavin continues to thrive in school and at home. Over the years, he has had a few breakthrough seizures, and he also has had bouts with cyclical vomiting syndrome (a condition similar to migraines), but he bounces back quickly and has had no developmental regression. His family continues to be amazed at just how well he is doing. His only medicine is cannabis.*

CHAPTER 2

The Endocannabinoid System

To those who don't "believe" in cannabis as medicine, I ask, "Do you know about the endocannabinoid system and what medical conditions are associated with its dysfunction?" If they cannot answer this question, they are not knowledgeable enough to comment on cannabis as medicine. I joke with my patients that I have no opinion about my car's engine, but my husband has many thoughts on it. I know nothing about car engines (nor am I interested), but my husband knows a lot. I am not qualified to make any statements about which engine is good or bad. Likewise, if you don't know about the endocannabinoid system, you are not qualified to have an opinion about cannabis as medicine until you educate yourself! I also joke that the medical use of cannabis is not a religion to believe in (unless you are Rastafarian) but based in science. Once you understand the science behind the use of medicinal cannabis, belief is irrelevant.

Here is just about everything you need to know about the endocannabinoid system: In 1964, Dr. Raphael Mechoulam and his colleagues at the Hebrew University of Jerusalem were interested in studying plants with reported medicinal effects.[1] They isolated THC from the cannabis plant and found it to be responsible for the plant's intoxicating effects. It took another twenty-four years to understand how and where THC worked in the human brain and body. In 1988, Dr. Allyn Howlett and her colleagues at Saint Louis University Medical School discovered the first cannabinoid receptor. Using advanced scientific techniques with radioactive dye attached to synthetic THC, the researchers were able to trace the path of THC to find where it worked.[2] They saw that it selectively attached to a specific receptor—previously called an "orphan" receptor because no one knew its function—located on the membranes of certain cells. A receptor works like a "lock" on the cell membrane, waiting for a specific "key" to bind to it. When the chemical key binds to the receptor, it triggers a chemical reaction in the cell, resulting in a change in the message that the cell is sending. We have other lock-and-key receptor systems in our brains and bodies, such as endorphins that bind to opioid receptors, dopamine that binds to dopamine receptors, and many others. The cannabinoid receptor happened to be discovered in the quest to understand how THC works to make people intoxicated.

Scientists hypothesized that we do not have these receptors for the THC key from the plant but rather we must make our own cannabis-like key that works at the receptor site. All other receptors found in humans have keys we make from within. Understanding this, researchers began looking for our "internal key." In 1992, the first of numerous "inner cannabis" compounds was discovered.[3] It was named "anandamide" by the scientists who discovered it. "Ananda" is the Sanskrit word for "bliss." Its scientific name is N-arachidonoylethanolamine, or AEA for short. The following year, researchers discovered a second cannabinoid receptor, primarily located within components of the immune system.[4] In 1995, a second "inner cannabis" compound was discovered and was named 2-arachidonoylglycerol (2-AG).[5] These compounds were given the umbrella term "endogenous cannabinoids," or "endocannabinoids" ("endo" is Greek for "inside" or "within"). Numerous other endocannabinoid compounds have since been discovered, although anandamide and 2-AG are the most researched.

The discovery of cannabinoid receptors and endocannabinoids caused tremendous excitement in the scientific community, and research into "cannabinoid science" exploded. Scientists named this system of receptors and the endocannabinoids that interact with them the "endocannabinoid system."

How Does the Endocannabinoid System Work?

The endocannabinoid system is made up of endocannabinoids, endocannabinoid receptors (two confirmed and others suspected), and the enzymes that make and break down the endocannabinoids.

This diagram shows two neurons where they meet at an area called the "synapse." The presynaptic neuron is sending chemical messengers

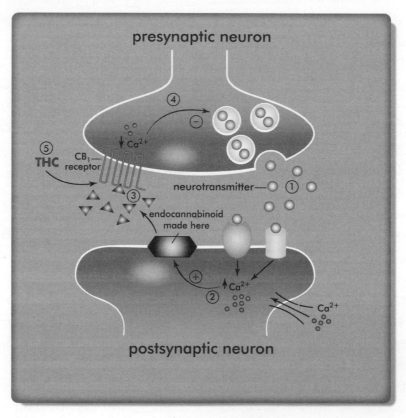

The endocannabinoid system.

called "neurotransmitters," and the postsynaptic neuron is receiving the neurotransmitters' messages.

Here's how the mechanism works:

1. When there is too great a flow of neurotransmitters (called neuro-excitation) from the presynaptic cell, an imbalance occurs, causing a disturbance in the postsynaptic cell, resulting in...
2. An increase of calcium flowing into the postsynaptic cell, causing the cell to make an endocannabinoid key (represented by the triangle in the drawing).
3. The postsynaptic cell then sends the endocannabinoid key back to attach to the cannabinoid receptor lock on the presynaptic cell.
4. This key-in-the-lock binding triggers a chemical reaction in the presynaptic cell that results in a dampening down of the flow of neurotransmitters, thereby correcting the imbalance.

A phytocannabinoid such as THC can substitute for an endocannabinoid—both are keys for cannabinoid receptors and can result in changing the imbalanced neurotransmitter message.

Why Do We Have an Endocannabinoid System?

When our cells are functioning properly and maintaining a healthy equilibrium, we are in what is called a state of homeostasis. **Very simply, the job of the endocannabinoid system is to regulate the flow of chemical messages that are sent between cells, with the goal of maintaining homeostasis.** When we experience inflammation, illness, infection, or chemical or traumatic insults, our endocannabinoid system goes into action, trying to restore balance amid the cellular messages.

Endocannabinoids are made and released by our cells on demand when we need them.[6] They do their job by binding to cannabinoid receptors, triggering a cell to change its message, and subsequently they are broken down by enzymes. They are what we call "short-lived" molecules. Human endocannabinoid levels in the bloodstream have been measured in the lab and in clinical trials, but currently this test is not available commercially. Studies show that emotional and physical stressors elevate levels of anandamide and other endocannabinoids with the goal of homeostasis.[7]

The endocannabinoid system is the most widespread receptor system in the human body. It regulates many of the most important physiologic pathways, including:

- Gastrointestinal activity
- Cardiovascular activity
- Pain perception
- Maintenance of bone mass
- Protection of neurons
- Hormonal regulation
- Metabolism control
- Immune function
- Inflammatory reactions
- Inhibition of tumor cells

As you can see, your endocannabinoid system is involved in just about every chemical process in your body! The Italian researcher Vincenzo Di Marzo noted that "the endocannabinoid system is essential to life" and affects how you "relax, eat, sleep, forget and protect."[8] Scientific evidence has proven that your endocannabinoid system is "switched on" when you need protection — for example, when certain diseases strike, such as cancer; neuropathic and inflammatory pain; multiple sclerosis; intestinal disorders; post-traumatic stress disorder; traumatic brain injury; hemorrhagic, septic, and cardiogenic shock; hypertension; atherosclerosis; and Parkinson's disease.[9] Endocannabinoids can lessen the negative effects of an illness by working to maintain a balance of cellular signals, minimizing and mitigating pathological processes.

You don't "feel" your pancreas releasing insulin, nor do you "know" when your thyroid releases thyroid hormone, even though these essential actions are happening all the time. In much the same way, you don't feel your endocannabinoid system working, but your cells make and use the endocannabinoids to keep the multiple systems in your brain and body functioning correctly, maintaining homeostasis of cell function. If your endocannabinoid system is not working properly, you may have an imbalance, which can manifest as a medical condition. There are no pharmaceutical medications that directly address an endocannabinoid dysfunction. However, **the cannabis plant contains a "treasure trove" of compounds that interact with the endocannabinoid system, helping to restore balance to the cellular messages.**[10]

Your Endocannabinoid System Is Different from Mine

People who use cannabis can have different experiences despite using the same dose, chemovar, or preparation. Other factors, such as mindset and the environmental setting, can influence response, especially when THC is used. Why does this happen? These different responses reflect differences in the baseline endocannabinoid system function of the person who is using cannabis. If you have a normally functioning endocannabinoid system, you may have a different response to cannabis than someone who has an imbalance in his or her endocannabinoid system. A great example of this is people who suffer from ADHD. Patients with ADHD have difficulty focusing, completing tasks, organizing tasks, and sitting still—all of which makes it hard to succeed at school and work. We know these patients suffer from an imbalance in a number of their neurotransmitters. Published reports and clinical experience with patients in my practice who struggle with ADHD show that cannabis medicine can help them focus, stay on task, remember things, and sit still for longer periods of time.[11] Someone who does not have ADHD and uses cannabis might report that cannabis makes them unable to concentrate or remember things—just the opposite of the ADHD patient. We now know that every person responds to cannabis based on numerous factors, with the status of their underlying endocannabinoid system as one of the main variables.

I often tell my patients that I wouldn't prescribe insulin to someone who doesn't suffer from diabetes. The person with diabetes has a poorly functioning pancreas that doesn't produce insulin, whereas a nondiabetic person has a perfectly functioning pancreas. Similarly, a person with ADHD has an imbalance in neurotransmitters stemming from endocannabinoid dysfunction.[12] In the same way a person with diabetes gets back into balance by taking insulin, a person with ADHD may find balance — better focus and function — by taking cannabis medicine, as it targets the cells sending the imbalanced neurotransmitter, fixing the message and ultimately restoring homeostasis.

Using medicine that targets the underlying imbalance should be the goal of all medical treatment. The discovery of the endocannabinoid system and the medical conditions associated with its dysfunction are now recognized and accepted by the medical community; therefore, we must recognize cannabis as a legitimate medicine.

Receptor Locations

The locations of the two cannabinoid receptors have been mapped out and explain the many diverse effects of cannabis.[13] Certain locations have Type I receptors (CB_1), some have Type II receptors (CB_2), and others express both types of receptors. Additionally, injury and inflammation can induce certain cells to express CB_2 receptors.

CB_1 receptors are located in areas of the brain related to:

- Pain sensation (areas of the brain: amygdala, also spinal cord)
  - The location of cannabinoid receptors on cells that perceive pain explains why so many patients report pain relief with cannabis use.

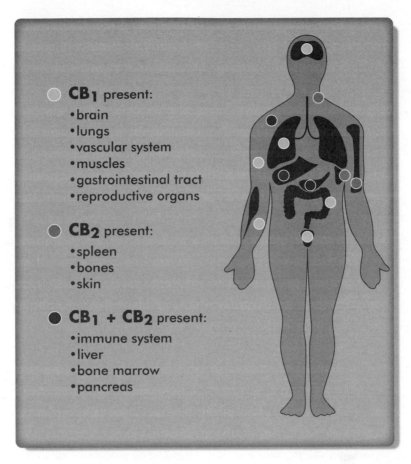

CB₁ present:
• brain
• lungs
• vascular system
• muscles
• gastrointestinal tract
• reproductive organs

CB₂ present:
• spleen
• bones
• skin

CB₁ + CB₂ present:
• immune system
• liver
• bone marrow
• pancreas

Location of receptors.

—Some patients report that pain disappears completely, some report a dulling of the pain sensation, and some report that pain is unchanged but they are not focused on it.

• Memory and learning (areas of the brain: caudate nucleus, hippocampus, putamen)

—For some patients, such as those with ADHD, the effects of cannabis can enhance memory and learning.

—Patients may report that with cannabis use they are able to focus and complete a task, retain what they have read, and be more productive and creative at home and at work.

—Acute doses of THC-rich cannabis can interfere with the ability to remember and learn.

- Emotion, such as anxiety, depression, fear (areas of the brain: cerebral cortex, amygdala)
  —One of the main conditions I see in my practice is anxiety and/or depression. Cannabis is well-known to alleviate anxiety but can in some cases increase it. In my clinical experience, if one has anxiety with cannabis use, it is usually due to a specific chemovar or a dosing issue (too much!), although there is a small subset of the population who may not metabolize THC well, resulting in anxiety with all THC use.

- Motor control and coordination (area of the brain: cerebellum)
  —Cannabis (THC specifically) has been shown to interfere with motor skills due to cannabinoid receptors located in the cerebellum, more so in new or inexperienced users; however, some patients with cerebellar disorders report benefits with cannabis use.

- Appetite (area of the brain: hypothalamus)
  —Cannabis (THC specifically) can increase appetite in some users due to the receptors in the part of the brain that, when triggered, increase appetite; this can be a positive side effect for those who are on chemotherapy or who are underweight.
  —Not all cannabis users experience hunger with THC use, but some patients, especially those who are obese, report this as a negative side effect.

- Nausea/vomiting (area of the brain: dorsal vagal complex)
  —Numerous research studies in animals and humans have shown that both THC and CBD, as well as other phytocannabinoids, act to inhibit nausea and vomiting.

- Pleasure and reward (area of the brain: substantia nigra)
  —THC is known to promote feelings of euphoria and reward, as there are cannabinoid receptors in the areas of the brain that regulate gratification and the perception of pleasure.

CB$_2$ receptors are located in areas of the body related to:

- The immune system
  - CB$_2$ receptors located in the various parts of the immune system have the job of maintaining immunologic homeostasis, meaning these receptors work to keep the immune system balanced. Many immune-related cells have these receptors: monocytes, macrophages, B cells, T cells, and cells in the spleen and tonsils.
- The peripheral nervous system
  - Increased levels of CB$_2$ receptors are found in the nerves of your body after an injury and help decrease the sensation and perception of pain.
- The skeletal system (effects on bone)
  - CB$_2$ receptors are located in bone and have been shown to decrease osteoclast activity (osteoclasts are the cells that break down bone) and increase osteoblast activity (osteoblasts are the cells that build up bone).

Areas that express both CB$_1$ and CB$_2$ receptors:

- Heart
  - The binding of THC to CB$_1$ receptors in the heart can cause an increased heart rate in new or inexperienced THC users. This effect disappears with more regular use.
  - CB$_2$ receptors, when activated, appear to protect the heart from injury (a cardioprotective role).
- Liver
  - Binding of a cannabinoid to the CB$_1$ receptors in an injured or sick liver can cause fibrosis (development of scar tissue).
  - Binding of a cannabinoid to the CB$_2$ receptors in an injured or sick liver counteracts the progression of fibrosis and works as a protectant.
- Gastrointestinal system
  - Both types of receptors are located in the nervous system of

the gut, called the enteric nervous system, where they inhibit gastric secretions, decrease gut inflammation and pain, and reduce gastric motility.

- Pancreas
  - CB_1 receptors are mainly expressed in non-insulin-producing pancreatic cells, while CB_2 receptors are found in all pancreatic cells.
  - The endocannabinoid acting as a CB_2 receptor (2-AG) decreases insulin secretion.
- Reproductive system
  - Cannabinoid receptors in the female reproductive organs regulate fertility, maternal–fetal signaling, and development of the placenta and embryo.
  - Cannabinoid receptors in the male reproductive organs regulate Sertoli cell survival, spermatogenesis, sperm–oocyte interaction, and the blockade of polyspermy.
- Skin
  - Both types of receptors have been found in the skin, specifically keratinocytes, and in the epithelial cells of hair follicles, sebocytes, and eccrine sweat glands. They are also found in the nerve fibers of the skin. In these locations, the cannabinoid receptors likely work to regulate skin inflammation and pain sensation.
  - CB_1 and CB_2 receptors in adipocytes (fat cells) function to make more adipocytes (a process called adipogenesis), increasing energy storage. They are also are involved in lipogenesis (the formation of triglycerides).

No Risk of Fatal Overdose

There are no cannabinoid receptors in the area of the brain that controls breathing and heart rate. This explains why there is no possibility of a fatal overdose with phytocannabinoids, nor has one ever been documented. In contrast, there is an abundance of opioid receptors in the respiratory control center in the brain. When high doses of opioid compounds, such as heroin, methadone, or oxycodone, bind to opioid receptors in the respiratory control center of the brain, the respiratory drive can be suppressed and may lead to respiratory arrest and death. This is not an issue known to occur from phytocannabinoids.

Additional Endocannabinoid Targets

Very importantly, endocannabinoids also work outside the endocannabinoid system at various other targets in the brain and body. These targets include:

- *GPR55,* or G protein-coupled receptor 55, which regulates pain and production of endocannabinoids
- The *TRPV,* or transient receptor potential vanilloid, a family of protein ion channels that are involved in inflammation and pain response
- *PPARs,* or peroxisome proliferator-activated receptors, which regulate the translation of genes involved in metabolism and energy homeostasis, and also confer cardioprotection and neuroprotection

More information about each phytocannabinoid's specific non-cannabinoid receptor targets are discussed in chapter 4.

Endocannabinoid System Dysfunction

Dysfunction of the endocannabinoid system is like the proverbial chicken and egg. When the endocannabinoid system is functioning well, homeostasis of many of the brain's and body's physiologic processes is maintained. We now know that chronic medical conditions can stress the endocannabinoid system to the point of dysfunction—that is, it is not able to continue to maintain balance—leaving the person with the chronic illness and struggling to get back into homeostasis. However, a dysfunction within the endocannabinoid system itself can cause chronic medical conditions. Underactivity or overactivity of the endocannabinoid system has been linked to disease states and is the focus of much research throughout the world. Understanding how the dysfunction of the endocannabinoid system can cause disease or can result from disease is crucial to the use of cannabis as medicine.

Endocannabinoid Deficiency Syndrome

In 2003, Dr. Ethan Russo, a board-certified neurologist and psychopharmacology researcher, posed an excellent question in a scientific paper, asking if a deficiency of endocannabinoids—the compounds that are made on demand in our brains and bodies to maintain homeostasis—can lead to disease. He hypothesized that having lower levels of these compounds, which would diminish the ability to maintain homeostasis, may lead to medical conditions such as migraine headaches, fibromyalgia, irritable bowel syndrome, and other "treatment-resistant" conditions, noting that many patients with these conditions had improvement of their symptoms with cannabis.

Since that article was published, a multitude of scientific studies have demonstrated that an impairment or dysfunction of the endocannabinoid system can be the cause of significant and difficult-to-treat medical conditions.[14] This deficiency may be genetically determined, meaning a person was born with it (congenital), while another person may develop it later in life (acquired). Chronic stress, poor diet, poor sleep, and chronic pain have all been shown to negatively impact endocannabinoid system functioning and can lead to endocannabinoid dysfunction.

Endocannabinoid system dysfunction has been found in the following medical conditions:

- Anxiety and depression[15]
- Autoimmune diseases[16]

- Cardiovascular disease[17]
- Complex regional pain syndrome[18]
- Eating disorders[19]
- Epilepsy[20]
- Failure to thrive in newborns[21]
- Fibromyalgia/myofascial pain syndrome[22]
- Huntington's disease[23]
- Irritable bowel syndrome[24]
- Migraine headaches[25]
- Multiple sclerosis[26]
- Nausea and motion sickness[27]
- Parkinson's disease[28]
- Schizophrenia[29]

Endocannabinoid Overactivity

In addition to an endocannabinoid deficiency, there can be dysregulation of the endocannabinoid system at the other end of the spectrum, namely overactivity. One example is the role of the endocannabinoid system in appetite, digestion, and energy metabolism.

Researcher Dr. Vincenzo Di Marzo reported in 2008 that overactivity of the endocannabinoid system may be associated with obesity and type 2 diabetes.[30] Studies found that overweight/obese individuals and those with type 2 diabetes have abnormally elevated blood levels of endocannabinoids, which may be due to lower levels of the enzymes that are needed to break down the endocannabinoids. Preliminary studies showed that overweight/obese people do not make enough of these enzymes, resulting in the endocannabinoids hanging around longer at the receptor, continuing to activate them.[31] This results in increased hunger, which increases body weight, which then increases endocannabinoid levels, which then increases hunger, and so on, creating a vicious cycle of endocannabinoid dysfunction. When obese men who had elevated endocannabinoid levels were enrolled for one year in a lifestyle-modification program requiring healthy eating and physical activity, their abnormally elevated endocannabinoid levels decreased, their weight and waist circumference were reduced, their triglyceride levels decreased, and their healthy cholesterol levels increased.[32] More research is needed, but it appears that maintaining a healthy weight through a balanced diet and regular exercise helps to keep the endocannabinoid system functioning normally.

The Story of Rimonabant[33]

Rimonabant is a synthetic drug that works as a CB_1 receptor inverse agonist, which means it binds to the receptor but causes the opposite effect. Rimonabant, by causing the opposite effect of endocannabinoids and THC at the CB_1 receptor, blocks hunger and influences metabolism. It was tested in placebo-controlled studies in thousands of overweight and obese patients, some with diabetes, high cholesterol, low HDL and high triglycerides (TGs), and was found to have numerous benefits, including sustained weight loss, reduction of TGs, increase in HDL, and better blood-glucose control. Unfortunately, this drug also caused a number of significant and unacceptable side effects, including depression, suicidal ideation, nausea, and anxiety. Although rimonabant became available in Europe in 2006, it was removed from the market in 2008, as its risks were shown to outweigh its benefits. Researchers are still investigating synthetic compounds that block CB_1 receptors as potential treatments for obesity and type 2 diabetes.

Upregulation and Downregulation of Cannabinoid Receptors

The number of cannabinoid receptors can change in response to what is going on around them in the brain and body.[34] Scientists call an increase in the number of cannabinoid receptors "upregulation" and a decrease in the number "downregulation."

Some disease states are associated with the upregulation of receptors:

- Animals with seizures have shown an increase in cannabinoid receptors in certain parts of their brains.[35]
- Animals with Crohn's colitis-type illness have upregulated cannabinoid receptors in their intestines.[36]
- Animals that suffer with nerve pain have upregulation of cannabinoid receptors in certain parts of their brains.[37]
- Animals with sleep deprivation show an increase in cannabinoid receptors in their brains.[38]
- Autistic children were found to have an increased number of CB_2 receptors on their white blood cells (autism often includes an element of immune dysfunction).[39]
- Cannabinoid receptors were upregulated in individuals with depression who committed suicide.[40]

One theory is the increase in cannabinoid receptors is a compensatory or protective mechanism: you have more receptors because your cells are looking for endocannabinoids to help restore balance. Upregulation can be maladaptive in some instances, such as increasing cellular fat deposits in liver disease.

Cannabinoid receptors can also downregulate — that is, there are fewer receptors available for cannabinoid binding. Usually in the case of being overactivated, cannabinoid receptors move from their location on the cell wall and "hide" inside the cell itself, a process called internalization. This too is thought to be a protective mechanism. When internalized, the receptor cannot be activated by cannabinoids. This process explains how tolerance to THC develops.

Tolerance

Research has determined that chronic heavy users of THC-rich cannabis have a decrease in the number of cannabinoid receptors.[41] This downregulation explains how these users develop tolerance to the effects of cannabis. Tolerance is also regionally selective, meaning that different parts of the brain can develop tolerance while other parts of the brain may not. For example, one of my patients who started using cannabis for multiple sclerosis found excellent relief of her spasticity from THC-rich cannabis. Initially, she experienced some memory loss but found that after a few months of use, this effect was no longer an issue. During this time, she never lost the beneficial effect on the symptom of spasticity.

Tolerance to THC may not occur if THC dosing is kept low—usually under 10 milligrams per dose. However, if tolerance does develop, the patient often will have to increase the amount or potency of THC in order to get the same effect. Although this is not dangerous, a loss of the medical effect and the higher financial cost of using more and higher-potency cannabis is not ideal. If a patient can abstain from cannabis use, the receptors will "come out of hiding" and become available again, resolving the issue of tolerance. Studies show that abstention from cannabis use for approximately twenty-eight days results in a return of normal numbers of cannabinoid receptors.[42] However, for patients who rely on cannabis medicine for chronic conditions, abstaining for this length of time may not be possible, as quality of life may be negatively impacted. I recommend using the lowest dose of THC that gives the desired effects. **If there is loss of beneficial effects, taking regular breaks from using THC-rich products is helpful in maintaining receptor availability.** Taking one or two days off per week or one week off every two to three months will minimize the downregulation of cannabinoid receptors, and the response to the medical effects of THC can be maintained. Adding CBD or other phytocannabinoids to the regimen may also help to minimize THC tolerance.

It is important to know that THC is the only phytocannabinoid understood to cause tolerance.

It's Not a Miracle, It's Science

Many of my patients who were suffering prior to cannabis treatment recollect feeling quite desperate by the time they came to see me. Struggling with a chronic illness and trying different therapies for years without any improvement in quality of life can change a person profoundly, causing depression, anxiety, and a sense of hopelessness. After finding relief with cannabis, many think it is a "miracle treatment" and certainly it may feel that way. But I must state that it is *not* a miracle, it is science. If your endocannabinoid system is not functioning well, simply put, you are out of balance. If dysfunction of the endocannabinoid system is the culprit, prescribed medications that do not work within this system miss the target and relief is often not achieved. Chronic illness leads to chronic stress, sleep deprivation, and other issues that negatively impact the endocannabinoid system, keeping it out of balance. For many patients, using cannabinoid medicine targets the root cause of the medical condition and healing can begin. For some, the effects are immediate; for others, it may take time for the system to get back into balance. Once the endocannabinoid system is functioning well, often less cannabis can be used to maintain homeostasis. Commonly, patients report that when they initially started using cannabis, they took higher doses, and after a few months, their dosing requirements went down. It may take time to achieve this if you have been sick and under stress for a long time. Using other natural modalities that have been shown to help the endocannabinoid system stay balanced, such as a healthy diet, regular exercise, and mindful stress-reduction techniques (e.g., meditation, tai chi, and yoga) in addition to cannabis, can be the solution.

Sophie's Story

Sophie was one of the first patients in California to use the famous Charlotte's Web CBD oil in 2013. I wrote about Sophie in my first book and include her story here, with an update.

I went to medical school from 1986 to 1990 and did an internship from 1990 to 1993, completely unaware of the incredible discoveries of the cannabinoid receptors and the endocannabinoid system. By 1995, the first two endocannabinoids were discovered, but cannabis medicine was still unknown to most physicians. When, in June of that year, three-month-old Sophie was diagnosed with infantile spasms, a rare seizure disorder with a particularly grim prognosis, the neurologists began a course of high-dosage steroids and benzodiazepines. By the time Sophie was nine months old, her development had plateaued, she was on three antiepileptic medications, and the seizures kept coming. Her neurologists in New York City could find no reason for her epilepsy and diagnosed her with cryptogenic infantile spasms. Over the next nineteen years, Sophie was treated with twenty-two drugs and two courses of the ketogenic diet, along with countless alternative therapies, including osteopathy, Chinese herbs, and acupuncture. Her spasms evolved into mixed seizures—atonic drops, tonic-clonic, partial complex, and absence—but no medication helped stop them. She suffered from serious side effects, and her quality of life was sometimes unbearable.

Elizabeth, Sophie's mother, told me that her old life ended on the day Sophie was diagnosed, and her new life began, a life of sleepless nights and days filled with intense caregiving, witnessing the constant suffering of her daughter, and navigating all the systems of care that having a sick and disabled child demanded. Sophie is severely disabled as a result of the seizures and the medications. While she can walk, she needs complete assistance with all life tasks, including feeding and diapering. She is nonverbal and needs a wheelchair because she tires easily and has seizures unexpectedly. She has hurt herself countless times, knocked out permanent teeth, gotten stitches, broken her leg and hand and nose as well as suffered contusions and scrapes.

Even as Elizabeth became a nationally recognized advocate for children with special healthcare needs, she never gave up hope that there was something that might help Sophie, and as the years went by, she became more and more convinced the traditional treatments for refractory epilepsy were nothing but a crapshoot. When she started hearing about cannabis and its effects on seizures, she began to explore the cannabis laws in California. In December of 2013, Sophie was one of my first patients to get quality-tested, whole-plant, CBD-rich cannabis oil. Within two weeks of starting the oil, Sophie had the first seizure-free day of her life, followed by a period of several weeks with no seizures. She began to smile and appeared relaxed and comfortable for the first time in decades.

I think often about the birth of and early diagnosis of Sophie—how her life and treatment virtually coincided with our initial forays into researching and learning about the endocannabinoid system. Elizabeth doesn't waste time thinking what Sophie's life and the life of her family might have been like if they had been able to try cannabis back when she was first diagnosed. While she shared with me how angry she feels when she's contacted by parents of young children on four or five medications yet still seizing, she is encouraged that more families in the epilepsy community are seeing the effects of cannabis medicine and fighting for access to it. She is at peace knowing Sophie's quality of life is now dramatically better, and her whole family rests easier.

Update: *It's been six years since Sophie first began taking cannabis, and while not seizure-free, she has far fewer seizures, and those she does have are shorter and less intense. She recovers from them more quickly and hasn't needed a rescue medication since she began taking cannabis. Elizabeth reports that they slowly weaned Sophie off most of one of the two medications she had been on for a decade, and the second medication entirely. While withdrawal was difficult, the CBD and added THC-rich oil lessened those symptoms. Sophie's overall health and well-being have been enhanced as well, with fewer illnesses and dramatically better sleep.*

CHAPTER 3

The Safety Profile of Cannabis

I n 2015, the acting chief of the US Drug Enforcement Administration said, "If you want me to say that marijuana's not dangerous, I'm not going to say that because I think it is. Do I think it's as dangerous as heroin? Probably not. I'm not an expert." Months later, he said in a briefing to reporters, "What really bothers me is the notion that marijuana is also medicinal—because it's not. We can have an intellectually honest debate about whether we should legalize something that is bad and dangerous, but don't call it medicine—that is a joke." He went on to say, "There are pieces of marijuana—extracts or constituents or component parts—that have great promise, but if you talk about smoking the leaf of marijuana—which is what people are talking about when they talk about medicinal marijuana—it has never been shown to be safe or effective as a medicine."[1] Political posturing aside, the former chief of the DEA has probably never heard of the endocannabinoid system.

Despite the lies, political agendas, and propaganda, science shows that **medicinal cannabis can be entirely safe when used responsibly.** Over the past hundred-plus years, numerous large investigations into the safety of cannabis have been published. Here are some highlights:

- *1894:* The *Report of the Indian Hemp Drugs Commission* was an Indo-British study of cannabis usage in India. The commission researched cannabis use for two years and wrote a report over three thousand pages long, concluding that "moderate use of hemp drugs appears to cause no appreciable physical injury of any kind," "moderate use of these drugs produces no mental injury," and "moderate use produces no moral injury whatever."[2]

- *1944:* New York City mayor Fiorello La Guardia, angered by the passage of the Marihuana Tax Act of 1937, commissioned the New York Academy of Medicine to research claims that smoking cannabis was dangerous and addictive. After five years of research, the academy published their report, stating that "the practice of smoking marihuana does not lead to addiction" and "the use of marihuana does not lead to morphine or heroin or cocaine addiction." Additionally, numerous human clinical studies were performed, reporting "definite evidence in this study that the marihuana users were not inferior in intelligence" and "they suffered no mental or physical deterioration as a result of their use of the drug."[3]

- *1972:* The National Commission on Marijuana and Drug Abuse was created as part of the Controlled Substances Act to research cannabis abuse in the US. Its final report, entitled *Marijuana: A Signal of Misunderstanding,* was presented to Congress and recommended ending marijuana prohibition. The report noted, "There is little proven danger of physical or psychological harm from the experimental or intermittent use of the natural preparations of cannabis," and went on to say, "The use of drugs for pleasure or other non-medical purposes is not inherently irresponsible; alcohol is widely used as an acceptable part of social activities."[4] The Nixon administration ignored the findings of the commission and designated cannabis as a Schedule I controlled substance, the most restrictive category of all, defining these compounds as having "no currently accepted medical use in the United States, a lack of accepted safety for use under medical supervision, and a high potential for abuse."[5]

- *1988:* Sixteen years after the National Organization for the Reform of Marijuana Laws (NORML) filed a petition with the US Drug

Enforcement Administration to reschedule cannabis from a Schedule I to a Schedule II controlled substance, which would allow doctors to prescribe it and researchers to study it, DEA chief administrative law judge Francis L. Young wrote in his ruling that "[m]arijuana, in its natural form, is one of the safest therapeutically active substances known to man. By any measure of rational analysis marijuana can be safely used within a supervised routine of medical care." He also wrote, "It would be unreasonable, arbitrary and capricious for DEA to continue to stand between those sufferers and the benefits of this substance in light of the evidence in this record." He stated that there was no evidence of lack of accepted safety with medical supervision and he recommended rescheduling it.[6] However, a DEA administrator named John Lawn rejected the recommendation, and a 1994 court of appeals sided with the rejection, leaving cannabis as a Schedule I substance.

- *1999:* The Institute of Medicine of the National Academies published a report called *Marijuana and Medicine: Assessing the Science Base.* The report concluded that "except for the harms associated with smoking, the adverse effects of marijuana use are within the range of effects tolerated for other medications."[7]

- *2015:* US surgeon general Dr. Vivek Murthy stated, "We have some preliminary data that for certain medical conditions and symptoms, that marijuana can be helpful," and went on to say that he believed US marijuana policy should be driven by science: "We have to use that data to drive policy-making."[8]

- *2017:* The National Academies of Sciences, Engineering, and Medicine published a review of relevant scientific research on cannabis called *The Health Effects of Cannabis and Cannabinoids: The Current State of Evidence and Recommendations for Research,* for which an expert committee conducted an extensive search of the scientific literature, reviewing more than ten thousand articles. The major limitation of this report is that the reviewed studies used synthetic cannabinoids or single-molecule cannabinoids, not "real-world cannabis," which is used by the majority of medical cannabis patients. Despite this limitation, the major findings were:

— "In adults with chemotherapy-induced nausea and vomiting, oral cannabinoids are effective antiemetics."

— "In adults with chronic pain, patients who were treated with cannabis or cannabinoids are more likely to experience a clinically significant reduction in pain symptoms."

— "In adults with multiple sclerosis (MS)-related spasticity, short-term use of oral cannabinoids improves patient-reported spasticity symptoms."

— "The evidence is unclear as to whether and how cannabis use is associated with heart attack, stroke, and diabetes."

— "The evidence suggests that smoking cannabis does not increase the risk for certain cancers (i.e., lung, head, and neck) in adults."[9]

It is crucial at this point to make a distinction between those using cannabis as medicine (i.e., medical patients) and those using high doses of THC for recreational purposes. The vast majority of studies assessing the safety and risks of cannabis have explored the effects only of the recreational use of chronic and/or high doses of THC. Medical cannabis patients use other cannabinoids in addition to THC, with mostly low doses of THC, as higher doses are not necessary to achieve the desired medicinal effects. This type of use has not been investigated in depth; however, preliminary studies of patients on medically supervised cannabis regimens that include proper dosing and multiple cannabinoids are showing that cannabis is safer than most pharmaceuticals and at least as effective for certain conditions.

Acute Toxicity

No lethal dose of cannabis has ever been reported. In the past, scientists employed the "LD50" as a measurement to compare the lethality of different substances. The LD50 is the dose at which 50 percent of those taking a specific drug would die, and it is expressed in the number of milligrams of the drug consumed per kilogram of body weight. This dose refers to an acute toxicity, meaning the lethality of one dose, not cumulative doses over time. The lower the LD50, the more toxic the substance. For example, the LD50 for aspirin is 200 milligrams per kilogram and the LD50 for common table salt is 3,000 milligrams per kilogram, showing that an acute overdose of aspirin is much more deadly than an acute overdose of table salt.

Scientists have had a difficult time trying to find the LD50 for THC. Extrapolating from animal data, which reports that the LD50 of orally ingested THC is over 1,000 milligrams per kilogram, it is thought that a 150-pound (70-kilogram) adult human would have to take 70,000 milligrams of THC, or over five thousand times the typical dose.[10]

The Centers for Disease Control (CDC) compiles yearly mortality data that shows deaths from alcohol, tobacco, and other substances. The latest CDC data reports that in the US in 2017 there were 70,237 deaths from drug overdoses, with 67.8 percent (47,600) due to opioids. There were 35,823 alcohol-induced deaths in the same year. The CDC also reports 480,000 deaths due to tobacco every year (1,300 per day). The CDC no longer has a category for cannabis deaths, as there have been none reported.[11]

An acute overdose of THC, although not fatal, can be quite unpleasant and may consist of feelings of paranoia, anxiety, panic, nausea, headache, vomiting, a racing heart, hallucinations, and a perceived sense of death. For some patients, an overdose of THC causes only severe sedation. All of these symptoms wear off and do not leave any lasting effects, except the desire to not have another similar experience. Overdoses are easily avoided by always knowing what you are taking and starting with a low dose before slowly increasing your dose over time. Other cannabinoids, such as CBD, CBG, and CBC, have no known lethality and in fact, with an acute overdose, have very few adverse side effects other than possible sedation and stomach upset.

Chronic Toxicity

There have been numerous animal studies investigating the potential long-term toxic effects of cannabinoids on the brain and other organs of the body. As mentioned, most of these investigations used acute and extremely large doses of THC in animal subjects in order to produce damage. As the vast majority of medical cannabis patients do not take large amounts of THC, these laboratory findings are irrelevant for those using cannabis medically.

In July 2016, researchers from New Zealand published a report on the effects of long-term cannabis use (presumed recreational use, although some may have been self-medicating) by 1,037 individuals who were followed for twenty years. Cannabis was not associated with detrimental health effects except for poorer periodontal health (thought to be a result of smoke passing through the oral cavity). However, tobacco use in this cohort was associated with worse health in eight of twelve outcomes, including periodontal disease, poorer lung function, increased systemic inflammation, and worse metabolic health. In fact, the researchers reported, "[W]e found no association between cannabis use and cardio-vascular risks (e.g., high blood pressure and worse cholesterol levels)," and "[t]he absence of associations between cannabis use and poor physical midlife health could not be attributed to better initial health, more physical activity, better diet, or less alcohol abuse," implying that long-term use of cannabis is safe.[12]

As to whether the effects of long-term exposure to cannabis causes persistent cognitive deficits in adults, the tremendous methodological difficulties inherent in this type of study are obvious, as the many variables are quite difficult to control. One study from 2001 that attempted this investigation recruited sixty-three current heavy cannabis users and seventy-two control subjects. Subjects underwent a twenty-eight-day washout from cannabis, called the abstinence period. On days 0, 1, and 7 of abstinence, the heavy users scored significantly below the control subjects on a battery of neuropsychological tests. By day 28, there were virtually no differences between the groups in any of the test results.[13]

In 2015, Dr. Marc Ware and his group at McGill University in Quebec, looking to determine the safety of chronic medical cannabis use, studied 215 approved medical cannabis patients using THC for chronic non-cancer pain and 216 controls with chronic pain who did not use THC. They assessed side effects as well as neurocognitive, pulmonary, liver, kidney, hematologic, biochemical, and endocrine functioning, plus efficacy for both pain and mood. They found that medical THC use was not associated with serious side effects but in some patients was associated with nonserious side effects, such as drowsiness, dizziness, and nausea. Neurocognitive function was improved in both cannabis users and the control group. There was no impact of medical cannabis use on measures of hematologic, biochemical, liver, kidney, and endocrine function among seventy-eight patients followed over one year. They also found "significant improvements in pain intensity and the physical dimension of quality of life over one year among the cannabis users compared with controls; there was also significant improvement among cannabis users in measures of the sensory component of pain, symptom distress, and total mood disturbance compared with controls."[14]

In 2016, Dr. Staci Gruber and her team — called MIND: Marijuana Investigations for Neuroscientific Discovery — at McLean Hospital in the Boston area reported that medical cannabis patients who were tested extensively before initiating cannabis and at three months of use showed improvements in executive function. They also reported "reduced sleep disturbance, decreased symptoms of depression, attenuated impulsivity, and positive changes in some aspects of quality of life. Additionally, patients reported a notable decrease in their use of conventional pharmaceutical agents from baseline, with opiate use declining more than 42%."[15] A second article published by this group documented brain findings through functional magnetic resonance imaging (fMRI) of medical cannabis patients. Following three months of cannabis treatment, patients demonstrated improved task performance accompanied by changes in brain activation patterns that resembled the brain patterns exhibited by healthy controls, suggesting a potential "normalization" of brain function. The authors noted that these effects were different from findings of recreational users, who were shown to have decrements in task performance accompanied by altered brain activation.[16]

Adverse Side Effects

Side effects from medical cannabis use are mild, temporary, and dose dependent. Low doses of THC (less than 10 milligrams) are well tolerated by most adult patients, but as with all drugs, some people are more sensitive to the effects than others. This is why we have the saying "Start low and go slow" when discussing the dosing of THC for new or inexperienced patients. Every person has what I call a "ceiling dose" of THC. This is the dose at which one begins to feel uncomfortable. Medical patients should aim to use doses under this level to minimize any unwanted side effects. It is important to understand that the correct dose of THC should not have any significant side effects and that combining other cannabinoids, such as CBD, with a proper dose of THC will minimize side effects and can enhance medicinal benefits.

Adverse side effects from an overdose of THC include:

- Anxiety
- Dizziness
- Drowsiness
- Dry mouth
- Dysphoria (a sense of unease)
- Hallucinations
- Headache
- Increased appetite
- Paranoia
- Racing heart

- Red eyes
- Vomiting

CBD is often touted as not having any side effects; however, this may not be true for someone who takes very high doses. One of the biggest concerns is drug–drug interactions since CBD is metabolized in the liver, where many other pharmaceuticals are metabolized. (More on this in chapter 5.)

Adverse side effects from high doses of CBD may include:

- Diarrhea
- Drowsiness/sedation
- Reduced appetite

There are now claims that CBD can harm your liver. This comes from the clinical studies of a pharmaceutically made 99 percent pure CBD product called Epidiolex (from GW Pharmaceuticals). In order to gain approval by the FDA, researchers conducting the Epidiolex clinical trials gave very high doses to patients on anticonvulsant medications, looking for any possible side effects. These doses were significantly higher than the real-world doses used by patients taking natural CBD products. In using these high doses, the researchers reported that the combination of Epidiolex and a drug called valproic acid, which can cause liver issues on its own, may result in elevated levels of liver enzymes. The elevated levels returned to normal with discontinuation or reduction of Epidiolex dosing, or with reduction of valproic acid dosing, evidence that this effect on the liver is reversible. However, I have not seen similar issues in any patients taking CBD under my care, except in one child with cancer who was being treated with four liver-toxic chemotherapies at the same time; when chemo was stopped, the levels went back to normal while the child was still taking CBD.

Side effects from other phytocannabinoids have not been researched, as they are only newly available for use by medical patients. Clinically, I have seen few or no side effects in patients using CBDA, CBG, CBN, delta-8-THC, THCA, or THCV.

In 2018, Israeli researchers published results from a retrospective study of 901 elderly patients (over sixty-five years of age) who used medical cannabis for at least six months, many of them using THC-rich products. The most common indications were pain and cancer. In addition to finding statistically significant efficacy for pain reduction and improvement in quality of life, this study found that cannabis treatment was not associated with a high number of adverse events in the short and medium term of the follow-up. Only a small number of patients stopped the treatment due to adverse events, which included dizziness in 9.7 percent, dry mouth in 7.1 percent, and somnolence in 3.9 percent.[17] Outside of a study, in real-world use of cannabis, side effects can often be minimized or eliminated with adjustments in dosing, cannabinoid profiles, and timing or method of use (covered in chapter 5).

Cannabinoid Hyperemesis Syndrome

CHS, first described in 2004, is a syndrome associated with chronic and high-dose THC-rich cannabis use. Symptoms include cyclical episodes of vomiting, nausea, and abdominal pain, as well as, in over 90 percent of cases, compulsive bathing in hot water, which can relieve the symptoms. THC affects the part of the brain that controls thermoregulation (temperature), and in this syndrome, the compulsion is to seek warmth. People who use cannabis often will try to use more cannabis to control the symptoms, especially the nausea and vomiting; however, in CHS this paradoxically makes the symptoms worse. If a person with CHS seeks care in a hospital emergency department, they often get the "million-dollar" evaluation because the symptoms are similar to other, more serious conditions, such as appendicitis, bowel obstruction, pelvic inflammatory disease, gallstones, pancreatitis, gastroenteritis, and cyclical vomiting syndrome (CVS). Most emergency physicians are now aware of this condition, which has helped with earlier and more accurate diagnosis, as chronic heavy use of THC combined with a report of compulsive bathing in hot water are clues that CHS is the cause of the trouble. Cessation of THC use and abstinence are the primary treatments for CHS. Only a small percentage of patients who are chronic heavy users develop CHS. It is thought to occur in a subset of the population that may be genetically susceptible, but at this time, the mechanisms of how CHS causes these paradoxical symptoms and why CHS happens to some and not others is unknown.

One of my patients, a young woman suffering with severe, chronic ankle pain after a traumatic injury requiring reconstructive surgery, started using highly concentrated THC to treat her pain (not on my advice!). She developed symptoms of CHS and had six separate ER visits before she was properly diagnosed because she was afraid to reveal her cannabis use to the physicians attending to her. When I met with her for a follow-up visit, we discussed THC overuse and a possible genetic predisposition to developing CHS. She was reluctant to start using other pain medications, so I recommended abstention from cannabis for one month and restarted her on cannabis but with a high-ratio CBD:THC product instead. She did not have a recurrence of CHS, although there are reports that in some people even a small amount of THC can cause CHS to recur.

Tolerance, Dependence, and Addiction

As discussed in the previous chapter, tolerance occurs after frequent, usually high-dose use of THC. The cannabinoid receptors downregulate—that is, they internalize into the cells and thus are no longer able to bind to endo- or phytocannabinoids. However, not all tolerance is undesired. Some patients may become tolerant to memory impairment or to sedating effects while still achieving pain relief. Cancer patients who are using cannabis for its anticancer effects often take high doses of THC, which can cause difficult side effects—brain fog, dysphoria, sedation, anxiety—but the development of tolerance over time allows these patients to continue with high doses. For all other patients, tolerance is easily managed with these strategies:

- Be thoughtful about your use. If you feel well and don't need to take a dose of THC, don't take it until you feel it's necessary.
- Keep THC doses low and intermittent if possible.
- Add other cannabinoids, such as CBD, to your regimen.
- Take a break from cannabis if you are a daily user: skip using it one to two days per week or take one week off every few months if you feel tolerance is building.

Cannabis dependence is defined as a "problematic pattern of use leading to clinically significant impairment or distress."[18] Symptoms of dependence include using THC-rich cannabis in larger amounts or over a longer period than needed or intended; making unsuccessful attempts to reduce or control use; and/or spending excessive time in the acquisition of, use of, or recovery from effects. The risk of THC dependence in recreational users has been found to be about 8.9 percent.[19]

Cannabis addiction is defined similarly to other addictions: compulsive drug seeking and intake, loss of control in limiting intake, and the emergence of a negative emotional state when access to the drug is prevented.[20] A cannabis withdrawal syndrome has been clinically described and includes symptoms of irritability, anger, anxiety, sleep disturbance, depressed mood, and decreased appetite, as well as sweating, headache, and shakiness.[21] Symptoms occur one to two days after discontinuation of THC use and can last one to two weeks.

As a cannabis specialist for over a decade, I can report that I do not see significant toxicity, dependence, or addiction when cannabinoids are used responsibly under medical supervision. Both dependence and addiction are issues related to recreational use. To be frank, patients suffering with medical conditions that interfere with their quality of life are just not interested in having side effects, dependence, or addiction issues from cannabis.

CHAPTER 4

The Medicinal Effects of Phytocannabinoids

The Science Explained

When I first started working in the field of medical cannabis in 2008, California dispensaries carried only products that were rich in THC. No one, other than some cultivators in various countries and scientists in laboratories around the world, was talking about or using CBD or other phytocannabinoids. Around 2012, when lab testing of cannabis became available, I heard from colleagues about rare CBD-rich plants cultivated in Northern California. However, dispensaries still did not carry any CBD products. In 2013, CNN aired a documentary called *Weed* in which Dr. Sanjay Gupta, a prominent neurosurgeon, talked about how he had changed his negative opinion about medical cannabis after learning about the endocannabinoid system. The documentary featured a little girl with Dravet syndrome, a devastating genetic pediatric epilepsy, who after having hundreds of seizures every month, responded to CBD-rich cannabis. The Colorado suppliers of this girl's CBD oil were subsequently inundated by desperate parents from all over the world, creating a long waiting list for access to this oil. It was at this time that CBD started appearing in dispensaries, and I began treating children for epilepsy with these products. I also began encouraging my adult patients with chronic pain and cancer to try adding CBD to their cannabis regimens. Since then, other phytocannabinoid products have become available, including THCA, CBDA, CBG, delta-8-THC, and THCV.

Unfortunately, research on the medical benefits of cannabis is still prohibited in the US due to the continued Schedule I status of all cannabis compounds, including CBD. Because cannabis laws are now enacted in almost every US state, as well as thirty countries, patients are using cannabis despite significant gaps in our knowledge. For example, we still do not know which cancers may respond to cannabinoid treatment, how many milligrams of CBD are needed to decrease inflammation in the gut, or if cannabinoids can really prevent dementia. As a physician who works with patients facing serious and sometimes life-threatening illnesses, it is frustrating to have a dominance of studies on the effects of cannabis in animals and very few in humans.

This chapter summarizes what we know about each phytocannabinoid currently available for patient use, although apart from THC and CBD, most phytocannabinoids still are not widely available. The latest scientific research is included, as well as clinical indications, my clinical experience, and reports from patients. We cannot say that an effect documented in laboratory test tubes or in experimental animal studies will be the same for humans, so I caution you to interpret the scientific findings carefully. Dosing, methods of delivery, and other details about how to use cannabis as medicine are discussed in chapter 5.

NOTE: It is important to make a distinction between the terms "psychoactive" and "intoxicating." A psychoactive substance is simply one that changes a person's mental state. Caffeine and nicotine are psychoactive. An intoxicating substance is one that alters a person's mental state with diminished physical or mental control. CBD is psychoactive but not intoxicating. THC is psychoactive and also can be intoxicating, depending on the dose taken.

Basic Concepts

In order to understand how cannabis plant compounds have medicinal effects, it is important to understand some basic scientific concepts. As described previously, receptors are located on the membranes of many of our cells and work like locks, waiting for a specific compound key to bind to them. Upon binding (also called "activation"), a chemical reaction is triggered inside the cell. THC has its well-known effects due to this direct binding to the cannabinoid receptors. Sometimes phytocannabinoids will bind to different sites on a receptor, causing a different chemical reaction. One of the ways CBD works is through this mechanism. Cannabinoid keys can also block receptors, turning off a cell's actions, or they can bind and cause the opposite effect, which is called "inverse activation." Additionally, cannabinoids can block enzymes that break down our endocannabinoids—meaning that our own endocannabinoids can hang around longer, giving more of an effect; this is referred to as "inhibition of uptake."

Delta-9-Tetrahydrocannabinol (THC)

THC is the most prominent cannabinoid in the cannabis plant. It was first discovered in 1942, but its chemical structure was not discovered until 1964, when it was also found to produce intoxicating, or "high," effects.[1]

Some people think THC is not medicinal, that it is just for getting high, but there is no question that THC has amazing medicinal properties, and with proper and responsible use, many different symptoms can be managed. I often read in medical journals that the intoxicating effects of THC are "unwanted," and although that may be true for some people, many of my patients report significant and life-changing relief with THC-rich cannabis. This does not make these patients "potheads." Remember, people with chronic and serious illnesses often suffer with endocannabinoid deficiency or dysregulation, meaning their endocannabinoid system is not working properly. **THC can and does correct this imbalance for many patients.** A person with an endocannabinoid dysfunction who finds THC-rich cannabis to be helpful should have access to this medicine, just as someone with diabetes or asthma should have access to the medications that benefit them. After talking with thousands of patients who have found excellent results with THC-rich cannabis medicine, I can definitively state that it is a safe and effective medication when used correctly. (As with all medicines, there are a few circumstances in which THC should be avoided; see chapter 6.)

One of the ways THC works is by binding directly to cannabinoid receptors, similar to the way endocannabinoids bind to these receptors. Remember that your endocannabinoid system works to maintain homeostasis of your cells. If your endocannabinoid system is working properly and experiences a trigger, such as illness, injury, or inflammation, your body's response is to make endocannabinoids to balance your cells' messages. As discussed in chapter 2, certain medical conditions are associated with an endocannabinoid deficiency, and anyone suffering with this deficiency cannot respond fully to cellular imbalance, as they do not make enough endocannabinoids to respond to the trigger.[2] Using THC can replace the missing endocannabinoids and restore a natural balance.

Scientific Research

In addition to interacting with the two well-known cannabinoid receptors located throughout the brain and body, THC interacts with numerous other receptors. Scientists call this ability to interact with many biological targets "compound promiscuity." It turns out that all of the phytocannabinoids are uninhibited in their actions. The mechanisms of action between THC and these physiologic pathways are quite complex but summarized here:

- *TRP channels (TRPV1, TRPV2, TRPV3, TRPV4, TRPA1, and TRPM8):* These are proteins located in the brain, heart, small intestine, lungs, skeletal muscles, and pancreas that are involved in the sensation of temperature, pressure, and pH, as well as smell, taste, vision, and pain perception.[3] Dysfunction of these proteins is implicated in neuropathic pain, cancer, inflammation, and respiratory disorders.

- *Glycine receptors:* Located throughout the central nervous system and spinal cord, these receptors are involved in inhibiting (dampening down) the transmission of messages related to motor coordination, pain transmission, and sensory processing. THC binds to these receptors, decreasing pain signaling.[4]

- *Serotonin receptors:* These are located throughout the central nervous system and gut, and are involved in cognition, mood, memory, body temperature, nausea, pain, and movement. The interaction between the endocannabinoid system and serotonin receptors is complex, with THC having different actions at the different subsets of serotonin receptors.[5]

- *PPARs:* These receptors are found in the nuclei of cells. In the liver and adipose tissue, they control the formation of fat cells and glucose metabolism. In the brain, they are involved in the regulation of inflammation and also new brain cell growth. PPAR activation by THC has been shown to have anticancer effects.[6]

- *GPR18:* This receptor, abundant in the central nervous and lymphatic systems, is considered "cannabinoid-receptor-like" and plays a role in lowering intraocular pressure as well as regulating metabolic disorders and cancer. THC directly binds to this receptor.[7]

- *GPR55:* Another receptor considered "cannabinoid-receptor-like," GPR55 is abundant in the brain, gut, pancreas, and adipose tissue, with evidence for clinical roles in energy metabolism, pain and inflammation, GI disorders, seizures, bone health, and cancer.[8]

- *Opioid receptors:* There is preliminary evidence that THC is an allosteric modulator of mu and delta opioid receptors, meaning THC can change the way endorphins and opioids attach to these receptors; however, the clinical significance remains unclear.[9]

Clinical Indications

What are the medicinal effects of THC?

- Anticancer
- Anti-inflammatory
- Antioxidant
- Improves sleep/sedating
- Neuroprotectant
- Reduces anxiety and depression
- Reduces/eliminates nausea and vomiting
- Reduces intraocular pressure
- Reduces spasticity and muscle spasms
- Relieves chronic pain
- Stimulates appetite

Note that many of these effects are discussed in part II, where ailments are detailed.

I have treated thousands of patients with THC-rich cannabis. Many of my adult patients commonly use THC at night, either smoked, vaporized, or via an edible product, to help with pain, sleep, and/or anxiety. The acute effects are gone by the following morning, and they report they are ready to take on the day. Some chronic pain patients find that taking multiple low doses throughout the day minimizes the need for other pain medications. Many cancer patients report that THC helps to enhance their appetite and decrease the side effects from chemotherapy, including nausea, vomiting, pain, and anxiety.

Some patients have such significant relief from their conditions with low-dose THC-rich cannabis that they think they are cured. Some also often find that once they are improved, low and intermittent doses of THC-rich cannabis keep their conditions under control. "I don't use as much as I used to" is a common phrase from my patients at their follow-up visits, indicating to me that they are feeling better and balance of the endocannabinoid system has likely been achieved. Some patients will feel so well that they stop using cannabis completely and may find that their medical condition does not return. Others find that ongoing use of THC maintains a balance and allows for the medical condition to be managed quite easily and without side effects.

One particular patient came to me with a long history of migraine headaches, which had started many years before when he was a teenager. His mother, grandmother, and three siblings all suffered from migraines as well. Trials of numerous other medications had not been successful, but he had complete resolution of his migraines for one year with the use of THC-rich cannabis. Thinking he was cured and no longer needed treatment, he stopped medicating with THC. Three months later, he came back to see me, reporting that the migraines had returned. A resumption of low doses of vaporized THC a few nights per week keep the headaches away, with beneficial side effects of less anxiety and better sleep. He reports no adverse side effects. This patient may have a genetic endocannabinoid deficiency causing his migraine condition, as evidenced by his family history and the medical use of THC resolving all symptoms.

Another patient who has had success with THC-rich cannabis is a woman who was going through menopause, which aggravated a mood disorder she had been diagnosed with in her twenties. She was struggling with anxiety, bouts of depression, anger, hot flashes, and very poor sleep. She had been prescribed hormone replacement medications but was reluctant to use them due to a family history of cancer. When this patient came to see me, she was what we call "cannabis naive" — that is, she had never used cannabis. She had numerous misconceptions and frankly was fearful about using THC, wanting to use only CBD. I educated her, but due to her fears, I started her on a product that was predominantly CBD. Over a period of two months, she titrated the dose from low to high with no benefits. At this point she agreed to try THC at night, starting with a very low dose of 1 milligram via a sublingual (taken under the tongue) tincture. Once she realized that she had complete control over the dosing, she felt more comfortable and found that 3 milligrams of THC taken about two hours before bedtime allowed her to get seven hours of restful sleep, followed by a day in which her mood was more stable. This patient has continued to find tremendous relief from her symptoms with this regimen for the past five years without having to escalate dosing or take other medications.

As discussed in chapter 1, the potency of THC-rich cannabis has increased over the last few decades. Additionally, highly concentrated forms of THC have appeared on the market. I have not seen issues with this increase, as patients using THC for medical purposes rarely over-medicate. They use trial and error to find the lowest dose that alleviates the medical condition. If they use more, they find that the higher dose can cause uncomfortable side effects or, with the development of tolerance to THC over time, the beneficial medicinal effects may be lessened or lost. When a patient reports having to increase to large doses of THC, tolerance may have developed. As mentioned in the previous chapter, abstaining for a few days to a week will diminish tolerance and allow the patient to lessen the amount of THC-rich cannabis needed while likely improving the medicinal effects.

There are a few things to keep in mind when using THC-rich cannabis medicine:

- Different people respond differently to THC. Some people feel significant effects and some do not; some like the way THC makes them feel and others do not.
- Patients should use the lowest dose that gives the desired effects so that tolerance can be limited.
- When taken orally, THC is converted in the liver to an active breakdown product called 11-hydroxy-THC (11-OH-THC). This compound is intoxicating and sedating, and has a long half-life, making edibles quite potent, long-lasting, and effective for nighttime use. Dosing is very important, as the conversion of THC to this compound cannot be predicted, hence the saying "Start low and go slow."
- Daily users of THC can take breaks, either skipping use one to two days per week or one week every few months to allow the number

of cannabinoid receptors to remain as close to normal as possible. Often people using doses under 10 milligrams do not develop tolerance, especially if CBD is included in the regimen.

- Patients should make sure to keep THC-rich cannabis medicine away from children and pets.
- The most common side effects from THC-rich cannabis are dry mouth, dizziness, sleepiness, rapid heartbeat, reddening of the eyes, coughing from inhalation of smoke or vapor, increased anxiety, and paranoia. Many patients are able to eliminate these effects by adjusting the dose, timing, and/or method of use.

THC-rich cannabis comes in many forms: raw flowers, which can be inhaled via smoking or vaporizing; vaporizer cartridges; edibles; transdermal patches; sublingual tinctures or extracts; topicals; capsules; and highly concentrated forms.

Cannabidiol (CBD)

Cannabidiol is the second most prominent cannabinoid in the cannabis plant. CBD was first discovered in 1940, and its chemical structure was elucidated in 1963.[10] As research into the multitude of medicinal properties of CBD continues to increase, more CBD chemovars and products are becoming available. Many medical cannabis patients who were primarily taking THC are now including CBD in their therapeutic regimens. Whereas THC binds directly to the cannabinoid receptor, CBD does not. This is why **CBD has no intoxicating effects and does not cause tolerance with repeated use.**

Scientific Research

CBD, like THC, interacts with the endocannabinoid system, but most of its therapeutic effects are from interactions with non-cannabinoid targets. In fact, CBD has been found to have sixty-five different sites of action![11] These sites can be broken down into four main categories: receptors, enzymes, ion channels, and transporters.

CBD interacts with many of the body's **receptors**. There is overlap with receptors that interact with THC; however, these two phytocannabinoids may have similar or different mechanisms of action at these sites:

- *Cannabinoid receptors:* CBD does not bind directly to the cannabinoid receptors like THC does; rather, it binds to a "side site" on the receptors, in turn affecting how THC binds to the same receptor.[12] This is called "negative allosteric modulation" of the cannabinoid receptors.

- *Glycine receptors:* CBD acts as a "positive allosteric modulator," which means it binds to a side site of the glycine receptors and enhances the body's own glycine, thus working to suppress inflammation and dampen the signal of neuropathic pain.[13]

- *GABA receptors:* CBD also acts as a positive allosteric modulator at these receptors, enhancing the body's own GABA, or gamma aminobutyric acid, resulting in antianxiety and anticonvulsant effects.[14]

- *Serotonin receptors:* Research shows that CBD binds to these receptors, modulating mood, pain, cognition, memory, nausea, and cardiovascular function.[15]

- *PPARs:* CBD also binds to these receptors, causing anticancer, neuroprotective, anti-inflammatory, and antidiabetic effects.[16]

- *Adenosine receptors:* When CBD binds to these receptors, it confers anti-inflammatory and neuroprotective effects.[17]

- *GPR55:* CBD blocks this widespread receptor (acting as a "receptor antagonist"), resulting in a decrease in neuronal excitation and conferring an antiepileptic effect.[18]

- *GPR18:* CBD is reported to weakly bind to and block this receptor, which is abundant in the central nervous and lymphatic systems. GPR18 is thought to play a role in intraocular pressure, metabolic disorders, and cancer, but the clinical significance is still unknown.[19]

- *GPR3, GPR6, and GPR12:* CBD is an inverse agonist at these receptors, meaning it binds to these receptors but causes an opposite effect.[20] These receptors play a role in neurodegenerative disorders (Parkinson's and Alzheimer's diseases), cancer, and infertility. The clinical significance is still unknown.
- *Opioid receptors:* There is preliminary evidence that CBD is an allosteric modulator of mu and delta opioid receptors; however, it is unclear how this translates to clinical situations.[21]

CBD also interacts with numerous **enzymes** in order to exert its influence in the body. Some of these enzymes and their effects include:

- Cytochrome P450 enzymes (influence metabolism)
- Mitochondrial electron transport chain enzymes (modulate brain energy metabolism)
- AANAT enzyme (involved in melatonin biosynthesis)
- FAAH enzyme (used in the breakdown of anandamide)
- COX and LOX enzymes (modulate inflammatory processes)
- IDO enzyme (mediates cytokine-induced sickness behavior)[22]

CBD interacts with **TRP ion channels** too, which are like pores in cell walls. Calcium, potassium, and sodium pass in and out of these channels, producing electrical signals that control the flow of neurotransmitters and other compounds made by the cells. TRP channels, as mentioned previously as a target of THC, are also targets of CBD and are implicated in the regulation of body temperature, pain, inflammation, cancer, and epilepsy.[23]

Lastly, CBD interacts with **transporter proteins,** which work to move chemical compounds throughout the brain and body. CBD is known to bind to transporter proteins in such a way as to block the reuptake of endocannabinoids, allowing them to have a longer effect at the cannabinoid receptors. This is one way that CBD helps to enhance the function of the endocannabinoid system.

Clinical Indications

What are the medicinal effects of CBD?

- Antibacterial
- Anticancer (CBD is antiproliferative, antimetastatic, and anti-angiogenic, so it doesn't just treat symptoms of cancer and cancer treatment — I discuss this more in the cancer section.)
- Anticonvulsant
- Anti-inflammatory
- Antioxidant
- Antipsychotic
- Neuroprotectant
- Promotes bone growth
- Reduces anxiety and depression
- Reduces/eliminates nausea and vomiting
- Reduces intraocular pressure
- Reduces spasticity and muscle spasms
- Relieves chronic pain
- Stimulates appetite

There are a few things to keep in mind when using CBD-rich cannabis medicine:

- CBD is alerting in lower doses and sedating in higher doses.
- CBD is well documented to be extremely safe for human use. Side effects are rare, usually occurring with very high doses, and can include diarrhea, sedation, and decreased appetite.
- CBD is metabolized in the liver, where many other pharmaceuticals are metabolized as well. This may lead to drug–drug interactions (discussed in chapter 5).
- CBD changes the flow of neurotransmitters in the brain, which affect a person's mental state, making CBD a psychoactive — but not intoxicating — compound.

- When patients use both CBD and THC at the same time, CBD changes the way THC binds to cannabinoid receptors. CBD may decrease the intoxicating effects of THC, depending on how much of each compound is taken. Knowing the ratio of CBD to THC, or CBD:THC, allows patients to determine potential intoxicating effects of the product; the lower the ratio, meaning more THC in relation to CBD, the more likely it is you will feel the effects of THC.
- CBD may help protect short-term memory loss and prevent the anxiety and paranoia that THC can sometimes cause.[24]
- CBD appears to be more effective when there is some THC, even a small amount, present in the product (remember the entourage effect).[25]
- When taken with THC, CBD blocks the breakdown of THC to its metabolite 11-hydroxy-THC, thereby decreasing some of the intoxication and sedation associated with this metabolite.[26]
- Patients using cannabis containing CBD do not develop tolerance. Studies of nabiximols (trade name Sativex, from GW Pharmaceuticals), a CBD:THC 1:1 plant-based pharmaceutical approved in Europe, reported no tolerance in 941 patients with a combined 2,213.98 years of exposure.[27] Clinically, I have not seen tolerance develop in patients using CBD products.
- There may be reverse tolerance with CBD in some patients, in which a patient responds better to a lower dose after being on a higher dose over time. I have a number of pediatric patients with epilepsy who have later required a reduction of their dose of CBD in order to maintain seizure control. Although it is unclear exactly why this may happen in some patients, the thought is that CBD use in time enhances the endocannabinoid system and other non-cannabinoid targets, allowing them to function better and resulting in a more balanced flow of neurotransmitters.

One of my longtime patients who has had great success with CBD-rich medicine came to me when she was eighteen years old. She suffered with rheumatoid arthritis, Crohn's disease, autism, and a seizure disorder. She was fed through a feeding tube, was nonverbal, and struggled with chronic pain. She began using a high-ratio CBD:THC tincture every eight hours, with the goal of treating her seizure disorder. She has had a greater than 90 percent reduction of seizures. Within the first few years, she was able to stop taking almost all other medications, which included anticonvulsants and biologics (injected medications that reduce inflammatory conditions), began eating by mouth, had the feeding tube removed, and became more engaged with her parents. Over time, the inflammatory markers on her blood tests became normal. The biggest change reported by her mother is that she is happier than she has ever been.

Another patient who reported excellent results with CBD-rich cannabis is an older woman who had severe traumatic injuries, including significant head trauma, after a car accident many years ago. After two years of rehabilitation, she continued to suffer from chronic pain and intermittent depression, which were not responding to conventional pharmaceuticals. She began using THC-rich cannabis, which eased her physical pain, but she did not find relief from her depressive symptoms. I encouraged her to add CBD-rich cannabis to her regimen, and she found a tremendous improvement in her mood. She uses two separate cannabis products, one CBD-rich in the morning and the other THC-rich at night. She has been able to discontinue pain medication and antidepressants since adding CBD to her regimen.

Like THC-rich cannabis products, CBD products are available in many forms, such as raw flowers, which can be inhaled via smoking or vaporizing; vaporizer cartridges; edibles; sublingual tinctures or extracts; topicals; transdermal patches; capsules; and highly concentrated forms.

Cannabinol (CBN)

Cannabinol is the third most prominent phytocannabinoid after THC and CBD. CBN was the first phytocannabinoid discovered at the end of the nineteenth century and was thought to be the main intoxicating compound in cannabis for many years until the discovery of THC.[28] It is found in trace amounts in the freshly cut cannabis flowers as well as in aged cannabis. As THC degrades over time, it oxidizes to form CBN.

Scientific Research

Cannabinol is less studied than THC and CBD, leaving us with many questions about its interaction with human physiology. Here is what we know so far:

- *Cannabinoid receptors:* CBN binds weakly to the CB_1 and CB_2 receptors, with stronger binding at CB_2.[29]
- *TRP channels:* Similar to how THC activates this family of proteins, CBN activates TRPA1 and blocks TRPM8, both of which are involved in pain, inflammation, and cancer.[30]

Clinical Indications

Although CBN is reported to bind weakly to CB_1 receptors, which should cause some intoxicating effects, three studies in which human subjects were given CBN in both low and high doses (ranging from 20 to 400 milligrams) reported no symptoms of intoxication.[31]

What are the medicinal effects of CBN?

- Antibacterial[32]
- Anticonvulsant[33]
- Promotes bone growth[34]
- Reduces intraocular pressure[35]
- Relieves pain[36]
- Stimulates appetite[37]

Two recent laboratory studies have shown that CBN can enhance the effects of other phytocannabinoids: the combination of CBN and THC was found to be neuroprotective in a model of Alzheimer's disease,[38] and the combination of CBN and CBC (cannabichromene) was analgesic in an animal model of chronic pain similar to fibromyalgia and temporomandibular disorders (such as TMJ syndrome).[39]

CBN also has been promoted as a sleep aid, although no studies support this claim. Human subjects taking isolated CBN did not report sedation; however, one study reported that CBN enhanced the effects of sedation caused by THC.[40] It is possible that patients who feel sedated from CBN are experiencing the effect from the THC or from terpenoids that remain in aged cannabis rather than the CBN itself. Despite the findings from studies, products containing higher amounts of CBN are gaining popularity for treatment of insomnia. Although some people may find CBN-rich products to be helpful in promoting sleep, THC-rich cannabis containing the sedating terpenoids is more effective for insomnia based on patient reports.

CBN products are available as tinctures, capsules, tablets, and tea. Also, CBN+THC and CBN+CBD combination products are on the market. Aged THC-rich cannabis flowers can be inhaled, as they will have a substantial amount of CBN.

Tetrahydrocannabinolic Acid (THCA)

THCA, first identified in 1965, is the main cannabinoid found in large amounts in raw, unheated, drug-variety cannabis flowers.[41] When THCA is exposed to heat (about 280–300°F), it is converted to THC by a process called "decarboxylation." There are two known forms of THCA— THCA-A and THCA-B—but the cannabis plant appears to make more THCA-A, therefore it is this form that has been the focus of studies and will be referred to as simply THCA.[42] Interestingly, THCA is thought to be one of the plant's defense mechanisms against insect predators.[43]

It has been difficult to study the effects of THCA, as it is considered to be an unstable compound that readily converts to THC. Any attempt to completely isolate THCA for research has failed since some portion of the THCA will convert to THC. Results from THCA experiments are therefore clouded by the persistent presence of a small amount of THC, making it hard to distinguish if findings are due to THCA or THC. Scientists are working to stabilize THCA by changing its chemical structure to limit the conversion to THC.

It is still unclear if THCA binds directly to cannabinoid receptors since results from laboratory and animal studies are contradictory. The current consensus is that THCA likely binds to cannabinoid receptors, albeit weakly. If this is true, THCA should be intoxicating, but patients who take THCA preparations do not report intoxicating effects. Researcher Guillermo Moreno-Sanz in a 2016 paper hypothesized that the most likely explanation for the contradictory findings is that THCA is unable to cross the blood–brain barrier (BBB) — the protective filter that prevents large molecules, certain immune cells, and disease-causing foreign invaders, such as bacteria and viruses, from entering the brain and spinal cord. Therefore, Moreno-Sanz proposes, THCA does not bind to cannabinoid receptors in the central nervous system.[44] It does, however, bind to the cannabinoid receptors located outside the central nervous system, conferring the therapeutic benefits.

Interestingly, THCA has been noted to reduce seizures in many pediatric patients. This effect has been investigated in only one experiment in mice,[45] but if the reports that THCA does not penetrate into the brain are true, how do we explain this effect? One hypothesis is that in certain conditions — such as epilepsy, ALS, multiple sclerosis, head trauma, schizophrenia, and systemic inflammation — the blood–brain barrier is compromised.[46] In these cases, THCA may be able to pass into the brain and interact with the endocannabinoid system and other targets, reducing seizures. Another hypothesis is that the antiseizure effects are caused by THC and other cannabinoids and terpenoids contained within the THCA preparation, not from the THCA itself. As you can see, more research is necessary to understand how THCA works for specific conditions.

Scientific Research

THCA, like other phytocannabinoids, has been shown to target numerous sites in the body:

- *CB₂ receptors:* As discussed previously, THCA likely binds to cannabinoid receptors located outside the central nervous system; these receptors are dense in the gut, where they play an anti-inflammatory role.
- *PPARs:* THCA binds to these receptors, causing anti-inflammatory and neuroprotective benefits in a laboratory model of Huntington's disease.[47]
- *GPR55:* Interestingly, THCA was shown to be the main phytocannabinoid influencing anti-inflammatory effects in the colon, mediated in part through this receptor.[48]
- *COX enzymes:* These enzymes produce prostaglandins, compounds that promote inflammation, pain, and fever.[49] Like CBD, THCA inhibits COX, decreasing production of prostaglandins.
- *TRP channels:* THCA binds to TRPA1 and blocks TRPM8, conferring anticancer effects.[50] These channels also are involved in pain and inflammation, but effects of THCA at this particular mechanism remain to be studied.

Clinical Indications

What are the medicinal effects of THCA?

- Anticancer[51]
- Anticonvulsant[52]
- Anti-inflammatory[53]
- Antispasmodic[54]
- Blocks anticipatory nausea (a type of conditioned nausea that occurs when a person who experiences nausea from chemotherapy develops nausea upon thinking about future chemo treatment)[55]

- Neuroprotectant[56]
- Potential antidepressant[57]

Patients use THCA for nausea, pain, inflammatory conditions, cancer, intestinal issues, autism, and seizure disorders. Some patients have reported excellent results from regularly drinking fresh juice made from raw cannabis flowers and leaves. This method of taking THCA is challenging, as a large number of plants are required to regularly juice fresh leaves. Fortunately, THCA-rich cannabis products have become more available over the past few years. These products should be kept in the refrigerator to minimize the conversion of THCA to THC. Contrary to recent claims, THCA does not convert to THC in the body.

One of my patients who suffered for years with irritable bowel syndrome and anxiety was using THC to treat his symptoms, obtaining only somewhat effective results. He would build tolerance to the THC, which resulted in him either taking higher, more expensive doses or taking breaks from THC, which then left his IBS untreated. He also had the unwanted side effect of severe "munchies," which led him to eating food that exacerbated his symptoms. We discussed his options and decided to have him try sublingual THCA, starting with 20 milligrams once a day. After about two weeks, he noticed decreased cramping, reduced abdominal pain, and less anxiety related to the condition. Occasionally if he eats something that aggravates his symptoms, he will increase his dose of THCA or use THC to rein in the flare-up. He has not had any further issues with tolerance or intoxication and has been able to remain on the same dose with good control of his IBS for almost three years.

I have not seen the development of tolerance to THCA in any patients. Toxicity has not been described, nor have I seen any significant unwanted side effects. Rarely THCA has caused anxiety or increased unwanted behaviors in some pediatric patients, but these effects seem to be related to the amount of THC within the preparation or due to the specific chemovar and have resolved quickly with a change in product.

THCA is available as a tincture in a carrier oil, which can be taken either sublingually or swallowed. Prefilled capsules, topical balms, and transdermal patches are also available. Some patients make their own capsules, filling them with a customized dose of tincture that works for them. Remember, THCA should be kept refrigerated to minimize conversion to THC.

Cannabidiolic Acid (CBDA)

CBDA was first discovered in 1940 and thought to be inactive.[58] Only recently has research begun to reveal its many medicinal benefits. CBDA is found in the raw cannabis flowers. When heated, it will convert to CBD through decarboxylation, similar to the conversion of THCA to THC. CBDA is nonintoxicating.

Scientific Research

Here is what we know so far about CBDA and its interaction with the brain and body:

- *Serotonin receptors $5HT_{1A}$:* These receptors play a role in controlling nausea and vomiting. CBDA, working through these receptors, is reported to be about a hundred times more effective than CBD at reducing nausea and vomiting in animals.[59] Combination THC+ CBDA at very low doses has a similar potency for nausea and vomiting.[60] Another study showed low doses of combination CBD+THC+CBDA suppressed vomiting in animals.[61] These same receptors are involved in anxiety. A recent study showed that stressed-out mice had a reduction in anxiety after a very low dose of CBDA was given.[62]
- *Anandamide:* CBDA blocked the uptake of anandamide, increasing its effects and thus enhancing the endocannabinoid system.[63]
- *2-AG:* Too much 2-AG (one of your endocannabinoids) is associated with obesity and insulin resistance; by inhibiting the synthesis

of 2-AG, CBDA may have therapeutic value in preventing these conditions.[64]

- *TRP channels:* CBDA acts at these channels involved in chronic and inflammatory pain as well as cancer. A study in mice found CBDA to be more potent than CBD for treating pain and inflammation. The same study showed that when given together, a combination of low doses of CBDA and THC was effective for pain and inflammation.[65]

- *COX enzymes:* These enzymes produce prostaglandins, compounds that promote inflammation, pain, and fever. Like CBD and THCA, CBDA inhibits COX, decreasing production of prostaglandins.[66] COX enzymes also have been shown to promote metastasis of breast cancer cells. CBDA was found in four laboratory studies to change gene expression by inhibiting COX, thereby decreasing metastasis.[67]

CBDA, like THCA, is considered an unstable compound in that it readily converts to CBD. Recently, researchers created a stabilized form of CBDA, called HU-580, or cannabidiolic acid methyl ester, in order to study CBDA without concerns of its conversion to CBD. Studies of HU-580 show antidepressant and antianxiety effects in mice.[68] Clinical trials in humans are lacking but certainly warranted, as CBDA appears to have multiple benefits at potentially low doses.

Clinical Indications

What are the medicinal effects of CBDA?

- Antianxiety
- Antidepressant
- Anti-inflammatory
- Potential anticonvulsant
- Reduces/eliminates nausea and vomiting
- Relieves pain

A patent filed in 2017 stated that CBDA reduced seizure severity of epilepsy in a rat model; however, the study was never published in a peer-reviewed scientific journal.[69] One of my pediatric patients with intractable epilepsy added CBDA oil to her existing regimen of CBD and THCA and experienced a further reduction of seizures; other patients have recently reported the same. In a 2019 study of a mice model of one of the most severe genetic pediatric epilepsies, called Dravet syndrome, CBDA increased the threshold for heat-induced seizures, making it less likely for the mice to have seizures due to high temperatures (a common seizure trigger for children with Dravet).[70] The CBDA doses used in this investigation were considerably lower than the human-equivalent recommended doses of CBD for seizures.

Another pediatric patient who struggles with two genetic conditions, both of which cause painful and debilitating bone abnormalities, was unable to attend school. She began a course of high-ratio CBD:THC oil (about 25:1) and titrated dosing up to hundreds of milligrams daily without any significant benefit (but high cost). At this point I changed her regimen to CBDA oil, and she had partial pain relief at a fairly low dose (about 8 milligrams). Increasing the dose did not confer more benefits, so I recommended adding in a nonintoxicating dose of THC (1 milligram to start, with instructions to increase slowly to find the best pain-relieving dose with no intoxication). Currently this patient is taking a combination 8 milligrams CBDA plus 3 milligrams THC twice a day (two separate products, both liquid extracts in oil) with such significant relief that she not only returned to school but also was able to participate in a school "marathon" in which she ran with her peers. She reports no side effects and no issues with tolerance. Her parents are thrilled with these results, especially since this combination is easily affordable.

Recent research shows that CBDA may be stimulating and alerting in its effects, similar to CBD's alerting effects in lower doses, so those new to CBDA should be aware it may disrupt sleep if taken in the evening.[71] It is available as a tincture and can be taken either sublingually or swallowed. Some patients make their own capsules containing the oil in the doses they determine to be effective. CBDA should be stored in the refrigerator to minimize its conversion to CBD.

Cannabigerol (CBG)

Cannabigerol is a phytocannabinoid that was discovered by Israeli researchers in 1964. CBG results from the decarboxylation of CBGA (cannabigerolic acid), the parent compound necessary for THC and CBD synthesis. CBG occurs in very small amounts in the cannabis plant, making it a minor cannabinoid; however, it is present in higher amounts in fiber varieties, and some of these plants will produce CBG almost exclusively. CBG is not intoxicating, but it is psychoactive in that it can affect mood.

Scientific Research

There has been a dramatic increase in research into CBG over the last few years. Similar to CBD, CBG has many sites of action in the brain and body, although much more research is needed.

- *Cannabinoid receptors:* Studies of CBG's actions at cannabinoid receptors report conflicting results. Depending on the dose and design of the laboratory investigation, CBG was found to both bind to and block CB_1 receptors and to bind to CB_2 receptors.[72] Patients taking CBG do not report intoxication, therefore it is unlikely to have significant binding at CB_1 receptors.
- *2-AG:* CBG blocks the enzyme MAGL (monoacylglycerol lipase) from breaking down the endocannabinoid called 2-AG, allowing it to have longer-lasting effects.[73]
- *Anandamide:* CBG inhibits the cellular uptake of anandamide, which increases anandamide's effects, enhancing the endocannabinoid system.[74]
- *TRP channels:* CBG activates TRPV1, TRPV2, and TRPA1, and blocks TRPM8, decreasing pain and inflammation and conferring anticancer effects.[75]

- *GABA receptors:* CBG blocks the uptake of GABA, the brain's main "calming" neurotransmitter, enhancing its effects.[76]
- *Serotonin receptors 5-HT$_{1A}$:* CBG blocks these receptors, which are involved in modulating mood, pain, cognition, memory, nausea, and cardiovascular function.[77]
- *PPARs:* CBG binds to these receptors, providing anti-inflammatory and neuroprotective benefits.[78]
- *Alpha-2 adrenergic receptors:* CBG binds to these receptors too, which are involved in blood pressure, pain, anxiety, and ADHD.[79]

Interestingly, CBG was shown to block CBD's antinausea effect in mice.[80] This hasn't been tested in humans, but potentially these two cannabinoids may counteract each other for this effect since CBD binds to serotonin receptors and CBG blocks them. However, a recent investigation found that the combination of CBD and CBG was more effective at decreasing neuroinflammation in a laboratory model of neurodegenerative disease (in particular, ALS) than either CBD or CBG taken alone.[81] Another very recent study in mice showed that CBG was able to lessen the decreased appetite and weight loss, and partially normalize the metabolic dysregulation, caused by cisplatin, a common and highly toxic chemotherapy drug. The authors of this study stated that CBG promoted "a wide-ranging pro-homeostatic effect."[82]

Clinical Indications

What are the medicinal effects of CBG?

- Antibacterial/anti-MRSA[83]
- Anticancer[84]
- Antidepressant[85]
- Anti-inflammatory[86]
- Antioxidant[87]
- Anti-psoriasis (inhibits keratinocyte proliferation)[88]
- Neuroprotectant[89]

- Promotes bone growth[90]
- Reduces bladder spasms[91]
- Reduces bowel inflammation[92]
- Reduces intraocular pressure[93]
- Reduces/eliminates nausea and vomiting[94]
- Stimulates appetite[95]

In my practice, the most common conditions responding to CBG are depression, autism, inflammation (from different causes), and psoriasis. One patient, a sixty-two-year-old man, was struggling with a ten-year history of severe depression, anxiety, and a terrible rash from psoriasis, a difficult-to-treat autoimmune condition. He also struggled with insomnia, which was aggravating all of his symptoms. I started him on sublingual CBG-rich oil, 20 milligrams twice a day, and a topical CBG applied twice a day to the rash. After one month, he reported that his insomnia, anxiety, and depression were all significantly better and his rash had improved by about 40 percent. At his three-month follow-up visit, he was still doing well with sleep and mood, but the rash persisted. We decided to switch to a combination CBG+CBD topical instead, resulting in further improvement. He also agreed to clean up his diet, avoiding processed foods and sugar, and at his one-year follow-up, his rash was almost completely resolved.

Another condition for which CBG may be helpful is autism spectrum disorder. Many of my patients with autism are taking some combination of CBD, THC, and THCA. When CBG became available, parents added it to the existing cannabis regimen to try to enhance the effects. In an informal survey, approximately 60 percent reported an improvement in their child's anxiety and overall mood. Approximately 30 percent reported an improvement in social interactions, focus, and speech. Very few side effects were reported, with the most common being increased anxiety, which resolved with discontinuation of the product.

CBG preparations are available as liquid extracts in a carrier oil, tablets, capsules, and topical balms. CBG-rich flowers are available for patients to vaporize. Since many of the CBG products on the market fall under the category of "hemp," meaning they are under 0.3 percent THC by weight and therefore are being sold online, it is recommended that patients obtain the COA (Certificate of Analysis) test results to be certain a product contains CBG and is devoid of pesticides and solvents. Clinically, most patients do not report sedating effects with CBG use; in fact, some report that it is alerting and stimulating, therefore I recommend daytime use when first trying CBG to avoid unwanted insomnia. However, some patients who have less anxiety with CBG use have reported an improvement in sleep.

Delta-9-Tetrahydrocannabivarin (THCV)

Delta-9-THCV is another minor phytocannabinoid that is present in drug-variety cannabis plants. It was first discovered in 1970 and named in 1971.[96] It is almost identical to THC in its chemical structure except it has two fewer carbon atoms. Interestingly, in the 1990s this compound was the focus of a number of studies not of its clinical benefits but of its usefulness as a drug screen to see if someone who tested positive for THC was using prescription synthetic THC (called dronabinol, brand name Marinol) or using natural (and presumably illicit) cannabis. It is no longer used for this purpose, as subsequent research in 2010 revealed this test to be unreliable.

Scientific Research

THCV has generated a large amount of interest due to the unique way it interacts with the cannabinoid receptors. Like the other phytocannabinoids, it has numerous sites of action. More research is needed to understand this interesting compound, as it appears to have some promising therapeutic benefits. The following findings are results from test-tube and animal experiments:

- *Cannabinoid receptors:* At low doses, THCV is a "neutral antagonist" at the CB_1 receptors.[97] This means it binds to the receptors and blocks other "keys," such as endocannabinoids and THC, from binding to them. At higher doses, THCV partially binds to CB_1 receptors. THCV binds to and activates CB_2 receptors but can also block these receptors, depending on the dose.[98]

- *TRP channels:* THCV activates TRPV1, TRPV2, TRPV3, and TRPV4, all involved in pain and inflammation, and blocks TRPM8, conferring anticancer effects. Its insulin sensitivity restoring effect is thought to be due to TRPV1 activation.[99]
- *Serotonin receptors 5-HT$_{1A}$:* THCV was found to activate 5-HT$_{1A}$, causing an antipsychotic effect.[100]
- *GPR55:* THCV weakly blocks this widespread receptor, involved in energy metabolism, pain and inflammation, anxiety, GI disorders, seizures, bone health, and cancer.[101]

Clinical Indications

THCV-rich cannabis has only very recently become available for patient use. Full understanding of its efficacy and potential side effects in humans remains unknown. In California, THCV-rich products also contain clinically significant amounts of THC, making it difficult to know which compound is responsible for the effects reported by patients.

What are the potential medicinal effects of THCV?

- Anticancer
- Anticonvulsant[102]
- Anti-inflammatory
- Antioxidant
- Antipsychotic
- Appetite suppressant
- Neuroprotectant
- Potentially improves glucose tolerance and increases insulin sensitivity
- Relieves pain

Pure THCV suppressed appetite and caused weight loss in mice that were fasting as well as mice that had eaten.[103] A cannabis extract with both THCV and THC did not have the same effect, likely due to the presence of THC; however, when CBD was added, the appetite suppressant effect returned. Additionally, THCV restored insulin sensitivity in obese mice.[104]

In two human trials, a pharmaceutical company investigated the effects of delta-9-THCV on type 2 diabetes. The first study showed that THCV significantly decreased fasting plasma glucose and improved pancreatic beta-cell function, as well as other parameters of glucose metabolism.[105] However, the second study failed to meet similar end points.[106] It is important to note that these trials used isolated THCV, not whole-plant THCV-rich extract.

Researchers who investigated cannabinoid effects on Parkinson's disease in a mouse model suggested the combination of CBD and delta-9-THCV as a potent neuroprotectant and antioxidant for this condition.[107]

THCV decreased neuropathic pain in a mouse model (reported in a patent).[108]

A 2016 report on ten male cannabis users reported that THCV was subjectively indistinguishable from the placebo, meaning they did not feel intoxicated. This report also looked at the combination of THCV+THC and found that 90 percent reported the "effects of THC to be subjectively weaker or less intense" in the presence of THCV. THCV also prevented THC-induced increased heart rate (meaning THCV likely blocked this effect) but worsened memory (meaning THCV may have potentiated the effect of THC on memory). It was well tolerated with no significant adverse effects.[109] Certainly more studies on THCV are warranted due to its potential therapeutic benefits.

If you recall the story of rimonabant from chapter 2, it was a synthetic form of THCV prescribed for weight loss and withdrawn from the market due to significant psychiatric side effects. THCV from the cannabis plant has the same effect on appetite but does not appear to have the same risks to mental health since it does not appear to negatively impact mood pathways in the brain.

THCV-rich cannabis is still somewhat difficult to find but is showing up in some medical cannabis dispensaries in the form of flowers, tincture, or tablets/capsules, although the current products have equal amounts of THC content.

Cannabidivarin (CBDV)

Cannabidivarin is a minor nonpsychoactive cannabinoid that was discovered in 1969.[110] Numerous animal studies have reported it to be an effective anticonvulsant by itself and additively when combined with CBD.[111]

Scientific Research

There is very little research on CBDV compared to other phytocannabinoids; however, the recent discovery of its anticonvulsant effects has triggered more interest in this compound. This is what we know so far about its interaction with our physiology:

- *Cannabinoid receptors:* CBDV does not bind to CB_1 or CB_2 receptors.[112]
- *DAGL:* CBDV blocks this enzyme, diacylglycerol lipase, which is involved in the synthesis of the endocannabinoid 2-AG.[113]
- *TRP channels:* CBDV activates TRPA1, TRPV1, and TRPV2; this is the mechanism thought to confer antiseizure effects.[114]
- *GPR55:* CBDV weakly blocks this receptor, involved in energy metabolism, pain and inflammation, GI disorders, seizures, and cancer.[115]
- *GABA receptors:* CBDV interacts with these receptors, which may explain its anticonvulsant effects.[116]

Recently CBDV was shown to "rescue behavioral and brain altera-tions" in a mouse model of Rett syndrome, a rare neurodevelopmental disorder with no known cure.[117] Per a recent patent filing, CBDV improved neuropathic pain in a mouse model of this difficult-to-treat condition.[118]

Clinical Indications

What are the medicinal effects of CBDV?

- Anticonvulsant
- Relieves neuropathic pain

As previously mentioned, multiple laboratory investigations report the anticonvulsant effects of CBDV in animals. A case report of a young man with severe epilepsy taking a homemade preparation of cannabis documented a significant reduction in his seizures when serum CBDV levels were high (although CBD and THC were also present in his serum, albeit at lower levels).[119] A recent clinical trial on single-molecule CBDV (not a whole-plant preparation) in adults with treatment-resistant focal epilepsy did not show significant differences when compared to the pla-cebo, but CBDV was found to be well tolerated.[120] Currently there are two clinical trials looking at CBDV for treatment of autism spectrum disorder.[121]

Delta-8-Tetrahydrocannabinol (delta-8-THC)

This minor cannabinoid, discovered around the same time as delta-9-THC, recently became commercially available for patient use. Delta-8-THC is an "isomer" of delta-9-THC, meaning it has the same molecular formula (21 carbon atoms, 30 hydrogen atoms, and 2 oxygen atoms) but differs slightly in the way the atoms are arranged in the chemical structure. Delta-8-THC has similar properties and pharmacological effects as delta-9-THC but with the benefit of less intoxication (about 50 to 60 percent less potent than delta-9-THC) for those patients who do not like or want this effect.[122] Additionally, delta-8-THC is more stable than delta-9-THC (i.e., it is less likely to degrade), giving it a longer shelf life.

Scientific Research

Full understanding of the benefits of delta-8-THC is lacking, as there is very little research into its physiologic activity in humans.

- *Cannabinoid receptors:* Delta-8-THC binds to these receptors, although with lower binding power than delta-9-THC.

A 2004 study in mice showed delta-8-THC caused increased food consumption and a tendency for improved cognitive function, without evidence of intoxication.[123] Another study investigating the effects of phytocannabinoids on acetylcholine—a very important neurotransmitter involved in motor function, memory, and cognition—found that delta-8-THC (as well as delta-9-THC) increased levels of acetylcholine and decreased its turnover.[124] This may have significant benefits in treating Alzheimer's disease, in which a deficiency of acetylcholine is known to play a large role.

Clinical Indications

The effects of delta-8-THC are quite similar to those of delta-9-THC; however, since delta-8-THC has not been available until recently, it is still unclear what dosing is most beneficial for these indications. As with other cannabinoids, starting with low doses and increasing to the desired effects is the best way to find the most benefits with the fewest side effects.

What are the medicinal effects of delta-8-THC?

- Antianxiety
- Anticancer[125]

- Neuroprotectant
- Reduces intraocular pressure[126]
- Reduces nausea and vomiting
- Relieves pain
- Stimulates appetite

In a 1995 study, researchers in Israel gave delta-8-THC to eight children on cancer chemotherapy treatments known to cause severe vomiting and found "the prevention of vomiting was complete," regardless of the chemotherapy given. This study reported that 480 doses were given over a two-year period with few or no side effects.[127] Doses of delta-8-THC were somewhat higher than doses of delta-9-THC used in similar trials. The patent filed after this investigation made the claim that delta-8-THC was 200 percent more effective at reducing nausea and vomiting than delta-9-THC.[128]

Clinically, a few of my patients have used delta-8-THC for nausea and for anxiety, taking it in the form of a 3-milligram sublingual tablet. These patients have reported efficacy with doses between 3 and 9 milligrams with very little intoxication. As we see more products containing this compound come on the market, we will have a better idea of its true therapeutic effects.

Cannabichromene (CBC)

CBC was discovered by Israeli researchers Raphael Mechoulam and Yehiel Gaoni in 1966.[129] CBC, like its phytocannabinoid cousins THC, CBD, and CBG, comes from the parent compound CBGA. A small amount of CBGA converts to cannabichromenic acid (CBCA), which, when exposed to heat, converts to CBC. CBC does not bind to cannabinoid receptors, although more research is needed to fully understand its actions.[130] CBC is not intoxicating and is usually present in small amounts in most cannabis plants, adding to the entourage effect.

Scientific Research

Although not as well studied as THC and CBD, CBC is known to have a few targets of action.

- *TRP channels:* CBC binds to TRPV1 and TRPA1, which are involved in pain signaling.[131]
- *Anandamide:* CBC inhibits the uptake of anandamide, allowing for longer-lasting effects.[132]

Clinical Indications

What are the medicinal effects of CBC?

- Anti-acne[133]
- Anticancer[134]
- Antidepressant[135]
- Relieves pain[136]
- Anti-inflammatory[137]
- Antibacterial[138]
- Antifungal[139]

Some interesting studies have investigated the interaction of CBC and THC. One study reported an enhanced anti-inflammatory effect when both compounds were used together and additionally found evidence of elevated THC in the brain of mice when CBC was present.[137] Another report found that mice that were given both compounds had less intoxicating effects from THC when CBC was given.[139] A 2013 study found CBC had a positive effect on adult neural stem progenitor cells, which play an important role in brain health and healing.[140] CBC appears to have many beneficial therapeutic effects, warranting further research into its full potential as medicine.

Summary

As you can see, the phytocannabinoid compounds found in the cannabis plant have many different sites of action within the human brain and body. They interact not only with cannabinoid receptors within the endocannabinoid system but also with many different receptors and other targets, causing changes in our biochemistry. Since our endocannabinoid system is involved in various parts of our physiology, the importance of understanding the actions of each phytocannabinoid becomes clear. As our knowledge grows with further research, patients will be able to select those phytocannabinoids that will benefit them most.

CHAPTER 5

How to Use Cannabis as Medicine

F iguring out how to use cannabis as medicine can be complicated for anyone who is new to it or inexperienced. As you learned in the previous chapters, several different phytocannabinoids and terpenoids make up cannabis chemovars and products. The essential concepts in this chapter—including how to read a COA, the different ways to take cannabis, and drug–drug interactions—will help you to understand the multitude of products and explain how to find a cannabis medicine regimen that is therapeutically beneficial while limiting unwanted side effects.

What's in Your Medicine?

All cannabis products used by medical cannabis patients should be tested in order to ensure quality, consistency, and safety. The report generated by a cannabis testing laboratory is called a **Certificate of Analysis, or COA**. Quite simply, the COA allows you to know with good certainty which cannabinoids and other compounds are in the product and if the product is clean and safe for you to consume. A "first-party COA" is the test performed by the company that grew the flower or made the product, and a "third-party COA" is one done by an independent laboratory.

A COA should include the following information:

- Profile and potency of cannabinoids
- Profile and potency of terpenoids
- Presence of residual solvents
- Presence of bacteria and fungi
- Presence of pesticides and fungicides
- Presence of heavy metals

Different states and countries have their own requirements for testing. For instance, California law requires testing to include all of the above plus moisture content for flowers. Arizona has not instituted required testing, Delaware requires testing only for pesticides, and Florida requires testing only for contaminants and potency. These laws are continually changing as states develop their medical cannabis programs, therefore it is best to check with the regulatory body in your state or country to find the latest testing requirements.

Cannabis can be tested in a number of ways, for instance gas chromatography (GC), high-performance liquid chromatography (HPLC), and mass spectrometry (MS). Unfortunately, different methods of testing may produce different results, and overall standardization is still somewhat lacking. As the cannabis industry matures, however, some states are mandating labs to be "ISO/IEC 17025 accredited," meaning they adhere to standard operating procedures and good lab practices with accountability for the data they report.

Cannabinoid Profiles

This COA lists the potency of the cannabinoids in "wt %" (weight by percent), "mg/g" (milligrams per gram), and "mg/mL" (milligrams per

Cannabinoid Profile			
Cannabinoids	wt %	mg/g	mg/mL
Delta-9-THC Total	0.50	4.99	4.74
CBD Total	5.99	59.90	56.95
CBG Total	0.01	0.12	0.11
Delta-9-THC	0.25	2.53	2.41
Delta-9-THCA	0.28	2.80	2.67
CBD	5.97	59.69	56.75
CBDA	0.02	0.24	0.23
CBG	ND	ND	ND
CBGA	0.01	0.13	0.13
CBN	ND	ND	ND
CBC	0.32	3.16	3.01
Delta-8-THC	ND	ND	ND
Cannabinoids	Pass		

Figure 1: COA showing phytocannabinoid potency results. (*Jeff Raber, PhD, of The Werc Shop*)

milliliter). The quantity of milligrams is most important since this is used for dosing.

As you can see in figure 1, above, there are 56.95 milligrams per 1 milliliter of CBD and 4.74 milligrams per 1 milliliter of THC, showing you that this is a CBD-dominant product. If you ingested 1 milliliter (which is about one-fifth of a teaspoon), you would be taking 56.95 milligrams of CBD and 4.74 milligrams of THC. Be aware that the total THC reflected in the top of the COA is the sum of THC plus THCA and the total CBD is the sum of the CBD plus CBDA. You can also see that this sample contains small amounts of THCA, CBDA, CBGA, and CBC. "ND" means "none detected."

NOTE: If you see a test result that lists only CBD content, it is very likely a "CBD isolate," which means there are probably no other phytocannabinoids in the product. I never recommend CBD isolates, as I have found that the full array of phytocannabinoids, a so-called whole-plant preparation, is more effective for serious conditions. Whole-plant products provide more robust therapeutic benefits, often at lower doses, due to the entourage effect and the synergy of the compounds.

Be aware that the cannabinoid content may vary from batch to batch, as it is very difficult to produce products with the exact same amount of cannabinoids in each batch. In California, cannabis potency on the label must be within 10 percent of the batch test result. For example, if a CBD-rich tincture has a label that claims "50 mg/1 mL," the batch test must show that the actual CBD is somewhere between 45 and 55 milligrams per 1 milliliter (10 percent in either direction). If the batch COA finds "40 mg/1 mL," this product would have to be relabeled before it could be sold to patients. This strict requirement ultimately protects patients from potential dosing errors.

Also be aware that some hemp products report a certain milligram amount of "hemp parts" or "hemp extract" on their labels. This is *not* the CBD content but the total cannabinoids in the product. The bottle should have a batch number or QR code that corresponds to a COA that can tell you which cannabinoids are present and how many milligrams of each phytocannabinoid are contained in the product. I advise patients to avoid products that do not have this information readily available.

Terpenoid Profiles

Remember that terpenoids are the essential oils found in the cannabis plant. These compounds give cannabis its odor and flavor, and contribute to the medicinal effects. Terpenoids work synergistically with each other and the phytocannabinoids, enhancing the entourage effect.

The COA lists the terpene profiles in terms of "mg/g" (milligrams per

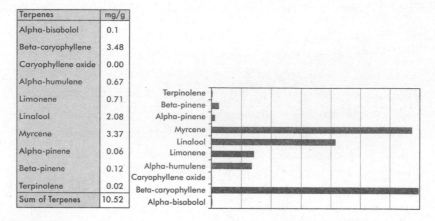

Terpenes	mg/g
Alpha-bisabolol	0.1
Beta-caryophyllene	3.48
Caryophyllene oxide	0.00
Alpha-humulene	0.67
Limonene	0.71
Linalool	2.08
Myrcene	3.37
Alpha-pinene	0.06
Beta-pinene	0.12
Terpinolene	0.02
Sum of Terpenes	10.52

Figure 2: Terpenoid potency results. (*Jeff Raber, PhD, of The Werc Shop*)

gram). As you can see in figure 2, the terpenoid profile of this product shows significant amounts of myrcene, linalool, limonene, alpha-humulene, and beta-caryophyllene, with a few other terpenoids in low amounts. This chemovar is likely to be anti-inflammatory and have benefits for mood and pain.

Testing for Residual Solvents

Solvents are often employed in the processing of cannabis extracts and concentrated preparations. Solvents that are not purged properly and remain in the end product are called "residual solvents." Butane, propane, pentane, and hexane—all of which are petroleum derivatives, highly flammable, and potentially carcinogenic—are used by some suppliers to make concentrates and extracts. Although some cannabis experts claim that professional butane extraction is safe and results in a clean product, the product may still contain an unwanted and potentially toxic residual solvent, especially if low-quality butane is used. I do not recommend products made with these chemicals unless analytical testing by a reputable lab reveals no residual solvents.

Ethanol, considered safe for most people, is also commonly employed as a solvent for concentrates and extracts. Chemically this solvent extracts chlorophyll along with the cannabinoids and terpenes, often leaving products with a darker color and a "grassier" taste, although some manufacturers will purge the chlorophyll to reduce this effect. Another commonly employed method is supercritical carbon dioxide (CO_2) extraction. No harmful solvents are used, resulting in zero possibility of residual solvents in the end product. CO_2 extraction is considered by many to be the cleanest and safest method, although it is an expensive process and may result in fewer terpenes in the end product. No matter the extraction process, all products used by medical cannabis patients should be tested for residual solvents before use.

Residual solvent amounts are often expressed in parts per million (ppm). Different states have set widely varied limits. For instance, California has a solvent residue limit of 5,000 ppm for solvents such as butane and ethanol,

Residual Solvent Detection				
Residual Solvent	LOD ppm	LOQ ppm	Action Threshold µg/g	Amount Detected µg/g
Acetone	5	16	5,000	ND
Acetonitrile	0.8	2.5	410	ND
Benzene	0.04	0.1	1	ND
Butane	5.5	17	5,000	ND
Chloroform	0.25	0.5	1	ND
1,2-Dichloroethane	0.1	0.3	1	ND
Ethanol	0.5	1	5,000	ND
Ethyl acetate	31	84	5,000	177.07
Ethyl ether	6	18	5,000	22,997.43
Ethylene oxide	0.5	1	1	ND
Heptane	33	90	5,000	ND
Hexane	0.5	1	290	ND
Isopropyl alcohol	7	21	5,000	22.18
Methanol	62	167	3,000	ND
Methylene chloride	0.5	1	1	ND
Pentane	6.4	19	5,000	ND
Propane	20	59	5,000	ND
Toluene	12.2	33	890	ND
Total xylenes	3	10	2,170	ND
Trichloroethylene	0.5	1	1	ND
Residual Solvent Results (Pass/Fail)				
All Cannabis Products		Fail		

Figure 3: Sample residual solvent results. (*Jeff Raber, PhD, of The Werc Shop*)
* µg/g = micrograms per gram; ppm = parts per million

Colorado set limits at 1,000 ppm, and Massachusetts is much lower at 12 ppm. Of course the best product is one that tests negative for all solvents.

As you can see in figure 3, this product, which was "homemade," failed testing due to very high levels of a solvent called ethyl ether. It tested positive for two other solvents as well, although both were below the state-determined "action threshold," which is the highest level allowed for any solvent. This is a real product that one of my patients was buying from an unlicensed distributor—an all too common example of non-chemists manufacturing cannabis products with the potential to make people sick. It is imperative that patients use only tested cannabis products from reliable and licensed manufacturers.

LOD, or "limit of detection," is the lowest quantity of a substance that can be detected by a specific instrument. It is expressed in parts per million (ppm). LOQ, or "limit of quantitation," is the lowest concentration of a substance in a sample that can be determined with acceptable precision and accuracy. It also is expressed in parts per million.

Testing for Bacteria, Fungi, and Mycotoxins

Cannabis can be contaminated with bacteria or fungi (yeast or mold) at any point in the growing or product-manufacturing process. Cannabis contaminated with bacteria or fungi can be dangerous, especially for anyone with compromised immune function. Bacteria and mold can be identified by plating, whereby prepared samples are placed on growth medium and incubated; any growth is counted and reported as "colony forming units per gram" (CFU/g). Another process, called "quantitative polymerase chain reaction" (qPCR), utilizes machinery that extracts DNA from the microbes, which is then genetically sequenced to identify the organism. States vary in permissible levels of microbial contaminants. Mycotoxins, such as aflatoxin and ochratoxin, are toxins produced by fungi and are known to cause serious illnesses. The limit for mycotoxins is usually 20 parts per billion (ppb), the same action level used by the FDA for food.

As you can see in the sample COA in figure 4, this product passed bacteria and mycotoxin testing, meaning that no pathogens were present.

Microbial Impurities		
Contaminant	Action Level (CFU/g)	Pass/Fail
E. coli	LLOD	PASS
Salmonella spp.	LLOD	PASS
A. fumigatus, niger, flavus, & terreus	LLOD	PASS

Mycotoxin Analysis					
	Action Level (ppb)				µg/kg
Mycotoxin	LOD ppb	LOQ ppb	Inhalable Cannabis	Cannabis Products	Amount Detected
Ochratoxin A	2.0	7.0	20.000	20.000	ND
Aflatoxin B_1	2.0	6.0	20.000	20.000	ND
Aflatoxin B_2	3.0	7.0	20.000	20.000	ND
Aflatoxin G_1	2.0	8.0	20.000	20.000	ND
Aflatoxin G_2	1.0	4.0	20.000	20.000	ND
Results	NT				

Figure 4: Sample microbial and mycotoxin results. (*Jeff Raber, PhD, of The Werc Shop*)
* CFU/g = colony-forming units per gram; LLOD = lower level of detection; ppb = parts per billion; µg/kg = micrograms per kilogram

Testing for Pesticides

The cannabis plant is like any other plant, prone to disease and infestation by pests. Pesticide chemicals, such as insecticides, herbicides, and fungicides, are used by some growers despite the fact that most people do not want these chemicals in their medicine. The COA typically will list the amount of pesticides if the product tests positive. As you can see in figure 5, this product—a concentrated THC oil—failed testing due to being over the limit of the pesticide malathion.

There has been no research investigating the side effects from inhaled or ingested pesticides specifically related to cannabis; however, other studies clearly show that pesticides have been linked to cancer; skin irritation; endocrine dysfunction; neurologic disorders, including Alzheimer's disease and ADHD; reproductive problems; and birth defects.[1] States where cannabis is legal for medical and/or recreational use have allowed for certain pesticides based on previous approval for use on food intended for human consumption.

Residual Pesticide	Action Level (µg/g)				µg/g
	Action Limit II	Action Limit II	LOD ppb	LOQ ppb	Amount Detected
Abamectin II	0.10	0.30	0.001	0.007	ND
Acephate II	0.10	5.00	0.039	0.131	ND
Acequinocyl II	0.10	4.00	0.518	0.760	ND
Acetamiprid II	0.10	5.00	0.008	0.030	ND
Aldicarb I II	LLOD	LLOD	0.009	0.030	ND
Azoxystrobin II	0.10	40.00	0.007	0.025	ND
Bifenazate II	0.10	5.00	0.003	0.010	ND
Bifenthrin II	3.00	0.50	0.003	0.011	ND
Boscalid II	0.10	10.00	0.008	0.026	ND
Captan II	0.70	5.00	0.434	1.450	ND
Carbaryl II	0.50	5.00	0.005	0.018	3.52
Carbofuran I	LLOD	LLOD	0.008	0.027	ND
Chlorantraniliprole II	10.00	40.00	0.027	0.071	ND
Chlordane I	LLOD	LLOD	1.080	3.600	ND
Chlorfenapyr I	LLOD	LLOD	0.550	0.504	ND
Chlorpyrifos I	LLOD	LLOD	0.010	0.036	ND
Clofentezine II	0.10	0.50	0.011	0.036	ND
Coumaphos I	LLOD	LLOD	0.032	0.109	ND
Cyfluthrin II	2.00	1.00	0.289	0.960	ND
Cypermethrin II	1.00	1.00	0.496	1.650	ND
Daminozide I	LLOD	LLOD	0.322	1.070	ND
Diazinon II	0.10	0.20	0.012	0.042	ND
Dichlorvos I	LLOD	LLOD	0.013	0.045	ND
Dimethoate I	LLOD	LLOD	0.007	0.002	ND
Dimethomorph II	2.00	20.00	0.003	0.009	ND
Ethoprop(hos) I	LLOD	LLOD	0.007	0.026	ND
Etofenprox I	LLOD	LLOD	0.008	0.026	ND
Etoxazole II	0.10	1.50	0.001	0.006	ND
Fenhexamid II	0.10	10.00	0.019	0.064	ND
Fenoxycarb I	LLOD	LLOD	0.005	0.018	ND
Fenpyroximate II	0.10	2.00	0.001	0.004	ND
Fipronil I	LLOD	LLOD	0.052	0.173	ND
Flonicamid II	0.10	2.00	0.005	0.015	ND
Fludioxonil II	0.10	30.00	0.012	0.041	ND
Hexythiazox II	0.10	2.00	0.004	0.015	ND
Imazalil I	LLOD	LLOD	0.036	0.122	ND
Imidacloprid II	5.00	3.00	0.006	0.109	ND
Kresoxim-methyl II	0.10	1.00	0.016	0.054	ND
Malathion II	0.50	5.00	0.005	0.017	5.51
Metalaxyl II	2.00	15.00	0.007	0.023	ND
Methiocarb I	LLOD	LLOD	0.004	0.015	ND
Methomyl II	1.00	0.10	0.008	0.027	ND
Mevinphos I	LLOD	LLOD	0.297	0.727	ND

DR. GOLDSTEIN	
Date Analyzed	
1/10/2020	
Sample Name	
ORIGINAL NECTAR THC	
0	
T&T #:	Batch #:
200110-160-DG-1-1	0

Pesticide Results (Pass/Fail)	
Inhalable Cannabis	FAIL

Residual Pesticide	Action Level (µg/g)				µg/g
	Action Limit II	Action Limit II	LOD ppb	LOQ ppb	Amount Detected
Myclobutanil II	0.10	9.00	0.127	0.280	0.11
Naled II	0.10	0.50	0.010	0.034	ND
Oxamyl II	0.50	0.20	0.010	0.034	ND
Paclobutrazol I	LLOD	LLOD	0.009	0.031	ND
Parathion methyl I	LLOD	LLOD	0.238	0.790	ND
PCNB II	0.10	0.20	0.970	3.200	ND
Permethrin II	0.50	20.00	0.025	0.069	ND
Phosmet II	0.10	0.20	0.004	0.014	ND
Piperonyl butoxide II	3.00	8.00	0.010	0.049	0.41
Prallethrin II	0.10	0.40	0.030	0.100	ND
Propiconazole II	0.10	20.00	0.029	0.099	ND
Propoxur I	LLOD	LLOD	0.004	0.015	ND
Pyrethrins II	0.50	1.00	0.439	0.618	ND
Pyridaben II	0.10	3.00	0.002	0.005	ND
Spinetoram II	0.10	3.00	0.000	0.530	ND
Spinosad II	0.10	3.00	0.001	0.004	ND
Spiromesifen II	0.10	12.00	0.000	0.001	ND
Spirotetramat II	0.10	13.00	0.014	0.047	ND
Spiroxamine I	LLOD	LLOD	0.008	0.029	ND
Tebuconazole II	0.10	2.00	0.001	0.005	ND
Thiacloprid I	LLOD	LLOD	0.010	0.034	ND
Thiamethoxam II	5.00	4.50	0.001	0.005	ND
Trifloxystrobin II	0.10	30.00	0.003	0.018	ND

Figure 5: Sample pesticide testing results. (*Jeff Raber, PhD, of The Werc Shop*)
* µg/g = micrograms per gram; LOD = limit of detection; LOQ = limit of quantitation; ppb = parts per billion

If the product contains pesticides and is made from concentrated extracts, the pesticides may also be concentrated. **I strongly recommend that you avoid these chemicals in your food and in your cannabis!**

What about organic cannabis? Many responsible cultivators are taking an organic approach. However, since cannabis is still federally illegal, the USDA does not recognize cannabis as a crop and certification agencies are prohibited from certifying cannabis crops as organic. Some terms cannabis providers may use to imply organically grown practices are "natural," "pesticide-free," and "locally grown." A number of private companies will certify cannabis cultivators and manufacturers that meet organic standards, giving them a "clean" designation, but until organic certification exists and pesticide testing is required by all states and countries, patients should seek out and use only cannabis that tests negative for all pesticides.

Heavy Metal					
	Action Level (ppm)				µg/g
Heavy Metal	LOD ppb	LOQ ppb	Inhalable Cannabis	Cannabis Products	Amount Detected
Cadmium	0.040	0.140	0.200	0.500	ND
Lead	0.010	0.030	0.500	0.500	0.04
Arsenic	0.060	0.200	0.200	1.500	0.01
Mercury	0.090	0.300	0.100	3.000	ND
Results	Pass				

Figure 6: Sample heavy metal testing results. (*Jeff Raber, PhD, of The Werc Shop*)
* LOD = limit of detection; LOQ = limit of quantitation; ppm = parts per million; ppb = parts per billion; µg/g: micrograms per gram

Testing for Heavy Metals

Cannabis plants are known to be bioaccumulators, which means they absorb minerals, including heavy metals, and nutrients from the soil. In fact, cannabis plants are such good bioaccumulators that they are used for phytoremediation, a process by which soil or groundwater can be cleaned by plants that pull their contaminants out. Famously, hemp was planted around the Chernobyl nuclear disaster site in the 1990s, and it significantly reduced soil toxicity. The four metals of most interest are arsenic, cadmium, lead, and mercury. These are known to be highly toxic, especially with prolonged exposure. There are no studies investigating heavy-metal poisoning from cannabis products; however, the FDA recommends that all medicinal products be tested due to the significant toxicity related to these compounds. Interestingly, cannabis labs across the country report a very low heavy-metal contamination rate (under 1 percent) for medical cannabis products. As you can see in figure 6, testing detected the presence of lead and arsenic, but the amounts were below the limits set by state regulations, allowing the product to "pass." It is recommended to use products that test negative for heavy metals in order to avoid any potential health risks.

The Different Delivery Methods

Many potential cannabis patients are turned off by the idea of smoking. You do not have to smoke cannabis to get the benefits! There are many different ways to use cannabis as a medicine, including by topical application, sublingual (under the tongue) tinctures, vaporization, and more. Different delivery methods may change the overall experience and effects, as each method alters the time to the onset of effects, the duration of the effects, and the effects themselves. Some patients prefer to use only one method; other patients vary the methods depending on factors such as the time of use (daytime versus nighttime), the expected duration of the effects, and the symptoms being experienced (such as anxiety or pain). Learning what to expect and experimenting with the various methods is the best way to know how you will respond.

Inhalation

With inhalation of THC-rich cannabis, the maximum blood concentration of THC occurs within minutes. The psychoactive and possible intoxicating effects can start from within seconds to a few minutes, reach a peak effect in thirty minutes, and taper off within one to four hours, depending on the dose. Inhalation of CBD is quite similar to THC, of course without the intoxicating effects if the product is low in THC.

The advantages of inhalation include a rapid onset of effects and easier dosing, especially for someone with nausea or pain. Since effects are felt fairly quickly, most patients can adjust their dose to the desired effect and avoid overdoing it, minimizing unwanted side effects. Exact dosing can be found easily with practice and can vary with depth of inhale, how many puffs are inhaled, and the potency of different products.

Vaporization is much preferred over smoking since it eliminates the toxins from the burning plant matter and reduces the resulting irritation to the lungs. Despite the belief that bongs or water pipes act as a "filter," they actually do not decrease the amount of tar or other particles in the smoke. In fact, water pipe or bong smokers inhale 30 percent more smoke to get the same effect as with a pipe or joint. The water traps THC without trapping very much tar, so the "hit" that is inhaled has fewer medicinal compounds and more toxins.[2] I do not encourage my patients to use bongs or water pipes.

Vaporizers are devices that heat up cannabis and emit a vapor that contains the medicinal compounds, ideally without the products of combustion, like tar, carbon monoxide, and particulate matter. Widely considered to be a "cleaner" way to inhale cannabis medicine, proper vaporization at temperatures between 315 and 420°F (160 and 220°C) produces significantly fewer by-products compared to combustion.

The advantages of vaporization of the cannabis flowers include:

- Smokeless inhalation
- The many chemovars to choose from
- A more efficient use of the medication
- A quicker onset of effects and easier dosing than non-inhalation methods
- Little odor
- Less toxicity for the lungs and airways
- Less risk of bronchitis and other respiratory symptoms (such as coughing, wheezing, tightness in the chest)

Vaporizers work by heating the cannabis flowers without burning them. They can create vapor by two different methods: with conduction, the cannabis flowers are placed on a surface that heats up like a hot plate, and compounds in the flowers touching or very near the hot surface vaporize; with convection, air is heated up and passed through the plant material, vaporizing the medicine. In both methods, the cannabis flowers should be ground up to improve the extraction of the medicine.

Patients have many choices of flower vaporizers, from large "desktop" versions, such as the very popular Volcano brand, to portable handheld devices. These devices are often referred to as "herbal vaporizers."

E-cigarette-type vaporizers became available around 2007 and have become extremely popular. Cannabis flowers are processed into a liquid form—usually an oil—which is placed into a cartridge or chamber and attached to a small pen-like battery. Be aware that these batteries do not have a temperature control and, for the most part, do not vaporize the oil but combust it. Concerns about cannabis oil cartridges used for vaporization include the risk of residual solvents, concentrated pesticides, and, more recently reported, possible contamination of the oil by a seepage of metals from parts of the cartridge.

The risks from long-term use of e-cigarette-type cannabis vaporizer cartridges are unknown. The recent association of these products with severe respiratory illnesses is a cause for concern. In August 2019, the CDC opened an investigation into vape-related hospitalizations after numerous previously healthy people developed acute and severe respiratory distress. Although the CDC reports a decline in these illnesses since September 2019, as of January 2020, more than 2,500 people have been sickened and almost 60 people have died. The CDC has named this condition EVALI, or "e-cigarette or vaping product use-associated lung injury." In the majority of EVALI cases, the vaporizer was not obtained from a legal, licensed medical cannabis dispensary. According to one study, people who vaporized THC purchased from illegal sources were nine times more likely to get EVALI.[3] The FDA reported that they found vitamin E acetate in the lung fluid obtained from the majority of EVALI patients; however, this contaminant was found in only 50 percent of samples tested. Other contaminants have been found, including medium-chain triglycerides and polyethylene glycol. According to reports, vitamin E acetate was added to illicit vaporizers in order to thicken the oil to make it last longer. One laboratory in California found that none of the two hundred vaporizer cartridges made by licensed manufacturers contained vitamin E acetate, but nine of fifteen (60 percent) from the illicit market tested positive for this chemical, as well as contained quite elevated pesticide levels.[4]

Since this public health crisis, I have encouraged my patients who want to inhale to switch to herbal vaporizers, as there are no cases of EVALI reported with the use of these with cannabis flowers. However, if a particular vaporizer cartridge has been very beneficial for a patient and they are reluctant to change using these products, I advise the patient to contact the cartridge manufacturer to ask about their manufacturing process and, very importantly, to only use products purchased through a state-licensed dispensary.

Ingestion

When cannabis is ingested through drinks, edibles, or capsules, the onset of effects begins after thirty to ninety minutes, but this varies widely from person to person, taking as long as three to six hours in some. The effects generally reach their peak in two to three hours and last for six to eight hours, depending on the dose.

THC absorbed through the intestinal tract will pass through the liver. This is called the "first pass effect." Much of the THC will be broken down into a cousin compound of THC, called 11-hydroxy-THC, which is intoxicating on its own, but when it's combined with THC, the potency of the intoxicating effects increases.[5] Ingestion produces different effects than inhalation for most cannabis users, who describe the experience as "more relaxing" or as a "body high," and report sedating effects. Many of my patients also find good sleep with low-dose THC edibles taken about one to two hours before they go to bed due to these sedating effects. However, some patients do not like the effects from ingestion. The different effects reported by patients between the methods of inhalation and ingestion are due to very little conversion of THC to 11-hydroxy-THC with inhalation and significant conversion with ingestion.

The advantages of ingestion are that smoke is avoided, there is no need for any equipment, such as a vaporizer, the duration of the effect is longer, and there is no odor. Edible forms of cannabis can be taken discreetly too. Due to the variation in bioavailability (how much your body absorbs) and in the products themselves, dosing of edibles is more difficult but can be managed if you start low and go slow.

Medical cannabis patients are advised to start with very small amounts (see dosing guidelines later in this chapter), especially for THC-rich edibles, wait for at least ninety minutes, and repeat the dose only if no effect is felt. Since ingested THC is metabolized in the liver to the more potent 11-hydroxy-THC, new or inexperienced users can easily overdo it. The effect from edibles can be quite potent, even with small amounts. In fact, the most common reason for cannabis overdose symptoms (increased heart rate, anxiety, excessive sleepiness, hallucinations, or paranoia) is the ingestion of too much of an edible THC-rich cannabis product. That being said, many patients do very well with edibles when they have been educated in the proper way to dose them.

What happens if you take an edible that contains both CBD and THC? CBD can partially inhibit the conversion of THC to 11-hydroxy-THC, reducing the overall intoxicating and sedating effects (when taken in proper dosing). The level of inhibition depends on the doses of each phytocannabinoid as well as your metabolism.

A recent study compared two doses of THC (5 and 10 milligrams) taken as capsules either with high-fat food or in a fasted state and found that food delayed the onset of effects but gave a longer duration of effects. Interestingly, the volunteers who took the 10-milligram capsule without food had more unwanted side effects when compared to the 10-milligram dose taken with fatty food. Additionally, this study showed a difference between men and women in that women had higher plasma THC levels after 5 milligrams without food.[6] This supports previous findings of differences between the sexes but may be attributable to the weight difference between men and women.[7]

In most states where medical cannabis is legally available, edible products are tested and labeled with the potency of THC, CBD, other cannabinoids, and occasionally with the terpenoid profile. Most states that allow edibles strictly control how many milligrams of THC are allowed per piece in order to minimize unwanted side effects and over-doses. Always check the wrapper for the potency information, as it is the only way to be sure that you are dosing correctly.

Cannabis tea, although ingested, does not fully convert CBDA and THCA to CBD and THC, respectively, meaning that ingestion will likely include raw cannabinoids as well as some decarboxylated (heated) cannabinoids. Juicing raw cannabinoids maintains the raw compounds. Some patients juice a large amount of freshly harvested cannabis flowers and leaves and freeze them in ice-cube trays to be used at a later date, added to smoothies or thawed and ingested. Ingested raw cannabinoids are rarely intoxicating.

Sublingual Tinctures

Cannabis tinctures or extracts have been made for hundreds of years. By definition, tinctures are alcohol-based liquid concentrates, and extracts are oil-based liquid concentrates. In the cannabis industry, however, the terms "tincture" and "extract" are often used interchangeably. Most patients use these products sublingually (under the tongue), where they are absorbed through the mucous membranes in the mouth. The medication goes directly into the bloodstream, bypassing the liver and avoiding the first pass effect described earlier. The medication's effects are usually felt within fifteen to sixty minutes and often last six to eight hours, depending on dosing. The standard measurement for tinctures is milligrams per milliliter, which is reported on the COA and some product labels as "mg per mL" or "mg/mL." (More on this later in the section on dosing.)

Another sublingual form of cannabis is the dissolvable strip, similar to breath strips. Patients often start with a small piece of the strip placed under the tongue. The dose may be repeated, with a wait time of at least sixty minutes before taking more if there is no effect.

Advantages of sublingual forms of cannabis are the avoidance of smoke, faster absorption than orally ingested forms, a minimal first pass effect in the liver, no odor, and discreet use. Patients can also control and customize dosing to their needs when using tinctures. For instance, if you have a 10-milligram THC edible but want to take only 1 milligram, it is difficult to be precise when cutting an edible into 10 pieces to get a 1-milligram dose. If you have a tincture with 10 milligrams THC per 1 milliliter, you can use a 1-milliliter syringe that allows for a 0.1-milliliter measurement (one-tenth of the syringe) to take 1 milligram. Additionally, patients who require higher doses of THC or CBD can use more concentrated tinctures to deliver larger doses in small volumes.

Pediatric patients and patients with disabilities may not be able to contend with certain delivery methods. I have found that tinctures work well for these patients, as they can be taken by mouth, hidden in food, or even given through a feeding tube. Concentrated tinctures are also advised, as a larger milligram dose in a smaller volume is easier when patient compliance is an issue.

Topical Application

There is abundant evidence that the endocannabinoid system is located throughout our skin, making it an attractive target for topical cannabinoid preparations. Cannabis can be made into ointments, salves, and lotions and can be applied to the skin to treat local pain, such as arthritis, or rashes, such as psoriasis or eczema. These preparations have been used in India and Latin America for thousands of years, with reports of significant relief from pain and excessive itching, plus they can be used to treat skin infections, including MRSA, a bacteria with strong resistance to antibiotics.

Intoxication from topical cannabis use is extremely rare. Blood and urine tests of patients using topical THC preparations exclusively, meaning no internal exposure, do not show presence of THC or its metabolites, allowing those who may be drug tested for employment purposes to use this method without repercussions.[8] Topical preparations containing one dominant or various combinations of phytocannabinoids are available.

A number of scientific studies researching the effects of topical preparations of cannabis demonstrated the following:

- THC, CBD, CBG, and CBN all blocked the development of psoriatic scales in a test-tube model of psoriasis.[9]
- Topical applications of THC helped mice heal faster from skin allergies.[10]
- A study comparing the skin's permeability with applications of delta-8-THC, CBD, or CBN found "the permeabilities of CBD and CBN were 10-fold higher than for delta-8-THC."[11]
- Multiple studies show that activation of the CB_1 receptor, by THC for instance, improves atopic dermatitis/eczema.[12]
- Five of eight patients (62.5 percent) with post-herpetic neuralgia had a mean reduction of pain by 87.8 percent with the use of a topical cannabinoid cream.[13]
- Five major phytocannabinoids showed potent activity against MRSA.[14]
- CBD gels in various doses applied to rats with arthritic knee joints found significant reduction of joint swelling, immune cell infiltration, and less thickening of the synovial membrane.[15]
- Topical cannabinoid cream significantly reduced pruritus (itching) in end-stage renal disease patients.[16]
- Topical THC and CBD given to three patients with pyoderma gangrenosum, a condition that causes large painful skin ulcers, decreased pain and allowed patients to significantly reduce their use of opioids.[17]
- A published report of parent-initiated use of topical CBD for epidermolysis bullosa, a debilitating and painful skin condition, reported faster wound healing, less blistering, and decreased pain in three pediatric patients.[18]

Many of my patients successfully use topical preparations for pain from arthritis, especially on the smaller joints, such as hands, feet, elbows, ankles, and knees. Some patients report relief from bursitis pain, plantar fasciitis pain, and scar tissue pain, as well as relief from neck, shoulder, and back pain. Some patients get relief with topicals for difficult-to-treat neuropathy. I have also successfully treated patients with contact dermatitis, psoriasis, and eczema. Additionally, there are anecdotal cases of patients applying cannabis to precancerous or small cancerous lesions with resolution of the lesions.

A few years ago I met with a woman in her eighties who was suffering from severe lower back pain. She had been offered a surgical option by her orthopedist but was told that at her age, full recovery would likely be at least six months to one year. After speaking with her primary care physician, she decided to try medical cannabis. When we met, she was somewhat adamant about using only topical, as she was cannabis naive and fearful of having intoxicating side effects. I explained that we could start with topical but that there were other nonintoxicating options if it was not effective. She began using a CBD-dominant salve, applied after a shower in the morning and repeated in the late afternoon. At her follow-up visit, she reported an 80 percent reduction of pain with no side effects! She was so happy with the results and fearful of running out of this effective preparation that she told me she purchased six containers at a time. I have a number of other elderly patients who have reported similar results, demonstrating the benefits of this method of use.

Topical preparations are not standardized and vary widely in ingredients, chemovars used, and potency. Sometimes patients have to experiment with a few different preparations to find the one that works best for their condition. Some patients report improved efficacy when they mix the cannabis preparation with over-the-counter topical pain relievers.

Since there have been a few cases of allergic reactions to topical cannabis products, you should read the ingredients carefully and test a small amount on an area of unaffected skin before using it for any medical condition. I also recommend avoiding the use of products that contain alcohol on open skin wounds since they may burn and aggravate the condition.

Rectal Suppositories

Although there are anecdotal reports of efficacy with cannabis suppositories, a review of the scientific literature shows poor absorption of phytocannabinoids through this route. Additionally, suppositories may cause significant harm to patients receiving chemotherapy and those who may have a compromised immune system. Chemotherapy can cause a breakdown in the mucous-membrane lining of the rectum, making it susceptible to tearing with suppository use and allowing deadly bacteria to enter the bloodstream.

Two studies trialing rectal THC-rich suppositories in monkeys reported THC is not absorbed rectally, as there were no circulating levels of THC in the bloodstream.[19] However, when a chemical compound called hemisuccinate was combined with THC, absorption was double that of oral ingestion of THC, indicating hemisuccinate helps THC pass into the bloodstream.[20] This chemically modified suppository was used in laboratory investigations only, is a patented product, and is not available to patients yet.

There are many anecdotal reports stating suppositories helped with cancer treatment, but most of these patients reported using other treatments too, including chemo and natural remedies, making it difficult to attribute benefits to the suppositories.

I rarely recommend THC-rich cannabis through the rectal route for systemic illnesses because we are still uncertain of the amount of medicine, if any, that gets into the system. However, there is some evidence that rectal suppositories can have benefits for rectal conditions, such as colitis (inflammation of the colon). In a 2012 study, mice with drug-induced colitis had a small but statistically significant reduction of inflammation with CBD suppositories.[21]

Unfortunately, there is no other research on rectal administration of cannabinoids. Clinically, I have treated patients suffering from hemorrhoids and anal fissures with THC-rich suppositories, resulting in a resolution of the problem without unwanted side effects.

Transdermal Patches

Transdermal patches containing cannabinoids are of great interest to both patients and scientists (evidenced by the numerous patents filed) because this method of delivery has some advantages when compared to oral delivery of cannabinoids. Compliance is easier for most patients, and first pass effect through the liver (THC converting to 11-hydroxy-THC, which may increase intoxicating effects) can be avoided. Additionally, patches may allow for a steady infusion of a drug to be delivered over time, minimizing a "peak" that might cause side effects.

One problematic issue with patches is that cannabinoids are fat-based compounds that do not mix with water, and the aqueous layer of the skin may interfere with absorption into the bloodstream. The addition of permeation enhancers (compounds that promote the flow of the drug through the skin) improves bioavailability. One study in mice reported that CBD in a formulation called an ethosome (a carrier composed of lipids, ethanol, and water) accumulated in the skin and underlying muscle within twenty-four hours and lasted at least seventy-two hours.[22] Animals pretreated with this product, which were then subjected to an injection of a pro-inflammatory drug, did not develop inflammation or swelling.

In a review of the ingredients of transdermal patches currently available through dispensaries, I noticed that some of these products contain numerous additives in order to promote permeation of the cannabinoids through the skin. Be sure to read the ingredients, as some of these compounds are not natural, may not be safe for prolonged use, and may cause allergic reactions. One patch lists diethylene glycol monoethyl ether (a solvent used in wood stains and industrial cleaners) and polysorbate 20 (a sugar alcohol treated with ethylene oxide, which is linked to a carcinogen). Another patch reports methyl salicylate on its ingredients list. This compound may be natural, derived from the wintergreen plant, or synthetically produced; however, the main issue is that once absorbed, the body converts it to salicylic acid, the active ingredient in aspirin. There may be added anti-inflammatory effects, but accidental poisoning has been reported from overuse of topical products that contain this compound. It is crucial to read the ingredients list of all transdermal patches to avoid unwanted chemical or allergen exposure.

Clinically, some patients report benefits from patches, especially for pain. A number of patients report feeling too intoxicated from patches that delivered higher than desired doses of THC. Combination CBD+THC and lower-dose patches are best for anyone inexperienced with this method in order to avoid unwanted effects. Remember too that CBD "hemp" patches available online are completely unregulated and may also contain ingredients that are not safe, necessitating a review of their COA.

A Comparison of the Most Common Delivery Methods

Remember to "start low and go slow"

	Inhalation	Ingestion	Sublingual tinctures	Topical application
Onset	Within minutes	60 to 90 minutes	15 to 60 minutes	Varies
Peak effect	30 minutes	2 to 3 hours	1 to 2 hours	Varies
Effect duration (varies based on dose and individual metabolism)	1 to 4 hours	6 to 8 hours	6 to 8 hours	Apply as needed to areas of pain or rash
Additional considerations	Vaporization is healthier than smoking. Dosing is easier since the effects are felt immediately.	No equipment is needed, there is no odor, and it's a discreet way to medicate. Dosing is more difficult than with other methods. Start with a small amount and titrate up as needed.	No equipment is needed, there is no odor, and it's a discreet way to medicate. Available as tinctures, extracts, and dissolvable strips.	Test for a possible allergic response by applying a small amount to a nonaffected area first. CBD absorbs better than THC. Repeat doses as needed.

Ratio and Concentration

A product's "ratio" is how much CBD that particular cannabis plant or preparation contains in relation to THC. For instance, a label may list "CBD:THC 5:1." This means it contains 5 parts CBD to 1 part THC. Said another way, it has five times more CBD than THC. If the product is labeled 20:1, it contains 20 parts CBD to 1 part THC, meaning it has twenty times more CBD than THC.

Sometimes a product has "CBD" somewhere on the label, but it does not list a ratio. If the label states the milligram amounts of both CBD and THC, you can calculate the ratio by dividing the milligrams of CBD by the milligrams of THC. If there is no ratio or "CBD" is not listed anywhere on the label, it is very likely a product high in THC with negligible amounts of CBD.

Knowing the ratio allows patients to determine whether the product will cause intoxication. In general, for inexperienced users, ratios over 10:1 CBD:THC—for example, 10:1, 15:1, 20:1, 25:1, or higher—will not cause intoxication. Ratios under 10:1 may cause some level of intoxication depending on the dose and the patient's tolerance to THC. The lower the ratio, the more THC relative to CBD and the higher the chance to experience intoxication. Remember, no matter what ratio is used, the presence of CBD in the product helps to buffer THC's intoxicating effects.

For the most part, there is no one ratio that works better than others for any particular condition since each individual's response to cannabis is unique. An example of this is children with autism. In my experience, after treating many children with this condition, approximately 50 percent respond to higher CBD:THC ratios, of about 20:1 up to 30:1, and approximately 30 percent respond to lower ratios, such as 1:1, 4:1, or 8:1. These patients have the same diagnosis but can respond differently to different ratios. We don't really know why this is, but it's likely because the response to cannabis is based on many factors, including genetics, the underlying disease process, absorption, and metabolism, all of which vary from person to person, despite some people having the same condition. The effects are also influenced by the other cannabinoids and terpenes in the product.

"Concentration" refers to how many milligrams of CBD and THC there are per milliliter (in tinctures or extracts). This information allows you to accurately dose cannabis oil products and to calculate the ratio if it is not on the bottle's label.

For example, a bottle of cannabis oil with 20 mg CBD per 1 mL + 10 mg THC per 1 mL will have a ratio of 2:1 (calculated by dividing 20 milligrams CBD by 10 milligrams THC). This oil has two times more CBD than THC. If you wanted to take 20 milligrams of CBD, you would take 1 milliliter. If you wanted to take 10 milligrams, you would take 0.5 milliliter. I recommend using 1 milliliter needleless syringes (available online), as these can help with dosing accuracy. They also have markings as low as 0.1 mL (one-tenth of 1 milliliter), allowing patients even more control over their dosing.

Edibles that contain CBD have ratios, but they do not have concentrations. Instead they are labeled with "total mg per package" and "total mg per piece" since most states in the US now have laws that limit each

1 mL syringe	Diluted or Low Concentration	Concentrated	Highly Concentrated (FECO or RSO)
0.1 mL 0.2 mL 0.3 mL 0.4 mL 0.5 mL 0.6 mL 0.7 mL 0.8 mL 0.9 mL 1 mL	5–40 mg/mL	50–100 mg/mL	200–900 mg/mL
	EXAMPLE 10 mg/mL	EXAMPLE 100 mg/mL	EXAMPLE 500 mg/mL
	0.1 mL = 1 mg 0.2 mL = 2 mg 0.3 mL = 3 mg 0.4 mL = 4 mg 0.5 mL = 5 mg 0.6 mL = 6 mg 0.7 mL = 7 mg 0.8 mL = 8 mg 0.9 mL = 9 mg 1 mL = 10 mg	0.1 mL = 10 mg 0.2 mL = 20 mg 0.3 mL = 30 mg 0.4 mL = 40 mg 0.5 mL = 50 mg 0.6 mL = 60 mg 0.7 mL = 70 mg 0.8 mL = 80 mg 0.9 mL = 90 mg 1 mL = 100 mg	0.1 mL = 50 mg 0.2 mL = 100 mg 0.3 mL = 150 mg 0.4 mL = 200 mg 0.5 mL = 250 mg 0.6 mL = 300 mg 0.7 mL = 350 mg 0.8 mL = 400 mg 0.9 mL = 450 mg 1 mL = 500 mg

Figure 7: Examples of differently concentrated cannabis oils. (FECO: full-extract cannabis oil; RSO: "Rick Simpson oil")

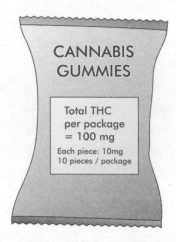

Figure 8: Example of cannabis edible product label.

edible piece to no more than 10 milligrams each, with a total of 100 milligrams allowable in one package.

Be aware that the ratio *does not* tell you the milligrams in a product. A 2:1 CBD:THC product may have 20 milligrams CBD + 10 milligrams THC, but it could also have any amount of CBD that is two times more than THC. For example, a product with 100 milligrams CBD + 50 milligrams THC and a product with 16 milligrams CBD + 8 milligrams THC both have 2:1 ratios of CBD:THC.

In summary, the ratio tells you whether or not the product might be intoxicating, and the concentration allows you to correctly dose tinctures or extracts.

Cannabis Oil Concentrations Vary

Cannabis oils can be divided into three types of concentrations, as shown in figure 7. Diluted- or low-concentration oils are usually from about 5 to 40 milligrams per milliliter. More concentrated oils have about 50 to 100 milligrams per milliliter, and highly concentrated oils—which are also called FECO, full-extract cannabis oil, or RSO, "Rick Simpson oil"—have 200 to 900 milligrams per milliliter.

I recommend using the diluted- or low-concentration oils for THC if

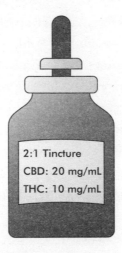

Figure 9: Example of cannabis tincture product label.

you are new or inexperienced with cannabis. This will allow you to accurately control how much THC you take and minimize side effects. This is also the concentration used most for children and elderly patients, especially when beginning a new cannabis regimen.

More concentrated oils between 50 and 100 milligrams are helpful for those who may want to take higher doses of CBD. For example, if you wanted to take 100 milligrams per day of CBD, you could take either five 1-milliliter syringes with 10 milligrams each of CBD or two 1-milliliter syringes with 50 milligrams each. Most people prefer to take less volume if possible.

FECO or RSO products are mostly used by patients who want to take very high doses of phytocannabinoids (often used to fight cancer). These oils are very thick and gooey, making them difficult to measure in exact dosages.

Cannabis Dosing: Start Low and Go Slow

There is a wide therapeutic range for cannabinoid dosing. Patients respond to certain chemovars or preparations in unique ways. Whole-plant cannabis medicine cannot be standardized because of the many variables involved, such as a patient's metabolism, the delivery method, the dose, the cannabinoid ratio, the makeup of the chemovar, and the product's formulation. **Dosing of cannabis is not "one size fits all." It is highly individualized and has been called "patient-determined, self-titrating" by many experts.**

A few years ago, a mother and adult daughter, both with long-standing debilitating migraine headaches, came to see me. The daughter had experimented with cannabis prior to her office visit, and she reported that if she vaporized THC-rich cannabis at the onset of the symptoms, the migraine did not progress and within thirty minutes all symptoms disappeared. She shared this information with her mother and encouraged her to try using the vaporizer in the same manner. Her mother found the migraine headache pain increased with vaporized THC, but sublingual application of a combination CBD+THC tincture significantly reduced her migraine symptoms. This example illustrates that even people with the same condition who are genetically related can respond differently to different delivery methods and different combinations of cannabinoids.

Patients have complained to me in recent years that there are too many cannabis products to pick from (what a difference from twenty years ago!) and they are overwhelmed when trying to choose their medicine. I teach them a simple approach that is methodical and allows them to find what works and what doesn't. I call it the "Rule it in or rule it out" method. Although it is simple in concept, it can be time-consuming. Be patient — you are asking a plant to change your chemistry! It is an effort for some, but many patients have stated that the end result — feeling better with no side effects — is worth the sometimes tedious process.

- Decide what delivery method you want to try first. Be aware that you may need to try a different delivery method depending on how you respond, but it is okay to start with a method that is most comfortable for you. Only try something new when you are at home and going to stay home for at least a number of hours in case of sedation or intoxication.

- Think about what effects you are looking for: do you hope for better sleep or pain relief or anxiety reduction? Knowing this will help you decide on whether to start with a THC-dominant product, a high-ratio CBD:THC product (CBD dominant), a low-ratio CBD:THC product (a combination of effects), or another cannabinoid, such as THCA, CBDA, or CBG. Of course which product you begin with may be influenced by what is available to you geographically and legally.

- Using the chart on the next page, categorize products by their COA or by their label information.

- Take a small dose (see the chart's dosing guidelines) and wait to feel its effects. Be patient, and only take another dose if the effects are not felt after two hours (unless you tried an inhalation method, in which case you can repeat the dose after thirty minutes if you feel no effects). It is better to take multiple small doses throughout the day rather than one large dose.

- Give yourself a few days at a certain dose before adjusting doses or switching products. Changes in your medical condition can take time. Remember that these compounds have many targets in the brain and body and need time to shift the unbalanced messages.

- Keep a journal of everything you try, with names of products, doses, and timing, so you can assess which products worked (or didn't work), which doses worked, and how long the effects lasted.

- If the product you try doesn't help, think about taking a higher dose. Almost every person who tries cannabis before coming to my office is underdosing, especially when it comes to CBD. If the product doesn't help after proper dosing, you have ruled it out.

- If the product helps, you can make small adjustments in the dosing, going higher or lower, looking for the "sweet spot" that gives you the desired effects without any unwanted side effects. If you can find this, you have ruled it in.

- If you find an effective dose of a product—one that helps without side effects—but you feel there is still room for improvement, add a second product with a different cannabinoid to see if the combination provides any benefits. Some patients find one product is effective and stick with that, and others find two or more work well in combination.

The following chart reviews the different categories of products and their potential effects:

	THC-rich products	High-ratio CBD:THC products	Low-ratio CBD:THC products
Phytocannabinoid composition and example ratios	THC with little or no CBD content Dosing based on THC	CBD:THC of 25:1, 18:1, 15:1, 12:1, 10:1 Dosing based on CBD	CBD:THC of 8:1, 4:1, 2:1, 1:1 Dosing based on THC
Intoxication level	*THC-dominant* effects Intoxicating, but very low doses may not be	*CBD-dominant* effects Not intoxicating for most, but can be with very large doses; low doses of CBD can be stimulating and higher doses can be sedating	*Combination CBD and THC* effects Can be intoxicating depending on THC tolerance
Conditions	Anxiety, appetite stimulation, autism, cancer, inflammation, mood, muscle spasms, nausea and vomiting, neuroprotection, pain relief, sleep	Anxiety, autism, cancer, depression, inflammation, intestinal disorders, mood, neuroprotection, pain relief, psychosis, seizures	Anxiety, autism, cancer, depression, inflammation, muscle spasms, nausea and vomiting, pain relief (especially nerve pain), sleep, spasticity

	CBG-rich products	THCA-rich products	CBDA-rich products
Phytocannabinoid composition	*CBG-dominant* effects	*THCA-dominant* effects	*CBDA-dominant* effects
Intoxication level	Not intoxicating	Not intoxicating for most, but high doses may contain enough THC to cause intoxication	Not intoxicating
Conditions	Anxiety, appetite stimulation, autism, bladder spasms, cancer, depression, inflammation, mood, nausea and vomiting, psoriasis	Autism, cancer, inflammation, intestinal disorders, nausea and vomiting, pain relief, seizures	Anxiety, cancer, inflammation, intestinal disorders, nausea and vomiting, pain relief

	CBDV-rich products	THCV-rich products	Delta-8-THC-rich products
Phytocannabinoid composition	*CBDV-dominant* effects	*THCV-dominant* effects	*Delta-8-THC-dominant* effects
Intoxication level	Not intoxicating	Not intoxicating for most, but high doses may be	Slight intoxication possible, depending on the presence of delta-9-THC
Conditions	Autism, neuropathic pain, seizures	Appetite suppression, cancer, inflammation, neuroprotection, pain relief, potential improvement of glucose tolerance and insulin sensitivity, seizures	Anxiety, appetite stimulation, cancer, glaucoma, nausea and vomiting, neuroprotection, pain relief

As you can see, there is a lot of overlap in the medicinal effects of these products. As previously mentioned, they are promiscuous compounds, working in many of the same places in the brain and body. Patients who have tried THC at some point in their lives are often less fearful of the effects of THC and therefore may choose products with more THC, whereas someone new to cannabis use may be nervous about THC's effects and may be more likely to start with higher-ratio CBD:THC products or one of the other nonintoxicating cannabinoids. If you have access to a physician who has experience with cannabis, discuss options that may be best for your condition. Don't forget: start low and go slow.

Dosing Guidelines for Adults

The following doses are guidelines only and may vary based on the medical condition being treated. Also, these doses are calculated for adults. Pediatric patients should not be using cannabis products without medical supervision, just as **medical supervision is recommended prior to starting any cannabis treatment.**

Remember, some products have combination cannabinoids that may influence dosing and response. Be sure to check the label and the COA of any product before using it.

- *THC-rich and low-ratio CBD:THC products (1:1, 2:1, etc.):*
  — 1 to 2.5 milligrams per dose for new or inexperienced patients.
  — If no effects are felt after one to two hours, repeat the same dose.
  — If you feel that you took too much, do not panic. Take a few deep breaths and remember that the effects will wear off soon. There is no danger to you. Distract yourself by watching TV, trying to nap, listening to music, or talking to a supportive family member or friend.
- *High-ratio CBD-rich products:*
  — CBD has a very wide range of dosing, much wider than THC.
  — A low dose is approximately 10 to 50 milligrams per day; higher doses are more than 50 milligrams per day.
  — In general, anti-inflammatory doses are about 50 or more milligrams per day.
  — It is very important to know that CBD may not decrease pain until inflammation has lessened, which may take days to weeks of daily use to achieve. (What I really mean here is, CBD is not magic and needs time to work!)
- *CBG-rich products:*
  — CBG has a wide range of dosing; however, many patients have found low doses to be effective.
  — A low-dose range is 2 to 20 milligrams; a high-dose range is 20 to 60 milligrams.
  — Some cancer patients may take up to 100 milligrams per day.
- *THCA-rich products:*
  — Clinically, patients using THCA products report benefits with low doses.
  — Dosing ranges from 2 to 10 milligrams to start, increasing to desired effects.

—Some patients have dosed as high as 200 milligrams per day with no reported side effects.

- *CBDA-rich products:*
    —Reports of CBDA being a hundred times more potent than CBD indicate that low doses may be effective.
    —Clinically, my patients start with low doses, about 2 to 10 milligrams, and titrate up to desired effects.
    —Some cancer patients report taking 50 to 200 milligrams per day.
    —Most CBDA products contain very little THC, therefore higher doses are rarely intoxicating.
- *CBDV-rich products:*
    —Studies report doses similar to CBD, starting at 10 milligrams and titrating up to desired effects.
    —Clinical trials for children with autism are using 10 milligrams per kilogram daily.
- *THCV-rich products:*
    —Most products currently available contain almost equal parts THCV and THC, therefore intoxication may occur at low doses.
    —Dosing starts at 1 milligram THCV, increasing to desired effects.
- *Delta-8-THC-rich products:*
    —Similar to delta-9-THC, this compound has a narrow range of dosing.
    —Dosing starts at 1 to 5 milligrams, titrating up to reach desired effects without side effects.
    —Clinically, patients using doses between 3 and 9 milligrams have reported decreased anxiety without feelings of intoxication.

Timing of Dosing

Some patients take one dose per day, others take two to three doses, and some take four or more doses. Once you start to feel the effects, pay attention to how long they last. Use this information to schedule your daily doses.

For example, one of my patients with chronic pain found a 4:1 tincture helped significantly, but the effects lasted only about six hours, after which her pain would flare intensely. The onset of effects of the next dose took one hour, leaving her in pain while she waited for relief. After she changed her dosing schedule to every five hours (during the day), she found more consistent pain relief. Interestingly, after about four months on this regimen, she found that her overall pain had decreased (likely she had less overall inflammation), and she was able to change the dosing schedule to every six hours.

With or Without Meals

As mentioned previously, eating a snack or meal containing fat at the same time as taking cannabis orally or sublingually (since some is swallowed) can help with absorption and minimize unwanted side effects, but it may delay the onset of effects. This is because cannabis is fat soluble. Try taking your dose with meals and then without meals, so you can make an informed decision based on your body's response.

A Few Important Things to Remember About Dosing

- Your dose of CBD can influence which product you should purchase, especially with high CBD:THC ratios. For instance, let's say you purchase a 1-ounce bottle that states the concentration is "200 mg CBD per 1 oz." If it turns out that you require a CBD dose of 100 milligrams per day, you will get only two days' worth from this bottle! This is not very cost-effective, and taking half a bottle of oil is not very palatable. If you figure out your monthly dose—for instance, 100 milligrams per day for 30 days equals 3,000 milligrams for a month—you can look for products with higher concentrations per bottle. There are some "medical cannabis masquerading as hemp" products on the market (discussed in chapter 1) that contain 3,000, 5,000, or 6,000 milligrams of CBD for those patients who require higher doses. Of course you must check the COA to make sure that these products are what they claim to be.

- When using tinctures, always shake the bottle well just before drawing up the dose.
- Remember to keep raw tinctures (THCA, CBDA) in the refrigerator.
- As previously mentioned, using a 1-milliliter needleless syringe makes dosing easy and accurate. Some patients "prep" syringes— that is, they prepare a week's worth of doses—to save time during the week. These syringes are available for purchase online.

Biphasic Effects

The term "biphasic" literally means "two phases." Studies show that phytocannabinoids have biphasic effects—that is, at low doses a phytocannabinoid may produce one effect but at high doses cause a completely opposite effect. A well-known example of this is THC's antianxiety effect at low doses and its increased-anxiety effect at high doses. A study in mice found that this biphasic effect is due to the way THC interacts with CB_1 receptors in different areas of the brain that control anxiety.[23] CBD too has biphasic effects, with low doses causing an alerting effect and higher doses causing a sedating or calming effect.

Each person has their own threshold of dosing where they switch from a low-dose effect to a high-dose effect. This is why patients should start low and go slow, but make sure to try higher doses too, ruling in or ruling out beneficial effects.

First-Time Use of THC-Rich Cannabis

Sometimes patients who have never used cannabis before may not feel any effect their first time. These patients may get frustrated and take more, which can result in an undesirable "overdose" effect (fast heart rate, excessive sleepiness, anxiety, and/or paranoia). If you try cannabis medicine and don't feel anything, you can take another small dose, but if you still don't feel anything, stop and try again the next day. No one knows exactly why some people don't feel the effects the first time, but the theory is, the first dose "readies" the liver enzymes to metabolize the cannabinoid.[24]

Sometimes with first-time use a patient may deny feeling any effects but the people around that patient notice the patient is acting differently. The adult son of one of my patients suffering from terrible side effects from breast cancer treatment reported at a follow-up visit that the first time his mother used cannabis (she took 2.5 milligrams THC sublingually) she got out of bed, where she had been spending most of her time, and began to make dinner. She was chatty and happy for the first time in months, and he said the whole family felt relieved that Mom was "back to normal." The fascinating part of this story is that when I asked the patient how cannabis made her feel, she said she didn't really feel anything; she just felt "normal." It was only after a few uses over the course of a week that she was able to notice the effects of the cannabis, telling me she liked the effects because she felt happier, had more energy, and was back to a more regular routine.

THC Overdose

Although we know there are no fatal overdoses with THC, you can take too much and have an unpleasant experience. Overdose is more common by the oral ingestion route since dosing by this delivery method can be inexact and the breakdown product of THC, 11-hydroxy-THC, is intoxicating and long-lasting. **There is no danger of respiratory arrest or death** as a direct result of using THC. Overdose of THC can cause rapid heart rate, altered time perception, paranoia, anxiety, impaired motor coordination, delusional thinking, excessive sleepiness, and/or a sense of impending death or perceived harm. If you take too much THC-rich cannabis and feel badly from it, reassure yourself that you are safe and that nothing bad is going to happen. Try to lie down and sleep or distract yourself with television. Taking CBD-rich cannabis may lessen the THC-induced overdose symptoms, but it can take some time to work. Patients may seek care in the ER and can be treated with benzodiazepines for the anxiety; once the cannabis wears off, there might be residual effects of lethargy and/or headache, but these will usually resolve quickly. Overdose may result in a patient's reluctance to use THC again, but THC overdoses can easily be avoided by taking only a small amount of measured THC-rich cannabis at a time and including CBD, which can buffer the intoxication of THC.

Medicinal Use vs. Recreational Use

I often explain to my patients that there are two ways to approach cannabis use. One is the recreational approach, and one is the medicinal approach. The goal of recreational use is to "get high." The goal of a medicinal dose is to treat a medical condition. For some patients there is overlap, and the sensation of feeling "high" is truly a sense of relief from physical and/or psychological pain. This is extremely valuable for many patients who are suffering, giving them much-needed respite and improvement in their quality of life. You do not, however, need to feel high to benefit from cannabis.

Using a CBD-rich medicine (higher CBD:THC ratio) or one or more of the other nonintoxicating cannabinoids will help to minimize and prevent intoxication, but if relief is not achieved, adding THC may be helpful and should not be feared. A medicinal dose of THC, simple to measure with tested products, can usually be found, and unwanted side effects can easily be avoided. Many of my patients using THC have found an effective dose for their medical condition that does not cause intoxication. It may take trial and error, starting with a low dose and increasing little by little to find the "sweet spot," but this goal can be achieved with some patience.

Drug–Drug Interactions

Many medications are metabolized in the liver and intestines through the cytochrome P450 system. This is an enzyme system that breaks down an estimated 60 percent of all pharmaceuticals. THC, CBD, and other phytocannabinoids are metabolized in this system as well, potentially changing the way other drugs are metabolized. There are two types of issues with a drug metabolized by the same enzymes as phytocannabinoids. The phytocannabinoids may block the metabolism of the other drug, causing it to build up and create unwanted side effects or toxicity. Alternatively, phytocannabinoids may increase the metabolism of the other drug, causing it to leave the body quicker than it should, possibly decreasing its effects. Conversely, the pharmaceutical may change the metabolism of the phytocannabinoids; however, studies investigating these effects are sparse. These are *potential* interactions and difficult to predict.

Another drug–drug interaction to consider is the combining of two drugs with similar effects, causing an additive effect. This is called "pharmacodynamic interactions." For instance, both THC and diazepam (Valium) can cause relaxation, sedation, and dizziness, and, taken together at the same time, may cause excessive sedation or unsteadiness, leading to a fall. There is no absolute contraindication in this example, but caution should be exercised any time THC is taken with other drugs, especially sedatives or hypnotics (sleep aids). Another well-known example is the combination of THC with alcohol, causing excessive intoxication, which can lead to accidental injury. This combination is highly discouraged. There can be benefits with some combinations; vaporized cannabis, for example, increases the analgesic effects of opioids without increasing the blood-opioid levels, meaning there is no increased risk of respiratory depression.[25]

Low doses of cannabinoids seldom cause issues with drug metabolism (although read more about this in the following list). Higher doses of CBD can cause interactions because CBD is metabolized by a few enzymes of the cytochrome P450 system, specifically one called *CYP3A4,* which is responsible for the metabolism of almost 30 percent of other medications. CBD is also metabolized by the enzymes *CYP2C9* and *CYP2C19.* This gets very complicated because there are many factors to consider when trying to predict potential interactions. **The best way to avoid issues with drug–drug interactions is to speak with your healthcare provider or pharmacist prior to starting cannabis medicine.**

In the meantime, here are a few tips to prevent drug–drug interactions, plus information about some of the more common interactions:

- Drug–drug interactions between pharmaceuticals and cannabinoids are more common if both drugs are taken via the oral route.
- Timing of dosing can matter. A study showed more interaction when CBD was orally ingested twenty minutes before the pharmaceutical was ingested.[26] Because of this one study, it is recommended to take CBD at least one hour after other pharmaceuticals. THC did not cause the same unwanted interaction. Unfortunately, without further research, we do not have enough information to know ideal timing for dosing.
- There are known drug–drug interactions with anticonvulsant seizure medications. This does not mean that cannabis and these pharmaceuticals cannot be taken together, but medical supervision and drug-level testing is advised. One known concern is the interaction of CBD with clobazam (brand name Onfi). Clobazam is converted by the enzyme *CYP3A4* to a second active drug called N-desmethylclobazam. CBD increases the production of this second drug, which may be beneficial since it is an anticonvulsant and a higher dose may be more effective; however, it may cause excessive sedation at higher doses. In 2018, Epidiolex, a pharmaceutical-grade product containing plant-derived CBD, was approved by the FDA for two rare, severe forms of pediatric epilepsy. In the Epidiolex clinical trial, 40 percent of patients on both clobazam and Epidiolex had to decrease the clobazam dose due to this side effect.[27]

- Another drug–drug interaction documented in studies of Epidiolex was with the anticonvulsant valproic acid (brand name Depakote), resulting in elevated liver enzymes. When the dose of either or both Epidiolex and valproic acid was reduced, the liver enzymes normalized.[28] Anyone taking CBD and valproic acid should be under medical supervision, and laboratory testing of the liver should be routine.

- Other known drug–drug interactions between CBD and seizure medications include eslicarbazepine acetate (brand name Aptiom or Zebinix), rufinamide (brand name Banzel), zonisamide (brand name Zonegran), and topiramate (brand name Topamax, Trokendi XR, or Qudexy XR). All changes of drug levels were "within the accepted therapeutic range."[29] Because of the risk of increased seizures with these drug interactions, patients with seizure disorders must have medical supervision when introducing CBD to their medication regimen.

- There is one case report of Epidiolex interacting with the blood thinner medication warfarin. The warfarin dose had to be lowered by 30 percent because the addition of high doses of Epidiolex in the treatment of this patient's seizure disorder interfered with the metabolism of warfarin, allowing it to build up and have increased effects, leading to excessive thinning of the blood.[30]

- THC also can affect warfarin. There are two case reports of THC use by patients on blood thinners causing increased actions of the blood thinner, with potential for excessive bleeding.[31] All patients on warfarin must be aware of these potential effects and weigh the benefits versus risks of using cannabinoids. Medical supervision is highly recommended in these cases.

- The newer blood thinners (dabigatran etexilate, rivaroxaban, apixaban, and edoxaban) are not metabolized by the same enzyme as THC; however, there is potential interaction with CBD.

For more information, visit ProjectCBD.org, an organization that offers the excellently written and well-researched *Cannabinoid-Drug Interactions Primer*.[32]

Patient Precautions

Treat your cannabis medicine the same way you treat any other medications. This medicine may affect other people differently, so do not share your medicine with family members, friends, or children.

Edibles may look appealing to children and animals, so make sure to avoid any accidental ingestion by keeping your medicine in a safe and secure location.

Do not try a new product unless you will be home or in another comfortable setting where you will have at least a few hours to see the full effects.

Do not drive or operate heavy machinery under the influence of THC. If you are using a nonintoxicating form of cannabis, always try it at home first to make sure your abilities will not be limited. Wait a number of hours to see how long the medicine lasts in your system so you are aware of the duration of the medication's effect.

It is recommended that you do not use alcohol at the same time that you take your cannabis medicines. The combination of cannabis with alcohol may lead to dizziness, increased risk of injury, poor judgment, and excessive impairment.

—◦◦◦—

Elise's Story

I met Elise in 2014 when she was twenty-six and severely debilitated by her chronic condition. I shared her story in my previous book and include it here, with an update.

Elise was diagnosed with juvenile rheumatoid arthritis (JRA) when she was sixteen. She would step off curbs while walking and notice that her heel would begin to swell. During the summer, she went bowling and noticed that not only her bowling elbow was swollen, but the other side as well. These were the little clues that led to the diagnosis, but it took about a year for the symptoms to become unbearable enough that she couldn't ignore them. She began getting sicker and sicker, with swelling in her knees and feet that prevented her from walking. The combination of pain and swelling caused enough nausea that she could no longer eat and began to lose weight. She was referred to a rheumatologist at a children's hospital but had to wait a couple of months for an appointment. When he finally saw her, the doctor admitted her immediately to the hospital, where she stayed for one week.

Elise said, "That was the beginning of being sick and the end of being well."

In the hospital, Elise was given a myriad of medications, including steroids. The medical team told her that she would be started on biologics (strong medications that affect the immune system) and would learn over time to give the shots to herself. She and her family read over the side effects and were frightened by them, but Elise was very sick, and they felt they had no choice. At one point a doctor told the family that the steroids shot into Elise's joints could cause calcification and fuse them. Elise had memories of her grandfather, with whom she had had a special relationship as a little girl. She remembered his hands, curled and deformed. She remembered his wheelchair. She thought of him when she was diagnosed. He too had had rheumatoid arthritis.

Despite the gravity of Elise's immediate condition and the diagnosis, the doctors were optimistic that she would go into remission. Unfortunately, Elise's response to the pharmaceuticals wasn't positive. She developed terrible side effects, and her pain increased. She was always sick and eventually couldn't walk or take care of herself. She began college but had to drop out and began using a wheelchair. She grew increasingly depressed as the pain and inflammation increased. She told me that she was in too much pain to do anything or go anywhere. Even a trusted osteopath who had treated her for years warned her that she was worried about Elise's life.

Elise's mother had been researching cannabis and wanted Elise to try it, but Elise wasn't interested. She believed the stereotype that people using it were just stoners. When her parents began suggesting she try a new pharmaceutical instead, she consented to come see me. Her exam showed severe deformities of her hand joints as well as swollen knees with very poor range of motion. She had only a tiny bit of hope that day when she came in, but she later told me she had immediately felt a connection to me and appreciated how honest I was about whether or not cannabis would help her.

She tried different chemovars and had mixed results at first, but in March of 2015, over ten years after her diagnosis, she began a new CBD-rich oil and noticed a drastic difference within weeks. Before starting the oil, Elise had felt so weak that she was afraid she wouldn't make it to her beloved sister's wedding. Her sister had been a support to her through all the years of Elise's illness, a best friend, and the only person whom Elise allowed to see how deeply the disease was affecting her. She told me that the two of them would cry together, her sister begging her to hold on and be at her wedding.

Elise knew that something good was happening when she reported that one morning she felt well enough to try to move from her wheelchair to the toilet by herself. When she succeeded, she was so shocked that she called her mother into the bathroom to witness what she reported was freedom for the first time in ten years! She had described herself as a sort of Tin Man from the The Wizard of Oz, with fused arms and no range of motion, but within weeks of starting the oil, she found the swelling and inflammation in her joints was going down. She could uncurl and open her fingers and elbows.

The effects of cannabis medicine on this young woman were profound. Where before the most basic of activities, like bathing or preparing meals, were so painful they were only to be dreaded, Elise reported that she could get into and out of the tub by herself, that she could wash herself and her hair with ease. Her independence grew tremendously, and she began cooking for herself as well.

"I'm trying to get some normalcy in my life," she reported. "For so long I couldn't do anything. I'm living again. I feel like this is the medicine that I prayed for yet didn't know existed. Finding cannabis was an answer to those prayers. I am so thankful to all those who shared their stories and encouraged me to try it. Everything shared was something that gave me hope that I could have a better life."

Elise also made it to her sister's wedding in June of 2015.

Update: *Elise continues to do well on cannabis. When I asked her if I could include her story in this book, she agreed. Her email to me speaks for itself:*

In May of this year I'll be thirty-two years old. Back when I was experiencing unbearable pain without any relief at twenty-six, reaching my thirties didn't seem very probable. I came to accept the likely fact of my life ending while I was still young after years of fighting with my own malfunctioning body and unruly immune system. I was devastated and furious at the same time but too weak to go on fighting much longer. Cannabis was a last resort for me, and I reluctantly tried it. This idea was solely thanks to my amazing incredible mom who tirelessly researched about it in a desperate attempt to find something, anything, that could help ease my pain and reduce the dangerous levels of inflammation throughout my whole body from JRA.

I can stand up and walk by myself a little when I'm not in a flare-up. Before this medicine, that wasn't remotely possible. I am physically stronger and surprisingly, remarkably more flexible than I would expect after having chronic inflammation since I was fifteen. My range of motion has drastically increased and this gives me greater physical independence in doing daily tasks like cleaning, cooking, dressing, showering, brushing my teeth, etc. When I was very sick I hated my body, I hated the agony it caused me, but as it's begun to heal, I find that I appreciate it.

Cannabis has reinvigorated my zest for creating. I've written since I was a child, but the years without pain relief made writing and drawing occur only on a sporadic basis. Now I write often, sometimes several times a day. It's wonderful also to have clarity of mind after such brain fog and fatigue for years. I attribute that to the whole-plant cannabis oil that my medicine is made from. As some coffee drinkers say they are "powered by caffeine," I would say that I am "powered by cannabis." My medicinal regimen includes: cannabis oil taken by mouth, edibles (I bake with my specific oil blend), topicals on my whole body, concentrates, vaping flower bud, and smoking.

This plant has given me my life back (and I might add, the will to live again as well). I am still figuring out how to do things again, how to adjust to being almost completely independent and make my own decisions about what to do with the rest of my life. Cannabis should be 100 percent available and legally accessible to everyone because if you have a body and a mind, chances are you might need medical care at some point in life and wouldn't it be beneficial to have it as a first option? I think so.

CHAPTER 6

Medical Risks of Cannabis Use

The patients who come to my office are seeking an effective solution to their difficult medical conditions. I rarely see major issues with cannabis use under my medical supervision. Every patient at every visit is asked if they experience side effects during its use, and the majority of patients report that they have none. Any side effects can often be resolved with changes in delivery method, products, chemovars, timing, or dosing. However, studies have shown medical risks of cannabis use in certain situations. These include possible increased risks to people with cardiovascular disease, pulmonary risks from smoking, risks from driving while under the influence of THC-rich cannabis, risks during pregnancy and breastfeeding, and risks to the pediatric population, specifically to developing brains. **It is important to note that the studies included in this book focused primarily on subjects using THC-rich cannabis without medical supervision, and the findings listed in this chapter do not apply to CBD-rich products or the other nonintoxicating phytocannabinoids being used by medical patients.**

Cardiovascular Risks Associated with THC Use

Heart tissue contains cannabinoid receptors, indicating the presence of the endocannabinoid system. Peripheral nerves also contain cannabinoid receptors, which are thought to regulate cardiovascular function. The current understanding is that low doses of THC, activating both CB_1 and CB_2 receptors, may have beneficial effects on heart health. However, a few studies have documented potential harms, specifically related to recreational THC use in certain individuals.

What we know about THC and its effects on heart rate and blood pressure is that

- THC causes an increase in heart rate, within minutes of use, by about 20 to 50 beats per minute, and the heart rate will return to normal after a few hours;
- THC can cause an elevation of blood pressure when one is lying flat, but there is a risk of blood pressure dropping if one stands too quickly;
- Research reports blood pressure decreases due to vasodilation of the blood vessels and overall relaxation with THC use;[1] and
- The cardiovascular effects of THC are more pronounced in a new or inexperienced user, whereas regular users of THC develop a tolerance to these effects.

Scientific Research

- Three studies showed a rare association with possible development of an abnormal cardiac rhythm with THC use.[2]
- A study from 1974 found smoking THC-rich cannabis was related to a more rapid onset of chest pain in patients with a history of chest pain when they underwent a stress test shortly after smoking a marijuana cigarette.[3] It's noted this effect may be due to the carbon monoxide in the smoke as opposed to a THC effect.
- One study showed an increased relative risk of developing a heart attack in the first hour after smoking cannabis (4.8 times increased risk over baseline).[4] Researchers suggested THC use might increase the risk of heart attack in susceptible individuals with coronary heart disease, although a 2013 report documenting eighteen years

of follow-up in these patients reported no statistically significant association between cannabis use and mortality.[5]

- There are a few case reports of young persons who have had a heart attack, arrhythmia, and even cardiac arrest after using THC-rich cannabis. Note there are only a few case reports in the scientific literature, and other factors, such as tobacco use, alcohol use, and previously unknown cardiac disease, may have played a role.[6]

- One study showed THC-rich cannabis use was associated with threefold greater mortality following acute myocardial infarction, with a graded increase in risk with more frequent use; however, another report concluded the opposite.[7]

- A 2015 report of the risk of cardiovascular disease (this definition included coronary artery disease, heart attack, heart failure, cardiac chest pain, and stroke) in 3,051 people revealed cannabis use was not significantly associated with an increased risk of cardiovascular disease.[8]

- A review of twenty-nine studies reported THC use, especially in high doses, increased the risk of stroke more than other cardiovascular diseases.[9]

- Studies in animal models reported CBD to be cardioprotective, beneficial for strokes, protective against drug-induced and diabetic heart problems (cardiomyopathy), and also protective for autoimmune myocarditis.[10]

The best approach in these situations is for those patients with known cardiovascular disease who are investigating the use of medical cannabis to discuss the latest scientific data, the risks, and the benefits with their personal physician, their cardiologist, and/or a knowledgeable cannabis specialist. If the decision to use medical cannabis is made, these patients should avoid smoking, choosing a different method of delivery, and use products that contain other cannabinoids in significant amounts rather than exclusively THC-rich cannabis in order to reap the benefits and minimize harm.

Pulmonary Risks of Smoking Cannabis

People have been smoking cannabis for centuries. In the 1970s, researchers and physicians developed methods to analyze lung function and determine the effects of tobacco smoking. Since cannabis was being used by many young people during this time, studies on its pulmonary effects were also performed. Interestingly, the findings between the effects of the two substances were quite different.

This is what we know about cannabis smoke:

- Similar to tobacco smoke, cannabis smoke contains ammonia, hydrocyanic acid, nitrosamines, and tar components, including phenols and naphthalene. Carcinogenic compounds, including benzopyrene and benzanthracene, are also in cannabis smoke.
- Very importantly, cannabis smoke does not contain nicotine and does contain phytocannabinoid compounds.
- Tobacco smoke causes bronchoconstriction (a narrowing of the airways), but THC-rich smoke and vapor causes bronchodilation (an opening of the airways).[11] THC and the terpene alpha-pinene are both known bronchodilators.[12]

Scientific Research

- Smokers of tobacco only, of cannabis only, and of both have increased incidence of respiratory symptoms, including chronic cough, phlegm production, wheezing, and bronchitis, when compared to nonsmokers.[13]
- Multiple studies document that chronic cannabis smoking (without tobacco use) is associated with an increased prevalence of bronchitis.[14]
- Symptoms of chronic bronchitis from smoking cannabis alone resolve with cessation of smoking.[15]

- Studies on lung function in chronic cannabis smokers are conflicted, with some studies showing no difference from nonsmokers and others showing mild airflow obstruction.[16]
- Two large studies failed to show an association between cannabis smoking and lung cancer.[17]
- A large study comparing 611 lung cancer cases, 601 upper-airway cancer cases, and 1,040 matched control subjects found no associations between cannabis use and risk of cancer; however, the study reports that the risk of cancer was clearly associated with tobacco use.[18]
- A study investigating the combined effects of tobacco and cannabis smoking revealed that smoking both tobacco and marijuana synergistically increased the risk of respiratory symptoms and COPD (chronic obstructive pulmonary disease, also called emphysema), but smoking only marijuana was not associated with an increased risk of respiratory symptoms or COPD.[19]

In summary, it appears that chronic smokers, whether tobacco or cannabis users, have an increased risk of developing respiratory symptoms such as chronic cough, bronchitis, wheezing, and increased phlegm. Studies do not show an increased risk of cancer with cannabis smoke despite the presence of carcinogenic compounds. It has been hypothesized that the presence of phytocannabinoid compounds in cannabis smoke may be protective against the development of cancer, but definitive research remains to be done.

To quote Dr. Donald Tashkin, a pulmonologist at UCLA and the world's leading researcher of the effects of cannabis smoke on the lungs, "The risks of pulmonary complications of regular use of marijuana appear to be relatively small and far lower than those of tobacco smoking. However, such potential pulmonary risks need to be weighed against possible benefits in consideration regarding medicinal use of marijuana."[20]

There are many different methods available to patients who want to use cannabis medicine. In an informal survey of my patients, approximately 80 percent who switched from smoking to vaporization found excellent results and no longer smoked. For those who wish to continue to smoke, higher-potency cannabis flowers achieve the same effects with less smoke exposure.

Risks of Driving Under the Influence with THC Use

Driving under the influence of any drug is of concern, especially for young people. A number of studies have explored the impact of cannabis— specifically THC, as it can be intoxicating—on motor skills and driving performance.

Scientific Research

- Driving simulator studies showed that cannabis can adversely affect certain driving skills—in particular, tracking ability, attentiveness, judgment of speed and distance, peripheral vision, and coordination at complex tasks.[21]
- A comprehensive survey of ten years of US accident data found that alcohol-free drivers with THC in their system had a slightly elevated risk of unsafe driving behavior but lower than that of drivers with legal amounts of alcohol in their blood.[22]
- Studies have found that THC is significantly more hazardous in the first one to two hours of acute intoxication.[23]
- Alcohol and THC used together increases the risk of fatal accidents.[24]
- A recent study using a driving simulator reported, "Cannabis was associated with slower driving, an increased tendency to drive below the speed limit, and increased following distance, whereas alcohol was associated with increased speed and time spent above the limit, but with no effect on following distance." The researchers analyzed blood levels of THC in these subjects, but there was significant individual variability, making it difficult to draw conclusions.[25]

Driving while under the influence of any intoxicating drug is a bad idea. Combining cannabis with alcohol is dangerous and increases the risk of accidents. Although cannabis patients may overcompensate while driving under the influence and actually be less at risk, it is illegal to drive while intoxicated. This is not advised in any circumstance.

Pregnancy and Breastfeeding with THC Use

The use of cannabis during pregnancy and breastfeeding is controversial. Research on cannabis use by expectant mothers is difficult for many reasons, including fear of legal repercussions and a multitude of other confounding factors (e.g., use of other substances, underlying health conditions, maternal nutrition, and level of prenatal care). A number of studies are summarized here; however, many gaps remain in our understanding of medicinal cannabis use during pregnancy and breastfeeding.

Scientific Research

- It is reported that THC crosses the placenta and enters the circulation of the fetus, reaching concentrations of 10 to 30 percent of the maternal concentration.[26]
- A recent review of studies investigating maternal cannabis use and child development reported the following:[27]
  - Maternal cannabis use does not appear to cause congenital birth defects.[28]
  - Low birth weight and smaller neonatal head circumference were associated with prenatal exposure to cannabis proven by positive maternal drug testing.[29]
  - Ultrasound images from thousands of pregnant women found an association between cannabis use and small but detectable lower birth weights and smaller fetal head circumferences but no association with adverse neonatal outcomes.[30]

—Increased neonatal ICU admissions were reported in babies with prenatal exposure to cannabis (by the mother's self-report or positive urine drug test), although tobacco was not accounted for in this report.[31]

—Longitudinal observation of children with prenatal cannabis exposure revealed normal physical growth at their first school entrance (age five to six) and adolescence.[32]

—Infants born to moderate to heavy THC-rich cannabis users had increased tremors and startle responses as well as sleep disturbances documented on EEG.[33]

—In May 2020, a comprehensive review of studies looking at prenatal cannabis exposure was published, reporting that in previously published studies, "the conclusions drawn sometimes extend too far beyond the actual data." The authors of this review took data from forty-five studies and compared them with a normative database, finding, "Of the 1,004 cognitive outcomes assessed, children with prenatal cannabis exposure performed more poorly on 34 (3.4%) and better on 9 (0.9%) when compared to controls."[34]

It is difficult to know if other variables not included in the research—such as unreported tobacco and/or alcohol use, poor diet, or exposure to chemicals (e.g., pesticides in food)—contributed to the contradictory findings in early studies. However, this latest review comparing exposed children to nonexposed controls is reassuring in that maternal cannabis exposure is unlikely to cause significant cognitive impairment in babies and children.

It is unknown if CBD use during pregnancy is safe. Since we don't have long-term studies on children born to CBD users, most experts recommend avoiding phytocannabinoids during pregnancy.

In special circumstances, such as severe morning sickness or other serious symptoms that cannot be safely treated with other medications, low, intermittent doses of cannabinoids may be recommended. By far, the largest risk I have seen as a cannabis physician is having a newborn taken away by Child Protective Services if either the mother or the newborn has a positive THC drug test during pregnancy or at the time of birth. Cannabis use still remains controversial in general, and use by pregnant women is especially frowned upon by society and the medical community. I have been involved in a number of cases in which the mother or infant tested positive for THC and the baby was removed from the parents' custody.

The Risks of THC Use in the Pediatric Population

Human brain development and the role of the endocannabinoid system throughout childhood and adolescence has been the focus of a number of scientific studies. The adolescent brain is different from the mature adult brain in its structure and in the way its neurotransmitters function. There is an increased sensitivity to changes and exposures in its environment, resulting in a vulnerability of the adolescent brain that is not present once the brain fully develops. Researchers have found that endocannabinoids are crucial in influencing how neurotransmitters in the developing brain promote proper circuitry and new brain growth. The endocannabinoid system goes through necessary changes during the adolescent years, with heightened cannabinoid receptor density and possible sensitivity. Interference with these changes, for example with the use of THC overactivating the cannabinoid receptor, may interfere with the development of the brain.[35] Normal endocannabinoid system functioning during these critical years is required for emotional and cognitive functions to mature correctly.[36] One researcher summed up the importance of the endocannabinoid system in the developing brain this way: "Endocannabinoid signaling is an important determinant of maturation of the adult brain ... [I]t seems quite likely that disruption of normative endocannabinoid signaling during adolescence may have long-standing consequences on adult brain function."[37]

Scientific Research

- Numerous animal studies have documented that THC or synthetic cannabinoids given to adolescent animals induce changes in emotional behavior, reward response, endocannabinoid levels, and impulsivity.[38]

- Studies in human adolescents (aged twelve to eighteen years) who are heavy users of THC-rich cannabis have shown that the interference with normal endocannabinoid system function may result in some long-lasting negative brain changes, especially in the areas of emotional and mental illness (particularly anxiety disorders), impulsivity control, memory issues, attention, decision-making, and lower overall and verbal IQ. First-time cannabis use after the age of eighteen years was not associated with lower IQ or neurocognitive performance.[39]

- Interestingly, recent studies of twins reported that "youth who used cannabis at age 18 had lower IQ in childhood, prior to cannabis initiation, and had lower IQ at age 18, but there was little evidence that cannabis use was associated with IQ decline from age 12–18," and "although cannabis use was associated with lower IQ and poorer executive functions at age 18, these associations were generally not apparent within pairs of twins from the same family, suggesting that family background factors explain why adolescents who use cannabis perform worse on IQ and executive function tests." The researchers concluded that the long-accepted premise that cannabis lowers IQ and impairs executive function was now in question, even when the amount of THC use reaches levels of dependence.[40]

- Although schizophrenia does not develop in the majority of teenagers who use cannabis, those with genetic susceptibility—such as schizophrenia or mental illness in a first-degree family member—combined with chronic heavy cannabis use at a young age, may have an increased risk of developing schizophrenia as a young adult. It is important to note that although there is a correlation, causation is difficult to prove since there are many variables involved in the development of psychiatric conditions.[41]

As you can see from the conflicting reports, questions remain as to whether THC-rich cannabis use during adolescence is harmful. The finding that "family background factors" would explain lower scores on IQ and executive function tests is relatively new and should be investigated further.

As a pediatrician, a medical cannabis specialist, and the mother of a teenager, I am opposed to healthy or otherwise "typically" developing children and adolescents using cannabis. I am also opposed to both cannabis and pharmaceutical use in children and adolescents with mild illnesses, such as occasional anxiety or sleep disturbance, when other treatment modalities, such as talk therapy, exercise, proper diet (especially diet!), sleep, hygiene, etc., can and should be used in these instances. However, children and adolescents who suffer from moderate to severe chronic medical conditions that either significantly disrupt their quality of life or are life-threatening or life-limiting should absolutely have the option of using cannabis under medical supervision.

Kiana's Story

I shared Kiana's story in my previous book and include it here, with an update.

> *When Nazy and her daughter, Kiana, walked into my office, I couldn't believe I was seeing the same child I had met two years earlier. When they initially came to my office, Kiana had already been on cannabis oil for a few months to treat her seizures, but her parents were frustrated by inconsistent results. They had seen some improvement with CBD, but they were exhausted with the constant chaos her medical conditions and the side effects of her medications were causing.*

Nazy and her husband live in the San Fernando Valley with their only child, eleven-year-old Kiana. When Kiana was born, the doctors suspected she had hypochondroplasia (a type of dwarfism), but it wasn't a definitive diagnosis, and it soon became evident that the baby had additional significant issues. At three days old, she was diagnosed with congenital hypothyroidism and immediately put on thyroid medication. Nazy remembers spending weeks in the hospital filled with anguish over what was unfolding as her baby underwent genetic testing, which was inconclusive. Eventually, Kiana went home and at four months old received her first vaccinations. That evening, Nazy noticed what looked to be a seizure, but her doctor assured her that it was unlikely and unrelated to the vaccinations. Nazy believes the doctors were used to her panicking and therefore dismissed her fears about seizures, and it wasn't until Kiana was nine months old that the doctor agreed the baby was experiencing seizures.

The family's life changed, Nazy told me, when Kiana went into a long, uncontrollable seizure (called status epilepticus) one morning while Nazy was driving. After Nazy called 911, Kiana was transported to the hospital and admitted to the intensive care unit. Over the next three years she was hospitalized multiple times, each time in status epilepticus. The only way the doctors could stop her seizures was to induce a coma, despite multiple treatments with multiple medications. By age nine, Kiana had tried fourteen different drugs in varied combinations, all of which gave her terrible side effects, particularly behavioral. Nazy suspected her daughter's extreme hyperactivity, disruptive behavior, head banging, screaming, and refusal to eat were due to the anticonvulsants she was taking, but her doctors dismissed her ideas and told her Kiana was a "very complex kid." Genome sequencing did not reveal any specific diagnosis, so the family was told Kiana had a refractory seizure disorder and hypochondroplasia. Brain surgery was recommended in lieu of other treatments.

Nazy was concerned about the possible risks of brain surgery and wanted to think about it before agreeing, so during the pretesting and despite the neurologists' conviction that there were no other options, she started researching alternative medicines and came across some articles about cannabis. Just when the hospital called to make a date for the surgery, Nazy insisted that she and her husband did not want the surgery and would try something different first. The doctors were upset with her, but she persisted. Around the same time the CNN documentary Weed *aired with the story of Charlotte, a little girl in Colorado whose life-threatening and uncontrollable seizure disorder was finally controlled with CBD oil. "I decided this was it," Nazy said.*

Ready to move to Colorado to try cannabis, Nazy discovered that she could obtain CBD oil in California. She started Kiana on the oil in August of 2013. Within one week, her daughter's behavior changed. She became calmer. Within two months, her seizures lessened in both severity and duration. During the first six months, Kiana was weaned off one of her seizure medications, and her parents saw even more improvement in both behavior and seizures. While she continued to take medication for her hypothyroidism, her thyroid levels stabilized where they were once quite varied.

Kiana's quality of life and that of her family improved so dramatically that it still feels almost unbelievable to Nazy and her husband. Despite years of speech therapy, Kiana was largely nonverbal, but within two months of taking cannabis medicine, she began talking. Nazy could leave the house with Kiana and take her on outings to the grocery store, to coffee shops and restaurants, without seizures, meltdowns, or disruption. The head banging and screaming stopped. She began eating again and even started feeding herself. Over the next eighteen months, her comprehension and alertness improved dramatically, and equally as important, she had long periods of seizure freedom. Her teachers and therapists were amazed by her progress and accomplishments. Nazy never imagined that Kiana would be able to read or write, and in that follow-up visit to my office, Kiana proudly wrote her full name and read a book to me.

"The quality of our life is astounding," Nazy told me that day in my office. "Kiana was like a zombie before, and I'd given up hope." While Kiana was weaning off the second anticonvulsant, she continued to show amazing progress at school and at home. She finally was living a good life. Her family can't imagine a day without cannabis medicine.

Update: *It's been five years since I first met Kiana and her parents. She continues to use cannabis for her medical conditions. Although not seizure-free, her seizures are significantly less frequent, shorter in duration, and less severe, and her recovery is quick. Now in high school, she is thriving, enjoying friendships, and learning new things. Incredibly, she is bilingual, speaking English and Farsi fluently. She is also a typical teenager, rolling her eyes at her mom when she is told what to do, telling her mother, "It's my life, Mom." Her quality of life has far exceeded anyone's expectations.*

PART II

Medical Symptoms and Conditions

The designation of cannabis as a Schedule I controlled substance has impeded research, but the discovery of the endocannabinoid system more than three decades ago has triggered an explosion of scientific investigation into cannabis as medicine. While scientists have learned a tremendous amount from this research, it is my patients' experiences that have truly informed me about medical cannabis.

In this part of the book, I review the scientific literature for each condition as it relates to cannabis. Some illnesses have been studied in depth, while others have not been studied at all. The challenging variables involved in the study of cannabis and the endocannabinoid system are almost too many to count. Most cannabis research was and still is performed on animals and often with very high doses, making it difficult to correlate findings with humans. Synthetic THC is commonly employed in these investigations (due to the Schedule I categorization of cannabinoids), but most cannabis patients use natural whole-plant cannabis containing hundreds of compounds, again making it difficult to interpret the results for clinical use. Different dosing methods—for example, intravenous and intraperitoneal injections used in animals—do not apply to human use. Research on the effects of CBD often uses isolated CBD, which is difficult to compare to CBD-rich whole-plant chemovars containing other cannabinoids and terpenoids. With this single-molecule treatment, the entourage effect is lost and a study's results will not reflect the use of "real-world cannabis." If patients recruited into a study have varying endocannabinoid system dysfunction, or lack of dysfunction, the outcome of the study may also be skewed.

The continued prohibition of cannabis research combined with the challenges of studying whole-plant cannabis, with its multitude of compounds, leaves much to be desired when randomized placebo-controlled trials are considered the gold standard. The lack of these trials has made many medical professionals skeptical. I once heard a physician say that a patient's report of less pain or better sleep is not evidence. I disagree. I think it is important to recognize that millions of patients around the world are finding benefits with medical cannabis.

Another important note is that cannabis trials, like all studies of medications, follow a protocol that uses predetermined dosing regimens. If a patient has a side effect, they have two choices: either continue with the trial or discontinue and drop out. If my patients have side effects, we work together to make changes to mitigate these unwanted effects. It is important to understand that a patient does not have to experience side effects when using cannabis. The vast majority of studies report that cannabis is well tolerated. Most side effects that are reported are mild to moderate, but be assured that medical cannabis patients predominantly do not experience side effects since their regimen is customized to their needs.

All of these factors must be taken into account when you are deciding whether to use cannabis. I find that patient experience often does not reflect the conclusions reached in studies, probably due to the variables I've just mentioned. Although I see people with many different conditions in my office, I find a thread of commonality among of them. Chronic illnesses that prompt a patient to seek out medical cannabis treatment have very similar basic symptoms: chronic pain, disruption of sleep, anxiety, depression, and an inability to participate in life—all of which can be treated effectively with cannabis. Although most conditions are not cured with cannabis, managing and sometimes eliminating these symptoms with a nontoxic natural medicine allows patients to experience an improved quality of life that is not controlled by illness. Being able to participate in life, at home and at work, as well as the elimination of suffering is what my patients report to me every single day. Cannabis is medicine.

Anxiety and Depression

Anxiety is the most common mental illness in the United States, affecting forty million adults over the age of eighteen. Major depressive disorder affects more than sixteen million adults.[1] These conditions often overlap, with almost half of those diagnosed with one disorder meeting the diagnostic criteria for the other. Anxiety disorders include generalized anxiety disorder (GAD), panic disorder, social anxiety disorder, separation anxiety, and phobias. Approximately 40 to 60 percent of those taking conventional medications for anxiety disorders and/or depression do not get full relief of their symptoms.[2]

With the recent increase in interest in cannabis and cannabinoid medicines, the scientific community is starting to recognize the importance of the endocannabinoid system's role in mental health. The authors of a 2016 review of the interaction between stress and the endocannabinoid system stated that there is a "compelling argument that endocannabinoid signaling is an important regulatory system in the brain that largely functions to buffer against many of the effects of stress."[3]

The areas of the brain that control anxiety, mood, and emotion — the amygdala, hippocampus, and prefrontal cortex — are dense with CB_1 receptors.[4] Studies show that disruption of the normal functioning of the endocannabinoid system can lead to anxiety and depression. Mice that are bred to be devoid of cannabinoid receptors have higher levels of anxiety than mice with cannabinoid receptors.[5] When scientists blocked the enzyme that breaks down anandamide (called fatty acid amide hydrolase, or FAAH) in mice, thereby increasing anandamide's actions, potent antianxiety and antidepressant effects were seen.[6] Similarly, mice that were bred without FAAH had less anxiety.[7]

Although research on the efficacy of cannabis treatment for anxiety and depression in humans is limited, evidence of endocannabinoid system dysfunction in these patients supports the idea that if this dysfunction can be targeted and corrected, symptoms will improve.

- Women with major depression were found to have significantly decreased levels of the endocannabinoid 2-AG when compared to women without major depression, suggesting an endocannabinoid deficiency in these patients.[8]
- The same researchers found that levels of the endocannabinoid anandamide were low in women who had reported anxiety, again suggesting an endocannabinoid deficiency disorder.[9]
- A significant increase in CB_1 receptors was found in the brains of individuals with a diagnosis of major depression who had committed suicide, compared to brain tissue of individuals who had died of other causes, suggesting an endocannabinoid system abnormality in those who suffer with severe depression.[10] Similar findings were discovered in alcoholic suicides as well.[11]
- People with major depression who had low levels of anandamide in their blood were found to have higher scores on measures of anxiety.[12]

Interestingly, *The New Yorker* magazine recently featured a story about a woman who has never experienced anxiety and cannot feel pain.[13] It turns out that she has a genetic mutation leading to less FAAH, making her anandamide "bliss" molecule hang around longer in her system. Scientists are studying her to see if her genetics will reveal an answer to the ongoing questions of human suffering from pain and anxiety.

In a 2017 review of the effects of medical cannabis on mental health, thirty-one studies with over twenty-three thousand participants were analyzed.[14] Included were eight studies of medical use that reported relief from anxiety as a primary or secondary benefit. Two reviews of nonmedical use (i.e., THC in higher doses) found a small association between THC and increased anxiety. In terms of depression, seven of nine studies of medical use reported mood improvement across different conditions, such as chronic pain, multiple sclerosis, and HIV. Four studies of nonmedical use reported increased risk of developing depression, especially with chronic, heavy THC use. However, two studies reported the opposite for nonmedical use, the first showing that cannabis users had a decreased likelihood of a major depressive event and the second reporting that cannabis users had a less negative outlook than nonusers.[15]

All of this information clearly shows that the endocannabinoid system is involved in the regulation of anxiety and depression, and dysregulation of this system may be an underlying cause. This makes the endocannabinoid system an attractive target for therapeutic treatment with phytocannabinoids for those suffering from anxiety and depressive disorders. Other receptors involved in mood regulation, such as serotonin and GABA receptors, can be targeted as well since they too interact with phytocannabinoids. Moreover it is clear that thoughtful and responsible medical cannabis use can result in benefits, while nonmedical use carries a risk of increasing symptoms.

Cannabis has been used to treat anxiety and depression for thousands of years. Multiple surveys of patients seeking care in medical cannabis clinics report anxiety and/or depression as their primary condition, as well as the ability to substitute cannabis for benzodiazepines and antidepressants.[16]

A recent case series reported on the use of CBD for anxiety and sleep and found almost 80 percent of participants reported a reduction in anxiety in the first month alone, with sustained reduction throughout the duration of the study.[17]

What do we know about how phytocannabinoids work to improve anxiety and depression?

- CBD, CBG, CBC, and CBN all act to inhibit the uptake of anandamide, allowing anandamide to last longer, resulting in antianxiety and antidepressant effects.
- THC essentially augments the action of anandamide, working directly at the CB_1 receptor, but dosing matters. Studies and patient reports show that low doses of THC relieve anxiety, but higher doses can trigger anxiety.[18]
- CBD can have antianxiety effects in both low and high doses, depending on the user's response.[19]
- Although the raw cannabinoids THCA and CBDA purportedly do not cross the blood–brain barrier, some patients report antianxiety

benefits. Remember that these products have not been heated and retain many other cannabinoids as well as terpenoids from the raw plant, which may be responsible for these effects. As discussed previously, in certain cases the blood–brain barrier may be compromised, allowing these compounds to pass into the brain.

Where to begin with cannabis treatment depends on a number of variables, but most patients who have used THC in the past with no negative experiences will often start with it to treat anxiety or depression. Low, intermittent doses of the appropriate chemovar can be very effective. The downside may be the development of tolerance if higher, more frequent use is needed. For some, the dose that gives the relief may also cause intoxication and/or sedation, making it difficult for the patient to work or drive. Many patients find that THC use only at night is effective in helping their anxiety or depression, assists with a good night's sleep, and does not affect driving or working since the intoxicating effects have disappeared by morning.

If you suffer from anxiety and/or panic, it is important that you do not overmedicate with THC-rich cannabis. If you take large doses frequently, not only will your cannabinoid receptors downregulate (decrease) and produce a loss of efficacy but also your endocannabinoids will lose their target of action, resulting in worsening anxiety.

If you do not want to take THC, CBD-rich products can be used. Most patients start with high-ratio CBD:THC products, such as 18:1, 20:1, 25:1, etc., and explore both lower doses (under 50 milligrams) and higher doses (up to 300 milligrams, or more, per dose). If you do not explore higher doses, you may miss finding your effective dose. If higher doses are not effective or too expensive, the next step is to try lower-ratio CBD:THC products, such as below 10:1. These can be quite effective, usually in doses that do not cause any intoxicating effects. If you find efficacy, you can continue on the same dose and product to see if the benefits persist over time. Making adjustments in the dose may become necessary, as you may find you don't need as much. If you find benefits but feel there is room for improvement, try adding another phytocannabinoid, such as CBG or CBDA (depending on your access to these products), to see if a combination of cannabinoids gives you better results. Terpenes that are calming and antidepressive in their effects include linalool and limonene.

This methodical approach, which takes time and patience, will help you figure out what works and what doesn't. Keeping notes on dosing, products, and your response will help you to "rule it in or rule it out." If you don't want to do this on your own, you should consult with a medical professional knowledgeable about cannabinoid medicines.

Many of my patients ask if they should discontinue their other anti-anxiety or antidepressant medications before trying cannabis. There is no right or wrong way to do this; however, my approach is to first try adding cannabis to the patient's current regimen, and if benefits are felt, we discuss weaning off the other medications. I strongly advise against "cold-turkey" discontinuation of any psychiatric medications, as there is no reason to experience difficulty when, once on cannabis and feeling better, you may be able to wean off them with minimal adverse effects.

—◦◦◦—

Cindy's Story

I wrote about Cindy in my previous book and include her story here, with an update.

A beautiful blond woman in her mid thirties, Cindy has three children under the age of five years old. She came to see me because she had been experiencing anxiety and difficulty sleeping since the birth of her second child. The symptoms were getting worse and were starting to affect her relationship with her husband and children. She told me she was irritable and felt out of control, constantly nagging at her husband and children. Her primary care physician had recommended using a daily antidepressant and an "as needed" antianxiety pill, but after reading about the side effects of these medications, she was reluctant to take them.

Prior to meeting with me, Cindy had shared her struggles with a close friend who happened to be a medical cannabis patient herself. Her friend explained how cannabis was helping with her anxiety, and she gave Cindy a CBD-rich edible to try. Cindy had experimented with cannabis a few times as a teenager and didn't care for the way it made her feel. Nervous about trying it again, she researched CBD on the internet, and after learning of the lack of intoxication with CBD-rich cannabis, she decided to try it on a weekend when her husband was home to help with the kids just in case she didn't react well.

Cindy said the result was one of the best days she'd had in years. Relaxed and in control of her emotions, she was calm when dealing with the children and felt markedly happy. She chose not to tell her husband she had taken CBD, but he came up to her later in the day and told her that she seemed more like the easygoing girl he had married. The positive results were so encouraging that Cindy's husband urged her to get medical cannabis approval from a physician.

When we first met, I educated Cindy on the endocannabinoid system, phytocannabinoids, and the various delivery methods for cannabis medicine. She found that a CBD-rich sublingual tincture used as needed for anxiety greatly improved her quality of life. Sleep also improved. She told me at a recent follow-up visit, "This treatment is so easy, just a few squirts of oil under the tongue and I'm more patient and loving to my children. I am in control of my emotions instead of being controlled by them. I'm happy again."

Update: *Since cannabis has been legalized for adult use in California, Cindy is no longer a patient, as she is able to access her cannabis medication without a physician's approval. During her last visit with me, she shared that since her children were all in school, life had gotten slightly less chaotic. She still used CBD as needed for anxiety, and she was still getting benefits. She had injured her knee playing tennis and was using topical CBD as well. She joked that she was now a "cannabis advocate," telling her friends and family members to try*

CBD if they mentioned any ailments to her. She reported that she sees cannabis as just another part of her healthy life.

Cindy likely has an endocannabinoid dysfunction that causes a dysregulation of her neurotransmitters, which resulted in anxiety and insomnia. The pharmaceuticals her doctor prescribed work to regulate neurotransmitters, but they come with a long list of side effects that can create new problems. Reluctant to take synthetic medication on a daily basis, Cindy found that "as needed" CBD-rich cannabis controlled her anxiety without any side effects. I have seen many patients like Cindy who function better and have no toxicity from cannabis, living pharmaceutical-free.

I am aware that many people negatively judge Cindy and people like her who have chosen to use cannabis medicine instead of pharmaceuticals. I wonder if they would question the judgment of a young person standing in line at a pharmacy, waiting to pick up multiple prescriptions that might cause terrible side effects. It is time we understand that we all have endocannabinoid systems, that there can be dysregulation in these systems that causes disease, and that these conditions can be effectively treated with cannabis medicine. The propaganda from the 1930s claiming that cannabis is the "devil's weed" is no longer acceptable, as the science of the endocannabinoid system is irrefutable. Cannabis must be an option for patients. Cindy has found relief with no side effects from a plant. It's as simple as that.

Appetite Stimulation

Cannabis use has long been associated with an increase in appetite, often called "the munchies." Joking aside, a number of studies done in the 1970s and 1980s showed that subjects given THC had increased intake of food, opting for snack foods over healthier options when given a choice.[20] Synthetic cannabinoids (such as dronabinol) have been shown to enhance appetite, cause weight gain, and stabilize body weight in

AIDS patients.[21] Additional research shows that cannabinoid receptors play a role in food consumption, with activation of CB_1 receptors resulting in hunger.[22] Other studies found that THC causes changes in our internal chemicals that regulate feelings of hunger.[23] For instance, THC increases ghrelin, the "hunger hormone" produced in the stomach and small intestine, which travels to the brain, where it turns on hunger.

Poor appetite may result from cancer treatment, side effects of medication, severe anxiety and/or depression, gastrointestinal conditions, and anorexia nervosa. Many patients report increased appetite as one of the many benefits of cannabis use, although not every patient feels this effect. Being able to feel hunger and have an interest in and enjoy food is normal for humans. It can be quite depressing when you can't eat and enjoy food. Cannabis can restore these feelings and enhance the quality of life for these patients.

Over the past few decades investigators have shown that cannabis and the cannabinoid receptors play an important role in the desire for food. Although there are only a few animal and human studies on this subject, they are consistent in reporting increased appetite with cannabis use:

- Rats injected with anandamide ate twice as much as rats given saline injections, but when the cannabinoid receptor was blocked, anandamide injections did not increase eating behavior.[24]
- Rats given low-THC cannabis extract had significantly increased food intake when compared to an extract without THC.[25]
- Men who smoked cannabis consumed 40 percent more calories than those who smoked placebo.[26]
- Oral THC given to Alzheimer's patients increased their weight.[27]

As I mentioned in chapter 4, THC binds to the cannabinoid receptors in our brains, but CBD does not act directly at these receptors. What I have found in my medical practice is that many patients who use THC-rich cannabis experience hunger and report that food tastes exceptionally good. Some patients—not all—may develop tolerance to the appetite-stimulating effects of THC. My patients using high-ratio CBD:THC cannabis products do not report the same feelings of hunger as some of those using THC-rich products, although some using low-ratio products (such as 1:1 or 2:1) do. Interestingly, some chronically ill patients, such as patients with severe epilepsy or those taking opiates, report that overall appetite is enhanced when CBD is used daily.[28] This may be due to better endocannabinoid system tone—that is, when the body's systems are working better, basic human functions, such as sleeping and eating, become more balanced, whereas studies looking at CBD-only pharmaceutically produced products taken in high doses for epilepsy report decreased appetite as a side effect.[29]

If you are a patient who experiences unwanted hunger with the use of cannabis, there are a few strategies you can try to avoid or control this effect, including switching to a different THC-rich chemovar or adding CBD to your cannabis regimen. You can also assure yourself that you are not really hungry and that the sensation of hunger is just a side effect of the cannabis medication. Drinking water and eating healthy snacks, such as apples or carrots, will help curb your appetite too. One of the best approaches is to not have unhealthy snacks in your house. If they aren't there, you can't eat them! Plus, THCV, which is becoming more readily available to cannabis patients, can suppress appetite.[30] Adding this to your regimen may have anti-hunger effects.

If you are worried about gaining weight with cannabis use, a number of recent studies reporting cannabis users are less likely to be obese than nonusers should put your mind at ease. Researchers found that "the prevalence of obesity is paradoxically much lower in cannabis users as compared to non-users, and this difference is not accounted for by tobacco smoking status and is still present after adjusting for variables such as sex and age."[31] Other studies support these findings, showing those who use cannabis have a smaller waist circumference and lower BMI (body mass index).[32]

Arthritis

Arthritis is a general term that refers to inflammation of the joints. More than 350 million people worldwide suffer from this debilitating and painful condition. Arthritis may result from normal or occupational "wear and tear" or may be a result of autoimmune disorders, such as rheumatoid arthritis and psoriatic arthritis. The main symptoms of arthritis are joint pain and stiffness. Over time, degeneration and destruction of the joint results. There are many conventional medications available, ranging from over-the-counter anti-inflammatories to prescription injections, but adverse side effects and minimal effectiveness is not unusual. Additionally, in 2012 the American Society of Nephrology (kidney specialists) recommended that anyone with diabetes, high blood pressure, heart failure, or evidence of chronic kidney disease should avoid taking nonsteroidal anti-inflammatory medications, as they can "elevate blood pressure, make antihypertensive drugs less effective, cause fluid retention and worsen kidney function in these individuals."[33] This leaves these patients with very few options for treatment of arthritis.

Arthritis sufferers make up one of the largest groups using phytocannabinoid medicines since they are effective in reducing pain and inflammation with minimal side effects. Two surveys found approximately 20 to 25 percent of patients who were using cannabis were doing so for arthritis.[34] Similarly, about 18 percent of patients seeking approval at a California medical cannabis clinic were seeking relief from arthritis symptoms.[35]

The endocannabinoid system is present in the tissues that make up our joints, making arthritis an excellent target for treatment. In fact, upregulation of cannabinoid receptors and increased endocannabinoid levels were found in rats that had osteoarthritis, showing that the endocannabinoid system tries to restore balance to an area of inflammation.[36] The joint fluid from patients with rheumatoid arthritis consistently has shown elevated pro-inflammatory compounds.[37] The goal of phytocannabinoid treatment is to reduce these pro-inflammatory agents through augmentation of the endocannabinoid system — assisting this system to decrease the inflammation that leads to pain, immobility, and destruction of the joints.

Numerous animal studies from the past two decades clearly show that cannabinoids impart potent anti-inflammatory effects, which can be beneficial in the treatment of arthritis:

- The administration of CBD after the onset of collagen-induced arthritis effectively blocked the progression of arthritis and had a potent antiarthritic effect. In this study, CBD blocked the formation of the pro-inflammatory chemicals, called cytokines, that are made in the body in response to a trigger, such as an infection, an injury, or a haywire immune system (autoimmune disease).[38]
- Daily administration of a synthetic cannabinoid was reported to protect joints from damage and to ameliorate collagen-induced arthritis in an experiment using mice.[39]
- Transdermal CBD application significantly reduced joint swelling as well as other measures of inflammation in a rat model of arthritis.[40]
- In another rat model of osteoarthritis, CBD dose dependently (meaning higher doses were more effective) decreased joint pain, increased use of the involved joint, reduced inflammation, and prevented future inflammation from developing.[41]
- In a randomized placebo-controlled study on dogs with osteoarthritis, oral CBD significantly reduced pain and increased activity over a four-week treatment period.[42]

Summarizing the available literature in the September 2005 issue of the *Journal of Neuroimmunology*, researchers at Tokyo's National Institute of Neuroscience concluded, "Cannabinoid therapy of rheumatoid arthritis could provide symptomatic relief of joint pain and swelling as well as suppressing joint destruction and disease progression."[43] Despite this strong statement, there are virtually no human trials on the benefits of cannabis for arthritis due to the continued (and ridiculous) prohibition of cannabis research. The only published trial is one from the United Kingdom using nabiximols (CBD:THC 1:1, Sativex), which found statistically significant improvements in pain on movement, pain at rest, and quality of sleep, and an improved rating in a measure of disease activity for patients with rheumatoid arthritis.[44]

All of the phytocannabinoids discussed in this book show anti-inflammatory properties. My patients with arthritis report that medical cannabis use provides pain relief, reduces the need for opiates and NSAIDs, improves mobility, and promotes better sleep. Choosing a regimen has gotten a bit more complicated since there are more phytocannabinoids available. Using the "Rule it in or rule it out" method previously described, start with one product and explore dosing and the timing of doses. If it does not help, change to another delivery method or a different cannabinoid profile. For instance, many patients with arthritis will start with topical preparations, containing either mostly CBD or some combination of CBD and THC, applied directly to the joints involved. I advise trying this twice a day, or more, for at least one week to see if there are any benefits. If not, taking cannabis internally can be tried next. Since some patients respond to high-ratio CBD:THC products, this is a good place to start if it is the only product legally available to you. If you do not feel better with lower doses, raise them, although remember that higher doses of CBD can be expensive. Lower-ratio CBD:THC, the raw cannabinoids THCA and CBDA, and also CBG, either alone or in combination, can be quite effective as well. If you are willing to go through the trial and error of sorting out what works best, you will likely find benefits. Remember too that many terpenoids, especially beta-caryophyllene, will help add anti-inflammatory effects.

I think it would be helpful at this point to share some of my patients' cannabis regimens as examples. All of these patients tried a number of different cannabis products before finding the regimen that was most effective.

- Tina, a fifty-eight-year-old mother of two and entrepreneur, struggled with disabling joint pain from autoimmune disease. The combination of topical CBD balm applied twice a day to painful joints in addition to a 4:1 CBD:THC tincture (about 32 milligrams CBD and 8 milligrams THC total per day—started lower and increased over two months) has reduced her joint pain significantly. She reports that she has been able to exercise more consistently and sleep is much improved.

- Jonathan, forty years old, was initially diagnosed with osteoarthritis when he developed joint pain in his thirties. After his symptoms became severe, he saw a specialist and was diagnosed with rheumatoid arthritis. He has had terrific results with higher doses of high-ratio CBD:THC oil taken sublingually during the day (100 milligrams CBD and 4 milligrams THC per day) and with vaporized THC flowers taken as needed for pain mostly in the evening.

- Stephan, an eighty-year-old former professional athlete with severe knee and ankle pain from osteoarthritis, uses high-potency CBD topical balm (with 400 milligrams per 1 ounce) numerous times daily and a low-dose 1:1 CBD:THC edible at night (2.5 milligrams CBD and 2.5 milligrams THC). He reports increased mobility, less pain, and better sleep.

- Genevieve, a thirty-seven-year-old stay-at-home mom of four, was a gymnast while in high school and college. She has arthritis pain in multiple joints in addition to back pain and has found THCA and CBDA tinctures (about 20 milligrams of each) taken together two or three times daily help decrease her pain from 8 out of 10 on a pain scale to a more tolerable 3 out of 10. She is currently in the process of increasing the doses to see if that will add benefits. She occasionally takes a 5-milligram THC edible before bedtime to help with sleep if her pain seems elevated.

- Amy is a sixty-eight-year-old accountant who was struggling with arthritis in her hips and knees. After losing weight, her arthritis improved, but she continued to have pain, which came on mostly later in the day. The combination of CBG (20 milligrams) and

CBDA (30 milligrams) taken together after breakfast and dinner gives her relief and improved mobility.

Asthma

It seems counterintuitive that cannabis would help people with asthma breathe more easily, but in 1973, Dr. Donald Tashkin and his colleagues at UCLA published a study in the *New England Journal of Medicine* showing that cannabis works as a bronchodilator, meaning it opens up the airways in both healthy and asthmatic people.[45] He also found that cannabis "succeeded in reversing experimentally induced asthma, in a manner that was comparable to what could be achieved with a standard therapeutic bronchodilator," which was widely used at the time. Dr. Tashkin's group showed that very low doses of THC were effective.[46]

Additional scientific studies have shown benefits of cannabinoids for asthma:

- A human study of 10 milligrams oral THC in six asthmatics and six healthy controls reported no significant benefits. I include this study to point out the biphasic effects in action — dosing matters! THC of 10 milligrams was likely too high of a dose, especially since Dr. Tashkin's research reports low doses were effective.[47]
- THC blocks a compound called acetylcholine, which works to maintain the muscle tone in the airways. This compound also causes tightening of the airways in an asthma attack. When THC binds to the cannabinoid receptor, it prevents the release of this compound and allows the airways to relax.[48]
- In an animal study looking at allergic asthma-like reactions, a synthetic cannabinoid reduced cough and shortness of breath as well as decreased inflammatory changes in lung tissue. These benefits were due to effects of the cannabinoid at both CB_1 and CB_2 recep-

tors present in peripheral nerves in the smooth muscle layer of bronchial tubes.[49]

The method of cannabinoid delivery for patients with asthma or other lung conditions should not include smoking. Beneficial cannabinoids are contained in combusted cannabis, but the smoke also contains numerous other compounds that aggravate the airway. Studies show chronic heavy cannabis smoking is associated with increased risk for bronchitis. Additionally, airway swelling, irritation, and inflammation have been reported.[50]

My patients with asthma who initially sought approval to use cannabis for other medical conditions have found, much to their surprise, their coexisting asthma condition is improved and they don't require as much asthma medicine. I have a few patients in my practice with very significant symptoms of asthma requiring them to take a number of daily medications, which often cause adverse side effects. For some, despite intensive treatment with the latest asthma medications available, they report ongoing symptoms and occasional flare-ups that require hospital visits. Adding cannabis (not smoked) has helped to improve control of the asthma symptoms, with fewer flare-ups, fewer hospitalizations, and occasionally less need for asthma medications. In my experience, patients treating asthma with cannabis are using THC-rich cannabis, mostly in low doses with vaporizers, sublingual tinctures, or edibles. Some patients find chemovars rich in the terpenoids pinene and limonene, which have bronchodilatory effects, to be quite helpful.

Attention Deficit Hyperactivity Disorder

ADHD is a neurodevelopmental disorder that unfortunately is quite common and on the rise.[51] This disorder affects a person's ability to regulate their attention, emotions, impulsivity, and hyperactivity. It can present in childhood or adulthood and can change from one type to another over a person's lifetime. There is also an increased risk of other psychiatric conditions, such as anxiety, depression, and substance-abuse disorders.

ADHD is divided into three types:

1. Predominantly inattentive presentation (ADD)
2. Predominantly hyperactive-impulsive presentation
3. Combined presentation[52]

The neurotransmitters dopamine, norepinephrine, and serotonin are thought to be dysregulated in ADD/ADHD.[53] Multiple genetic variations involved in these neurotransmitters have been found in people with ADHD. It is thought that the three different types may be explained by differences in the involved neurotransmitter. Dopamine sends messages within the parts of the brain that control reward and motivation (nucleus accumbens); planning, problem-solving, and attention (prefrontal cortex); and cognition and learning (dorsal striatum). People with ADHD of the hyperactive-impulsive type seem to have an overly efficient removal of dopamine, which interferes with dopamine's ability to exert its effects. Norepinephrine is involved in alertness, attention, and memory, and its deficiency is thought to be related to inattentive presentation, or ADD. The loss of impulse control and aggression seen in ADHD is hypothesized to be due to dysregulated serotonin. Stimulant medications are prescribed for dopamine-related ADHD, as they block removal of dopamine, allowing it to hang around the brain for longer periods. Non-stimulant medications target norepinephrine, allowing it to last longer. These medications, although quite effective for some, can have side effects of poor appetite, insomnia, high blood pressure, weight loss, tics, headache, and stomach upset.

There is evidence that patients with ADHD have genetically based endocannabinoid system dysfunction and altered anandamide breakdown.[54] As the endocannabinoid system is involved in balancing neurotransmitter messages, abnormalities in its function may contribute to ADHD symptoms.

There are some reports in the scientific literature of benefits from medical cannabis treatments:

- A twenty-eight-year-old with ADHD was able to function normally with high levels of THC, including passing a driving test. The researchers who reported this case stated, "There was evidence that the consumption of cannabis had a positive impact on performance, behavior and mental state of the subject."[55]
- A 2015 report of thirty patients with ADHD, considered treatment resistant, found medical cannabis to be effective and well tolerated.[56]
- A trial of thirty patients with ADHD given nabiximols (1:1 CBD:THC, Sativex) did not show statistically significant improvement; however, the overall testing scores were better in the group receiving the cannabinoid medicine when compared to the placebo group. Secondary outcomes reported for the group receiving the cannabinoids indicated improvement in hyperactivity/impulsivity and a trend toward improvement for inattention.[57]
- A January 2020 report from Technion, Israel Institute of Technology, stated that treatment with medical cannabis was associated with decreased ADHD symptoms and decreased medication use. Interestingly, higher amounts of the phytocannabinoid CBN correlated with fewer ADHD symptoms.[58]

In clinical practice, many adults report that THC-rich cannabis significantly helps with focus, impulsivity, and memory, and allows them to finish tasks. Other patients find that cannabis treatment works best in counteracting the unwanted side effects of their prescription ADD/ADHD medications, which are otherwise effective.

Patients report that stimulating THC-rich chemovars (often referred to as "sativa" chemovars) and those chemovars that contain higher amounts of pinene, a terpenoid that helps to increase focus and aids in memory, work well for their ADHD symptoms. For some, the less stimulating chemovars work better, especially when combating coexisting symptoms, such as insomnia and anxiety. I encourage adult patients to try different chemovars and products to find what works best for them.

I have found that some pediatric patients with ADHD respond to CBD-rich cannabis. Many of these patients have other coexisting diagnoses, such as seizure disorders, Tourette syndrome, or severe anxiety, that also improve with CBD treatment. Some children do well with higher CBD:THC ratios (for example, 25:1) and others show improvement with lower ratios. My approach for children and teenagers with severe ADHD symptoms is to start with high-ratio CBD:THC preparations, assess their response, and add THC in small amounts for the desired effects. Additionally, a few of my patients have improved with CBG and/or THCA.

John's Story

I wrote about John in my previous book and include his story here, with an update.

When John first came to see me at the age of nineteen, his mother accompanied him to the office. I noticed immediately and was touched by the close relationship between the two. John had been diagnosed with ADHD when he was eleven years old after the school reported to his parents that he was struggling with schoolwork and impulsivity in the classroom. He was prescribed a stimulant medication and remembers feeling terrible on it. "I felt like a zombie," he told me. His mother also disliked the effects of the medication and stopped giving it to him, saying that it made his personality disappear. Reluctant to try other medications, she pulled him out of school and homeschooled him until John graduated from high school.

Despite being nervous that he might fail, he started college and was introduced to cannabis recreationally by some new friends. He was shocked to find that, for the first time, he was able to actually focus on schoolwork. Impulsivity, which had been a big issue for him, disappeared. He says that his brain always felt like it was racing, and using cannabis slowed his thoughts to a "normal" pace. He was able to think and process information better than he ever had.

Since John felt that cannabis was helping him achieve in school, he decided to tell his mother. Initially upset, she was surprised to learn that many people had found the same results. She made a deal with him that if his grades were good for the semester, she would take him to get medical cannabis approval so that he could obtain and use cannabis legally, getting assistance from a physician to help him understand the best way to use it. He made straight A's that semester!

John's mother reported to me how skeptical she had been, but she was open to cannabis treatment because he had struggled for so long. When he was first diagnosed with ADHD, she shared, he felt stupid because his teachers were frustrated by his behavior and treated him differently from the other children in the classroom. With home-schooling and individual attention, he excelled, but she was concerned about his ability to function outside the home. Seeing him achieve in college with the responsible use of cannabis medicine assured her that he would be able to make it on his own. She is amazed and troubled that she never heard from other parents or John's doctors that cannabis could help her son combat his ADHD symptoms.

John reported that THC-rich cannabis in low doses (vaporized) before school helped him to focus and achieve with no intoxicating effects. He also reported that he felt less anxious and ready to take on any task. He skipped cannabis on the days he didn't need it to avoid developing tolerance.

Update: John has graduated college and is planning to apply to graduate school to study chemistry. He also is working at a job that does not require preemployment drug testing. John says that he sees cannabis as his medicine, nothing more or less, just a normal part of his day that allows him to function and achieve his goals.

Autism Spectrum Disorder

Autism spectrum disorder, or ASD, refers to a broad range of complex conditions that impact a person's communication, social skills, self-regulation, and behaviors. It is considered a spectrum disorder because each person is affected differently and to different degrees. The CDC reports that one in every fifty-nine children is affected by ASD, and boys are four times more likely to be affected. The core symptoms of ASD are impaired communication, impaired reciprocal social interaction, and restricted, repetitive, and stereotyped patterns of behaviors or interests.[59] Although two antipsychotic medications have been approved to treat the irritability associated with ASD, they do not address the core symptoms. Additionally, approximately 40 percent of children do not respond to these medications or to behavioral interventions.[60] Approximately 10 to 30 percent of people with ASD also have epilepsy.[61] Researchers report several overlapping pathways for both ASD and epilepsy.[62] Since the endocannabinoid system has been shown to be an important physiologic regulator of seizures, as well as highly involved in the control of emotional, behavioral, and social interactions, scientists are now looking into its dysfunction as an underlying cause and possible target of treatment for ASD.

A number of investigations have looked at the potential role of the endocannabinoid system's involvement:

- One study looking at the role of the endocannabinoid system in fragile X syndrome (a syndrome that causes learning disabilities, cognitive impairment, and features of autism spectrum disorder) found that the genetic defect causing this syndrome also caused abnormal endocannabinoid metabolism and activity. The same study found that pharmacological enhancement of endocannabinoid signaling normalizes this defect and corrects behavioral abnormalities in a mice model of fragile X syndrome.[63]

- Recent research has found evidence that acetaminophen may trigger autism by activating cannabinoid receptors.[64]
- In a rat model of autism, subjects that had prenatal disruption of their endocannabinoid system had behavioral abnormalities associated with autism spectrum disorder.[65]

Recently a number of human studies have shown that children with ASD have abnormalities in their endocannabinoid system compared to children without this disorder:

- A clinical study performed on children three to nine years old demonstrated that CB_2 receptors on white blood cells of the children with ASD were increased (thought to be compensating for low endocannabinoid levels) compared with matched healthy controls.[66]
- A 2018 study from Stanford University documented that children with ASD have lower levels of plasma anandamide compared to children without ASD. The authors reported that "anandamide concentrations significantly differentiated ASD cases from controls, such that children with lower anandamide concentrations were more likely to have ASD." This finding is quite important in that anandamide levels may be used as a biomarker to help diagnose ASD.[67]
- A 2019 study from Israeli researchers reported that children with ASD have lower levels of three endocannabinoids when compared to children without ASD. The study found that the lower levels were "not significantly associated or correlated with age, gender, BMI, medications, and adaptive functioning of ASD participants."[68]

A case study from Austria published in 2010 documented the use of dronabinol (synthetic THC with no CBD) in a six-year-old boy diagnosed with autism.[69] He received dronabinol therapy for six months with no change in other therapies or initiation of any other new treatments. An examiner and his parents rated his behaviors on a scale. He had significantly decreased hyperactivity, lethargy, and irritability. Stereotypic behavior and speech also improved. There were no reported adverse side effects. The dosing for this child was low, beginning with 0.62 milligram THC one time per day in the morning. By the end of six months, he was taking 1.2 milligrams THC in the morning, 0.62 milligram THC in the afternoon, and 1.86 milligrams THC at night for a total daily dose of 3.68 milligrams to achieve the reported improvements, with no evidence of intoxication.

Although two human clinical trials investigating the use of CBD for ASD have been approved in the US, neither had been started at the time of writing. However, a few findings from clinical trials in other countries are quite promising:

- In Israel, sixty children with severe ASD symptoms were given a 20:1 ratio of CBD:THC oil. Thirty-one (52 percent) responded well to this product; those who did not were switched to lower ratios (more THC relative to the CBD), resulting in another twenty children (69 percent) showing improvement. At the end of the study, 73 percent remained on treatment. The authors reported that the range of dosing was 1.2 to 6.4 milligrams per kilogram per day CBD and 0.07 to 0.51 milligram per kilogram per day THC for children who received three daily doses, and 0.2 to 3.4 milligrams per kilogram per day CBD and 0.08 to 0.36 milligram per kilogram per day THC for children who received two daily doses.[70]
- Also in Israel, 188 patients were treated with a 20:1 CBD:THC oil between 2015 and 2017. After six months, 82.4 percent remained in active treatment with the following results: 28 patients (30.1 percent) reported a significant improvement, 50 (53.7 percent) moderate, 6 (6.4 percent) slight, and 8 (8.6 percent) had no change in their condition. Treatment was considered well tolerated, safe, and effective.[71]
- An observational study in Brazil of patients with ASD (some with epilepsy) taking a cannabis preparation containing a CBD:THC

ratio of 75:1 reported that of the fifteen patients who adhered to the treatment, all but one showed improvement of ASD symptoms.[72]

Most of the families that come to my office seeking cannabis treatment for their loved one with ASD have tried multiple interventions and medications, including off-label (not FDA-approved for ASD) psychiatric medications that were prescribed despite no scientific evidence documenting benefits for ASD. This group of patients is challenging to treat because many are nonverbal, sensitive to small changes, and often have other medical conditions that must be taken into account. It is truly trial and error since this is a spectrum disorder, with each individual having a unique response to the various phytocannabinoids. It is important that families wishing to explore cannabis for the treatment of ASD have realistic expectations and understand that it is not a cure but another tool to help manage symptoms and improve quality of life.

A number of important aspects must be understood if CBD is going to be used to treat autism. Firstly, there are patients who respond well to low doses and those who require much higher doses, meaning trials of both low and high doses may be required to find what works (i.e., ruling both low and high doses in or out). If a child responds to a low dose, a high dose may not be needed. Secondly, cannabinoids can take some time to work, so being patient and not changing doses or products from day to day will help to assess benefits and side effects. Thirdly, the biphasic nature of cannabinoids (explained in chapter 5) must be taken into account because lower doses of CBD (less than 50 milligrams) can sometimes overstimulate someone with ASD, aggravating symptoms, while higher doses can be calming and focusing. If low doses exacerbate symptoms, higher doses should be tried. In one of the trials from Israel mentioned earlier, the researchers reported a wide range of dosing, from 15 milligrams three times a day (45 milligrams daily) up to 285 milligrams three times a day (855 milligrams daily), clear evidence that there is a wide range of therapeutic dosing for CBD.[73] Lastly, reverse tolerance (discussed in chapter 4) may occur, requiring the lowering of a dose that was previously effective.

Tincture preparations are recommended so that dosing can be titrated up or down more easily, allowing for "custom" dosing. If a patient refuses to take the oil (it can be unpalatable for some), it can be placed into empty capsules. One family that came to see me was using purchased capsules that contained 25 milligrams CBD. One capsule was too low of a dose and two capsules was too high of a dose. Tinctures allow patients to fine-tune and personalize dosing.

Edible products are occasionally more effective than tinctures. Most states that allow for THC edibles require them to be 10 milligrams or less. For instance, in California THC edibles come as 2.5, 5, or 10 milligrams. Some parents of children with ASD will cut the edibles in half or in quarters to start. There are also edibles that contain both CBD and THC in varying ratios. One of the benefits of edibles is that some patients get longer-lasting effects, allowing them to get through a school day without having to re-dose.

Many of my patients with ASD are on unique combinations of cannabinoids, found only through trial and error. Some take only high-ratio CBD:THC, some take THCA and THC together, some are taking 1:1 CBD:THC, some are on CBG and CBD, and so on. The "Rule it in or rule it out" method is helpful to narrow down the many choices; however, it is time-consuming and can be extremely frustrating. An excellent resource that is very helpful to families is the nonprofit Whole Plant Access for Autism (www.wpa4a.com). They are dedicated to providing high-quality scientific information and are committed to helping families figure out if cannabis might be helpful. I am on their advisory board and can confidently endorse their work.

Autoimmune and Inflammatory Conditions

The roles of the endocannabinoid system, endocannabinoids, and phytocannabinoids in immune function and inflammatory conditions is a popular area of research. Cells of the immune system release numerous compounds that create inflammation, which may be a normal response to a trigger, such as an infection or injury, or an abnormal over-response of the body, leading to inflammatory disease. This abnormal over-response is what is called autoimmune disease. The endocannabinoid system plays a protective role in regulating these responses and, as such, has been described as the "homeostatic gatekeeper" of the immune system, preventing overwhelming and imbalanced pro-inflammatory responses to harmful triggers.[74]

All immune cells make endocannabinoids and have cannabinoid receptors, usually more CB_2 receptors than CB_1 receptors.[75] In order to understand the role of these components within the immune system, scientists often use mice bred without a specific component to see what happens when that component is removed or altered. For example, mice bred without cannabinoid receptors have increased allergic inflammation, and mice bred without the enzyme FAAH, which breaks down anandamide (meaning anandamide hangs around longer and has a stronger effect), have more anti-inflammatory, less allergic responses.[76] This tells us that we need our endocannabinoid system to maintain homeostasis—balance—within our immune system and to control inflammation, now thought to be the root cause of so many illnesses.

Cannabinoids as anti-inflammatory agents have been researched in connection with many autoimmune diseases, including type 1 diabetes, rheumatoid arthritis, allergic asthma, multiple sclerosis, colitis, chronic liver inflammation, and cancers with inflammatory components.[77] They have also been investigated for use as suppressors of the body's over-response after a major injury. For instance, after a head trauma or heart attack, the body's immune system kicks in, sometimes adding to tissue damage due to the release of inflammatory chemicals. Multiple animal studies show cannabinoids can inhibit the severity of disease, reduce an over-response of the immune system, delay the onset of disease, and decrease inflammation.[78]

There are many examples of cannabinoid-induced anti-inflammatory effects; here are just a few important findings:

- *Brain inflammation:* Mice with a closed-head injury that were treated with a synthetic cannabinoid had decreased levels of inflammatory compounds in the brain with better recovery and clinical outcome than those that did not receive the cannabinoid.[79]
- *Intestinal inflammation:* Mice with inflammation in the colon (colitis) that received a synthetic cannabinoid had decreased colonic inflammation and fewer inflammatory cells on biopsy.[80]
- *Joint inflammation:* Mice with arthritis that received a synthetic cannabinoid had significantly reduced joint swelling and decreased serum levels of pro-inflammatory compounds.[81]
- *Cardiovascular inflammation:* Mice that had heart attacks after ischemia-reperfusion (tissue damage that occurs when blood flow is cut off and then reinstated) and received a synthetic cannabinoid had less heart tissue damage and reduced levels of inflammatory compounds.[82]

A very interesting 2018 study in patients with multiple sclerosis, one of the most common autoimmune conditions, affecting over two million people worldwide, documented that after four weeks of treatment with nabiximols (1:1 CBD:THC, Sativex), testing of the whole genome before and after treatment revealed suppression of the genes sending pro-inflammatory messages, especially in those patients who were classified as responders to the treatment.[83]

Another interesting example relating to cannabinoids and the immune system is a condition called graft-versus-host disease (GVHD). This is an immune condition that occurs after a transplant, wherein cells from the donor attack the tissues of the host who received the transplant. Multiple studies have shown involvement of the endocannabinoid system in GVHD, making it a target for therapeutic intervention.[84] In a trial of forty-eight patients who were transplant recipients, treatment consisted of 300 milligrams CBD taken orally, starting seven days before transplantation until thirty days after the transplant. Patients were followed for seven to twenty-three months. None of the patients developed

GVHD while taking CBD. The incidence of GVHD (by day 100 after the transplant) was 12 percent lower than expected when compared to control subjects not treated with CBD.[85]

Many patients using cannabis are treating conditions that have underlying inflammation as the root cause of the symptoms. Since medical conditions vary from person to person, and response to cannabinoid treatment varies as well, patients will respond to different cannabinoid profiles and doses. Some of my patients experience an improvement of their inflammation using only THC-rich cannabis, as evidenced by their reports of less pain and better mobility. Other patients are using CBD-rich cannabis in a daily high-dose regimen to try to suppress inflammation that occurs in autoimmune disease. Some patients are using CBD and THC combined in various ratios depending on what works best for their symptoms. CBG, CBDA, and THCA as anti-inflammatories are proving to be effective, either alone but more often in combination. Anti-inflammatory terpenes include beta-caryophyllene, myrcene, pinene, humulene, cineole, and citronellol.

———∾———

Lori's Story

Lori started feeling unwell in 2006, with vague symptoms of joint pain, insomnia, and anxiety. As time passed, her symptoms progressed to include lethargy, weight gain, migraine headaches, brain fog, and depression. She sought medical care and was erroneously diagnosed with Lyme disease despite inconclusive test results. She felt worse with Lyme treatment, which she was warned about, and after a full year of misery with continued symptoms, she was diagnosed with various other disorders, including fibromyalgia and irritable bowel syndrome. She struggled to get out of bed and function normally, often unable to do so.

A battery of tests revealed Lori was suffering from Hashimoto's thyroiditis, an autoimmune condition of the thyroid that explained many of her symptoms. She became convinced that conventional medications were making her worse, and she began to pursue alternative treatments, such as acupuncture and trigger-point massage. She stopped taking the prescribed pharmaceuticals and adopted a strict gluten-free diet. She began to feel better but still struggled with anxiety, joint pain, poor sleep, and migraines. It was at this point that she decided to try cannabis.

Lori was quite apprehensive when starting cannabis, afraid that THC would aggravate her anxiety, which was still somewhat out of control. She had read many online stories of patients experiencing life-changing results with high-ratio CBD:THC tinctures, and after we went over all of the options, she decided to try this first. She had no improvement with 25:1 or 18:1, even with high doses. I advised her to try 4:1 CBD:THC, as the higher amount of THC would likely have more of a direct effect on pain, sleep, and anxiety. She began with very low doses and titrated up slowly over a few months, sharing with me that she was beginning to sleep through the night, have less pain during the day, and experience a significant reduction in anxiety. Over the next eight months, Lori started to feel like her old self again. She has experimented with some of the newer products, including a blended tincture of CBDA and THCA, which eliminated her migraine headaches, and a CBG tincture, which helped to further control her anxiety.

All of Lori's symptoms point to an endocannabinoid deficiency, further aggravated by chronic anxiety and sleep deprivation. Unfortunately, until the medical community acknowledges the endocannabinoid system and its impact on illness, patients like Lori will continue to be misdiagnosed and given treatment that is not effective.

Lori has been a cannabis patient for over five years now, living her best life. She continues to adhere to a strict diet devoid of all inflammatory foods. She is able to put in long days at work as well as enjoy family and travel, and most importantly, she is in control of her life again. When I asked her about how cannabis helped her, she stated simply, "It saved my life."

Cancer

The American Cancer Society defines cancer as "a word used to describe more than 100 diseases in which cells grow out of control."[86] Although researchers have made significant strides in treatments, cancer continues to be the second most common cause of death in the US (heart disease is the first). Cannabis has been investigated for its use in combating the symptoms associated with cancer and its treatments. However, it is also being used to kill cancer cells, since phytocannabinoids have been found to have anticancer properties. The first three parts of this section will discuss the use of cannabis to help with specific symptoms associated with cancer and its treatments, and the final part will address its ability to help kill cancer.

Chemotherapy-Induced Nausea and Vomiting

The first report in the scientific literature of the effective anti-vomiting, or antiemetic, benefits of cannabis appeared in the *New England Journal of Medicine* in 1975.[87] Twenty cancer patients who did not respond to conventional antiemetic medication received either THC or placebo two hours before chemotherapy. The THC patients reported that they had less vomiting without any significant side effects. A slew of studies in the 1980s found cannabinoids to be effective for chemotherapy-induced nausea and vomiting (CINV), equal to or better than the antiemetics available at the time, leading to FDA approval of two synthetic THC medications for this indication: dronabinol and nabilone.[88] In 2001, a large review of thirty studies with a total of 1,366 patients comparing synthetic cannabinoids with placebo or approved antiemetic pharmaceuticals concluded the cannabinoids were highly effective compared to placebo and other medications, and patients preferred the cannabinoids over the other medications.[89]

The following are other important studies:

- A 1979 National Cancer Institute investigation compared the antiemetic effects of oral and smoked THC with oral and smoked placebos. Efficacy against nausea and vomiting was dose dependent, as higher doses correlated with decreased symptoms. Additionally, oral delivery was compared to inhalation, with evidence that inhaled THC was absorbed more reliably.[90]
- A 1988 report found 78 percent of fifty-six cancer patients who did not get relief from standard antiemetic therapy were symptom-free after cannabis use.[91]
- In 1995, Israeli researchers found delta-8-THC to be quite effective (with negligible side effects) in preventing nausea and vomiting in a group of pediatric cancer patients.[92]
- A 2007 study compared dronabinol (synthetic THC) to a newer antiemetic called ondansetron (brand name Zofran), and both in combination, in sixty-four patients on chemotherapy. The response was similar for both drugs alone and in combination; however, nausea intensity and vomiting/retching were lowest with dronabinol.[93]
- The National Academies of Sciences, Engineering, and Medicine (NASEM) in their 2017 report *The Health Effects of Cannabis and Cannabinoids: The Current State of Evidence and Recommendations for Research* stated that "[i]n adults with chemotherapy-induced nausea and vomiting, oral cannabinoids are effective antiemetics."[94]

Despite the benefits noted in these investigations and the abundance of anecdotal reports of symptom relief from patients documented by their physicians, the medical literature does not have any large, good-quality studies on the effects of whole-plant cannabis for CINV. Since the US government continues to prohibit cannabis research, we do not know if it is more effective than the newer group of available antiemetic pharmaceuticals. Many patients prefer to use cannabis not only because they find it to be effective for CINV but also because it adds the beneficial side effects of less anxiety, reduced pain, and better sleep. As a clinician, I have found that many cancer patients prefer to inhale cannabis when treating CINV. This appears to be due to the faster onset and the easy control of dosing when compared to other delivery methods. It can be difficult to swallow edibles or hold tinctures under the tongue when nausea or vomiting is present. These methods also have delayed onset of action, not ideal when you are experiencing severe nausea and vomiting.

Many of the phytocannabinoids have antiemetic properties, including CBD, CBDA, THC, THCA, and delta-8-THC. In my clinical experience, patients on chemotherapy seem to prefer THC, as it is quite effective and can be vaporized easily. I have witnessed only three patients obtain CINV relief with delta-8-THC, as it is new on the market and can be difficult to find; however, these patients reported benefits with it taken as a sublingual tablet preparation.

Anorexia and Weight Loss

Many cancer patients report lack or loss of appetite—called anorexia—and significant weight loss associated with cancer and its treatment. Weakness and wasting of the body—cachexia, in medical terms—is quite common and is notoriously difficult to alleviate. The well-known side effect of "the munchies" is one of the most common symptoms compelling cancer patients to seek out medical cannabis.

Over the past few decades, investigators have shown that cannabis and the cannabinoid receptors play an important role in the desire for food. A number of studies looking at their effects on appetite and weight gain are summarized in this section. Of note, these studies investigated the effects of oral ingestion of synthetic THC, not whole-plant THC-rich cannabis, making it difficult to draw conclusions, as most medical cannabis patients use the latter. Additionally, the criteria for inclusion in these studies varied; for instance, one study included patients who had lost 2.3 kilograms or more of weight over two months and/or had a daily intake of less than 20 calories per kilogram of body weight, and another included only advanced incurable cancers and an involuntary weight loss of 5 or more percent within the past six months, making it difficult to compare results since the participants were at different stages of illness.

- In an early study, seven of ten cancer patients given dronabinol (synthetic cannabis) increased their weight.[95]
- In a study of forty-two patients with cancer, dronabinol increased appetite and reduced the rate of weight loss.[96]
- Of eighteen patients with various cancers who received 2.5 milligrams of synthetic THC four times a day, thirteen reported improved appetite; however, seven had side effects (not unusual with synthetic THC).[97]
- A large study of 469 cancer patients with anorexia compared megestrol (a synthetic hormone that increases appetite) with dronabinol. Megestrol was more effective, but dronabinol increased appetite in 50 percent of patients.[98]
- THC-treated cancer patients were found to have improved and enhanced chemosensory perception and reported that food "tasted better"; premeal appetite and proportion of protein calories increased when compared to the placebo.[99]
- A 2006 study compared cannabis extract, dronabinol, and placebo in 169 advanced cancer patients and found no statistically significant difference in appetite. (Increased appetite was reported by 73 percent, 58 percent, and 69 percent of patients, respectively.)[100]
- A 2019 small study from Israel documented treatment of cancer patients with anorexia-cachexia syndrome who took THC-rich plant-derived cannabis capsules. Patients started on 10 milligrams once per day and increased to twice daily (note that this is four times the highest recommended starting dose of 2.5 milligrams). Of seventeen patients who started the treatment, only six completed the study, with three patients gaining 10 or more percent of their body weight. The other three remained at their starting weight. All reported an increase in appetite, and half reported better sleep and reduced pain.[101]

Clinically, many cancer patients struggling with these issues report that inhaled cannabis is extremely helpful for enhancing appetite, stabilizing weight (or slowing the rate of weight loss), and, importantly, enjoying meals rather than dreading them.

Cancer Pain

Moderate to severe pain is known to occur in 30 to 50 percent of all people with cancer, causing a decrease in quality of life.[102] Cancer pain may be nociceptive (caused by physical damage from the tumor), neuropathic (coming from either nerves involved in the cancer or nerve damage due to chemotherapy), or inflammatory (when tumors release pro-inflammatory chemicals). Patients may have mixed types of pain, creating challenges for treatment. Opioids remain the keystone for cancer pain; however, some patients experience inadequate pain relief and unacceptable side effects, including nausea and constipation, which are common. According to a 2008 study, nearly 50 percent of patients with cancer pain are undertreated.[103]

Animal studies have attempted to assess whether cannabinoids are effective for cancer pain and, if so, what underlying mechanisms of action are involved:

- In mice with paw tumors, synthetic cannabinoid-like compounds acting in synergy at both CB_1 and CB_2 receptors reduced pain.[104]
- Synthetic cannabinoids reduced both inflammatory and cancer pain in mouse models, with actions at both cannabinoid receptors.[105]

The number of studies on the use of cannabis for cancer pain in human trials is limited. Results are promising and show that cannabis treatment is effective without causing significant adverse side effects:

- Significant pain relief was obtained in cancer patients with higher doses of oral THC vs. placebo; pain relief peaked at three hours and was still near maximum six hours after the dose.[106]
- Another study compared two different doses of oral THC compared to two different doses of oral codeine in cancer patients. The

higher doses of each medication were found to significantly reduce pain when compared to the placebo.[107]

- Thirty-nine cancer patients who did not respond to chronic opiate treatment of pain received combination THC+CBD extract and reported decreased pain, improved sleep, and less fatigue with no development of tolerance or loss of effect over time.[108]

- A multicenter, double-blind, randomized, placebo-controlled, parallel-group trial study that compared a THC+CBD extract, a THC extract, and a placebo in patients with advanced cancer who were experiencing inadequate analgesia despite chronic opioid dosing found that the pain relief from the THC+CBD extract was statistically significant vs. the placebo. The THC alone showed no significant improvement vs. the placebo.[109]

I have evaluated hundreds of cancer patients using cannabis, and many of them find enhanced appetite, better mood, pain relief, improved sleep, and less fatigue. After years of disinterest in cannabis, a number of local oncologists are now referring their cancer patients to my office as they too are witnessing that cannabis can help patients tolerate the difficulties associated with cancer and cancer treatment. Opioids are now killing more people than car accidents, and these dedicated and responsible physicians are reluctant to continue prescribing them without considering alternatives that include cannabis.

Cannabis as a Cure for Cancer

This is a controversial topic. Since cannabis is classified as a Schedule I controlled substance, research on the anticancer properties in human clinical trials has been prohibited. As of the writing of this book, there is one published human trial on cannabis use as an anticancer compound, with a second trial in progress (both in Europe).

There exists, however, a significant body of scientific research that shows both THC and CBD as well as other phytocannabinoids have anticancer properties. These compounds cause cancer cells to commit suicide (called apoptosis), inhibit tumor growth, inhibit metastasis and cancer cell migration, and inhibit angiogenesis, which is the growth of blood vessels that feeds tumors.[110] Additionally, research shows that phyto-cannabinoids can work synergistically with certain chemotherapies and radiation to enhance anticancer effects.[111] Moreover, a number of studies document that cannabinoids can attenuate serious side effects from chemotherapy, such as neuropathy.[112]

The following is a short list of studies documenting the anticancer effects of cannabinoids on specific types of cancer. This is by no means a complete review of the scientific literature, as there have been thousands of articles published in the last three decades exploring the potential of cannabis as an anticancer agent. **It is important to note that these are not human trials**.

- *Breast cancer:* Whole-plant cannabis preparations were more potent than THC alone in producing antitumor effects in both test tubes and animal models of breast cancer.[113]
- *Colorectal cancer:* THC induced apoptosis in colorectal cancer cells through the activation of the CB_1 cannabinoid receptor.[114]
- *Glioblastoma multiforme:* THC decreased cell proliferation and increased cell death of human glioblastoma multiforme cells.[115]
- *Leukemia:* THC is a potent inducer of apoptosis in three leukemic cell lines at low concentrations and as early as six hours after exposure.[116]
- *Lung cancer:* CBD promoted lung cancer cell death through the enhancement of immune cell anticancer mechanisms.[117]
- *Melanoma:* THC use resulted in the activation of autophagy (cell self-digestion), loss of cell viability, and the activation of apoptosis of melanoma cells.[118]
- *Neuroblastoma:* Both THC and CBD impeded growth of neuroblastoma cells in test tubes and in mice implanted with tumor cells.[119]
- *Pancreatic cancer:* Cannabinoid receptors are expressed in higher levels in pancreatic tumor cells; cannabinoids killed pancreatic

cancer cells, inhibited growth, and inhibited the spread of tumor cells.[120]

- *Prostate cancer:* CBD induced apoptosis and enhanced the cancer killing of chemotherapy in mice implanted with prostate cancer cells.[121]
- *Skin cancer:* Synthetic cannabinoids induced apoptosis and inhibited growth of nonmelanoma skin cancer.[122]

In the only published human trial, Spanish researchers directly administered THC into glioblastoma multiforme cancer cells (this is a highly aggressive brain tumor with a very poor prognosis) in terminal patients and found it inhibited tumor cell proliferation without any adverse side effects.[123] A second trial still underway by a pharmaceutical company in the UK has reported initial results: twenty-one adults with glioblastoma multiforme were divided into a control group, receiving temozolomide chemotherapy only, and a treatment group, receiving temozolomide in combination with 1:1 CBD:THC (not whole plant). One-year survival for the control group was 44 percent, while one-year survival for the chemo-plus-cannabinoid group was 83 percent, with a median survival over 662 days, compared with 369 days in the control group.[124] It is no surprise that the company performing this important research filed a patent for this combination treatment.

In states with legalized medical cannabis, many desperate cancer patients are seeking cannabis to not only treat their symptoms but also directly treat their cancers despite the lack of human clinical trials. There are thousands of anecdotal reports of cancer patients using concentrated cannabis oils containing THC, CBD, and other cannabinoids, reportedly resulting in complete resolution of their cancers. Cannabis for cancer treatment is not FDA-approved nor is it considered standard of care by regulatory medical boards. However, patients who are not responding to conventional cancer treatments are using it.

I cannot supply dosing information for treatment of cancer in this book, as it is highly customized depending on the type of cancer, the stage of cancer, concurrent chemotherapy or immunother-

apy treatments, and other important considerations. But some of my patients have had incredible results. A number of them with advanced cancers who were told they had only a few months to live are living months or years beyond their prognosis with a good quality of life. I believe that cannabis treatment can extend life in certain cases and may eliminate cancer when given early in the course of the disease and in relatively high doses. However, cannabis is not a magical medicine that kills cancer overnight. The quickest I have seen evidence of tumor shrinkage presumed due to cannabis is approximately two months after it was added to a patient's treatment. Unfortunately, a few patients who achieved remission with cannabis, taken as the only treatment or added to conventional cancer therapy, subsequently relapsed when they stopped taking the oil, even years into remission. Because of this, I instruct patients that they may need to be on cannabis oil for life, albeit at lower doses, if it was effective in helping them achieve "no evidence of disease" status.

Although I am overjoyed when my cancer patients improve, as a scientist I am quite frustrated by the lack of human studies. We must allow clinical trials in humans in order to find answers to the very important questions of dosage, duration of treatment, and which cannabinoids to take for different cancers. All of these questions remain unanswered and continue to be a roadblock to patients seeking lifesaving cannabis therapy.

Alexander's Story

I wrote about Alexander's battle with cancer in my previous book and include it here, with an update.

> *Sixteen-year-old Alexander had been given only months to live when his parents brought him in to see me in April of 2015. I had come in on my day off, as my scheduler had notified me that this new patient had no time to wait for an appointment. In a wheelchair, cachectic, and wearing a brace around his neck for support after surgery to remove a*

tumor in that area, Alexander had to be lifted by his father and placed on the examination table. He had no energy, seemed quite ill and frail, and while his parents said very little and appeared extremely nervous, they were eager to know if cannabis might help their son.

I learned that morning that Alexander had been diagnosed with stage IV metastasized osteosarcoma (bone cancer) in early 2013 when he was thirteen years old. The path to diagnosis had been long and frustrating. Alexander had complained of leg pain for months, which his pediatrician had dismissed as "growing pains." When a lump appeared, he was finally sent to an oncologist, who diagnosed him with the bone cancer that had already spread to his lungs. Chemotherapy was started, and after a few months, he underwent surgery to remove the tumor in his leg. In early 2014, all of his scans were negative for cancer cells, but a few months later, a lung tumor was discovered, and he underwent another surgery. His mother shared with me that through all of this, Alexander remained "a trouper," and that while he had some down periods, he took everything that was happening to him in stride. "He's my hero," she said in a broken voice.

In January 2015, Alexander developed shoulder pain, and an MRI revealed new tumors next to his spine. He underwent multiple surgeries to remove these tumors and started having postoperative fevers, which did not resolve. One month later, another MRI revealed at least thirty metastatic lung tumors and another tumor next to the spine. At this point, Alexander had constant high fevers, wasn't eating, and was vomiting all the time. He was taking multiple narcotics for the near-constant pain. By April of 2015, when he came to my office, his parents had been told to "put Alexander's affairs in order," that he could expect to live for a few more months.

His parents had heard about cannabis oil from a friend, and they asked Alexander's oncologist about it. She was supportive and referred the family to me. I explained that cannabis would help their son with nausea, vomiting, appetite, and pain relief. I also explained that laboratory and animal evidence in the scientific literature showed both

THC and CBD kill cancer cells and stop cancers from growing and spreading, and that although human studies were lacking, I had had some success treating cancer patients with high-dose cannabis oil. I recommended a regimen of concentrated CBD and THC oils, taken under the tongue. Alexander started the regimen with low doses and titrated up to high doses over a period of a few months. His mother later admitted to me that she thought there was no way this tiny bit of oil could possibly help her son (although the volume of oil was small, the milligram dosing was high). Within three days, Alexander had perked up, and within a week, the fevers went away and Alexander didn't need to take nearly as many pain pills. He also began eating and gained back some of the weight he had lost. He had been on palliative doses of chemotherapy that were ineffective, and as he improved, his oncologist increased the doses. In July 2015, three months after starting the cannabis oil, Alexander had four scans to check on the cancer, and to everyone's surprise, his scans showed no evidence of cancer anywhere in his body. Another round of scans in November 2015 were also negative for cancer.

Update: *Alexander is now twenty-one years old, and repeated scans continue to be negative for cancer. Chemotherapy was discontinued in February of 2016. Alexander takes both CBD and THC in maintenance doses to this day.*

Alexander's story seems quite incredible, but there are a number of reasons why I believe his cancer responded to cannabis treatment. Studies have shown that osteosarcoma cells die when treated with synthetic cannabinoids.[125] Two additional studies in animals showed that when cannabinoids are added to chemotherapies commonly used for osteosarcoma, specifically doxorubicin and gemcitabine (both of which are quite toxic and only somewhat effective), their antiproliferative, antimetastatic, and antiangiogenic properties are enhanced, meaning the cannabinoids and chemo work synergistically to fight cancer by stopping cancer growth, inhibiting the spread of cancer cells, and blocking the cancer's ability to grow its own blood vessels.[126] We do not know if Alexander's cancer responded to cannabis alone or to the combination of chemo plus cannabis. However, knowing that Alexander faced a certain death, and knowing cannabis treatment is safe and nontoxic (certainly when compared to the chemo and surgeries he endured), his parents and I both felt that adding cannabis to his treatment regimen was worth trying.

Chronic Pain and Neuropathy

Cannabis has been documented as an effective pain reliever for centuries. Multiple surveys of medical cannabis patients report chronic pain to be one of the main reasons for using cannabis. The majority of chronic pain patients in these surveys were seeking an alternative to prescription pharmaceuticals and had tried numerous other treatment modalities, including physical therapy, surgery, acupuncture, and/or chiropractic therapy, prior to seeking cannabis treatment.[127]

Over the last decade in my medical practice, I have treated thousands of patients with arthritis, neuropathy, post-traumatic or post-surgical pain, chronic back pain, and other pain conditions. Many are able to reduce or discontinue use of pharmaceutical pain medications, including NSAIDs and opiates. My patients report over and over that when pain is controlled, sleep is better, anxiety is reduced, and functioning at home and at work is vastly improved. Some patients use one cannabinoid product and others use combinations of cannabinoids in order to achieve pain relief.

As mentioned in chapter 3, the National Academies of Sciences, Engineering, and Medicine (NASEM) published in 2017 the report *The Health Effects of Cannabis and Cannabinoids: The Current State of Evidence and Recommendations for Research*. Sixteen experts reviewed more than ten thousand of the most recent scientific articles, selecting those of the best quality, to determine if cannabis is an effective medicine. The committee concluded that "[i]n adults with chronic pain, patients who were treated with cannabis or cannabinoids are more likely to experience a clinically significant reduction in pain symptoms."[128]

A 2015 review of the current scientific literature documented 2,454 chronic pain patients in twenty-eight different randomized controlled trials, looking at fourteen studies of CBD+THC tincture (Sativex), four studies of smoked THC, five studies of nabilone (synthetic single-molecule THC), three studies of THC sublingual spray, two studies of dronabinol (another synthetic single-molecule THC), one study of vaporized cannabis, one study of oral THC, and one study of ajulemic acid (a synthetic cannabinoid derivative of THC). Chronic pain conditions evaluated in these trials included neuropathic pain, cancer pain, diabetic peripheral neuropathy, fibromyalgia, HIV sensory neuropathy, pain from MS or other neurological conditions, non-cancer pain, central pain, rheumatoid arthritis, musculoskeletal problems, and chemotherapy-induced pain. This review concluded that "the average number of patients who reported a reduction in pain of at least 30 percent was greater with cannabinoids than with placebo." Eight of the trials (seven with Sativex and one with smoked cannabis) reported that plant-derived cannabinoids were 40 percent more likely to reduce pain than placebo.[129]

In 2017, German researchers reviewed sixteen studies with 1,750 participants experiencing chronic pain and concluded, "Cannabis-based medicines may increase the number of people achieving 50 percent or greater pain relief compared with placebo," although those taking cannabis had more mild to moderate side effects.[130]

There are numerous published surveys of outcomes from medical cannabis patients suffering from chronic pain. These are retrospective reports, not randomized controlled trials; however, collectively they show that patients, when given legal access to medical cannabis, report significant efficacy for treatment of pain, and often they are able to reduce the use of other medications, including opiates. It is important to note that patients in many of these locations do not have access to the variety of different cannabinoid products available in California or Colorado, which may have limited their ability to fine-tune their regimen. For instance, New York State allows for only three types of cannabinoid ratios: high THC, high CBD, and 1:1. Other cannabinoids and products that might provide better efficacy, such as THCA or different CBD:THC ratios, may not have been available to survey participants.

- In a 2016 survey of 374 approved medical cannabis patients in Michigan, 185 patients who completed the survey were using cannabis for relief of chronic pain. The authors of this report found statistically significant decreases in medication side effects and in total number of medications taken, including opioids. Many of the respondents reported improvements in their quality of life.[131]
- A 2016 online survey of 1,429 medical cannabis users in 18 countries (77.8 percent from the US, 61 percent with chronic pain) reported 86 percent had improvement in symptoms, with 25 percent substituting cannabis for opiates.[132]
- A 2017 survey of 271 Canadian medical cannabis patients revealed that 71 percent (186 patients) were able to substitute cannabis for prescription drugs (63 percent), alcohol (25 percent), tobacco/nicotine (12 percent), and illicit substances (3 percent). Overall, 32 percent were able to substitute cannabis for opiates, 16 percent for benzodiazepines, and 12 percent for antidepressants; and 257 of the 271 respondents reported cannabis to be very effective at relieving symptoms. The researchers reported, "Our data suggested no relationship between age, amount of cannabis used, mode of administration, access or affordability on substitution effect."[133]
- A 2017 survey in New Mexico compared thirty-seven habitual opioid-using chronic pain patients approved for medical cannabis use with twenty-nine non-approved patients, also using opioids, and found that after twenty-one months, being enrolled in the cannabis program was associated with 17.27 higher odds of ceasing opioids, 5.12 higher odds of reducing daily prescription opioid dosages, and a 47 percent reduction of daily opioid dosages. Survey responses found statistically significant "improvements in pain reduction,

quality of life, social life, activity levels, and concentration, and few side effects from using cannabis one year after enrollment."[134]

- A 2018 report from the Cannabis Clinical Research Institute and the Institute for Drug Research, both in Israel, reviewed the use of medical cannabis in 901 elderly patients (over sixty-five years old) spanning a period of almost three years. They found 93.7 percent of respondents reported improvement in their condition, with a pain reduction from a median of "8 out of 10" to "4 out of 10." After six months, 18.1 percent were able to discontinue or reduce their use of opioid-based medications.[135]

- In a 2019 report of 204 elderly medical cannabis patients (over seventy-five years of age) in New York, 69 percent reported benefits, with 49 percent reporting improvement in chronic pain, 18 percent reporting improvement in sleep, 15 percent reporting improvement in neuropathy, and 10 percent reporting improvement in anxiety. Opioids were reduced in 32 percent of respondents. Adverse effects were initially reported in 34 percent, but once they changed dosing or product, only 13 percent reported side effects. Overall, 3.4 percent (seven patients) discontinued due to unwanted side effects.[136]

- A 2020 retrospective cohort study from a cannabis medical practice in California followed 180 patients with chronic lower back pain from one to eleven years, finding 50.8 percent were able to stop all opioid use. Of the twenty-nine patients who did not stop opioids, nine were able to reduce opioid use, three had no change, and seventeen increased their usage. Of all the patients, 48 percent subjectively felt cannabis helped them mitigate their opioid intake.[137]

What about using cannabinoids and opiates together? It appears that cannabinoid receptors and opioid receptors interact with each other, and the combination of these compounds is effective for analgesia while at the same time reducing the dangerous, and potentially deadly, side effects of opioids. As one author wrote, "A combination of low dose analgesics devoid of undesirable side effects would be ideal to replace high dose analgesics that cause unnecessary sedation, respiratory depression and constipation."[138]

Here are some recent findings from research investigating the interaction of cannabinoids and opioids:

- Multiple animal models document that cannabinoids enhance the pain-reducing effects of opioids, and vice versa.[139]
- In a rare human clinical trial of whole-plant cannabis performed at the University of California, San Francisco, twenty-one participants with chronic pain who were on morphine or oxycodone were given inhaled cannabis. Results showed the addition of cannabis did not increase the levels of opiates in the bloodstream (thereby no increase in the risk of overdose), but pain was significantly reduced. The researchers concluded that "vaporized cannabis augments the analgesic effects of opioids without significantly altering plasma opioid levels. The combination may allow for opioid treatment at lower doses with fewer side effects."[140] (This was an unusual study in that federal government agencies approved and allowed these patients to vaporize cannabis flowers in a hospital setting.)
- Healthy volunteers subjected to pain stimulus were given four different combinations of medications: THC and morphine, placebo and THC, placebo and morphine, or placebo and placebo. While neither drug was effective with placebo, the combination of THC and morphine revealed a synergistic analgesic effect.[141]
- Another recent study looking at the combination of gabapentin, a commonly used pharmaceutical for neuropathic pain, revealed the combination in mice of this drug with THC showed synergistic enhancement of pain relief.[142]

Patients with pain primarily from inflammatory conditions can find relief from all of the different categories of phytocannabinoids. Depending on someone's access to products, I recommend starting with high-ratio CBD:THC products or sometimes the raw cannabinoids THCA and/or CBDA. Using the "Rule it in or rule it out" method, patients start with a low dose and increase to reach the desired effects, understanding that they may need to either switch to another cannabinoid if the first product isn't working or add a second product to the first to enhance the effects. Some patients will take a higher CBD:THC ratio during the day to control daytime pain and a higher THC product at night to help promote sleep. It is important to note that THC has been shown to have twenty times the anti-inflammatory potency of aspirin and two times the anti-inflammatory potency of hydrocortisone, so it should not be left out or ignored if other phytocannabinoids are not fully effective.[143]

Patients with nerve-based pain (neuropathy) appear to benefit from the combination of CBD and THC in a 1:1 ratio, although some report 2:1 or 4:1 to be more beneficial. Raw cannabinoids may also help these patients. As previously mentioned, each person must use trial and error to find his or her "sweet spot" where symptoms improve or abate.

—✺—

June's Story

At seventy-seven years of age, June was reluctant and fearful to try cannabis. She came to see me with her adult son, who was concerned about her daily opiate use. After years of being quite active, she started having back and neck pain about fifteen years previously, and it was getting worse, interfering with her sleep and her ability to be independent. She had tried multiple different treatments over the years with little or no success. Her son had become frustrated that she was growing increasingly less mobile and had brought up the idea of trying cannabis. June confessed to being a product of the Reefer Madness generation, telling me she always thought marijuana was dangerous.

After explaining how phytocannabinoids might help her, and that she could try products that would not be intoxicating, she still seemed skeptical but was willing to try a high-ratio CBD:THC tincture. I explained to her that it would take time for the oil to correct the inflammation and imbalance she had been living with and to not give up too soon. She joked that since she had no expectations for it to be effective, she wouldn't be disappointed when it didn't help. June began with 10 milligrams CBD twice a day of a 25:1 CBD:THC tincture, increasing the dose in 10-milligram increments every four to seven days. Her son reported she initially had complained to him that the oil "wasn't doing anything," but by day 21, her family noted she was more active and complaining less of pain. By eight weeks, she had found significant reduction of pain and was able to cut back on her opiate use by 30 percent. She also reported improved sleep since pain was no longer waking her. By her one-year follow-up appointment, she had discontinued the opiates, using them only as needed on a bad day. She reported better mobility and was even able to start exercising again, joining friends for a daily walk. Her current regimen consists of a 25:1 CBD:THC oil, 50 milligrams in the morning with breakfast and another 50 milligrams with dinner.

Diabetes

Diabetes is a group of metabolic and autoimmune diseases that result in high blood sugar. Type 1 diabetes mellitus (DM)—sometimes called juvenile diabetes or insulin-dependent diabetes—occurs when the cells in the pancreas responsible for making insulin (the hormone that balances glucose levels) are destroyed by the body's own immune system. Type 2 DM occurs when insulin is produced but not used properly; this is also called insulin resistance. Patients with type 1 DM require insulin to survive. Type 2 DM, which is newly thought to be due to autoimmune mechanisms, can be controlled with dietary changes, oral medications, and sometimes insulin.[144] High blood sugar from either type of diabetes can result in severe organ damage, including blindness, kidney damage, nerve damage, and cardiovascular disease.

Type 1 Diabetes

Type 1 diabetes usually results from a genetic predisposition to immune dysfunction combined with an environmental trigger, most commonly a viral infection. Once triggered, the major components of the inflammatory system destroy pancreatic cells that produce insulin. You have already learned that the cannabis plant contains numerous anti-inflammatory compounds. Researchers have sought to understand if cannabinoid compounds may prevent and/or delay progression of insulin-dependent diabetes. A number of studies in mice have shown promising results:

- In an experimental model of mice with autoimmune diabetes, THC caused a reduction of high blood sugar and decreased the loss of insulin by suppressing the severity of the autoimmune response.[145]
- In a study of nonobese diabetic mice (an experimental model for type 1 diabetes), the development of diabetes was prevented when the mice were given CBD.[146]
- Mice with initial symptoms of diabetes that were given CBD had no progression of disease, had suppression of pro-inflammatory response, and had an increased anti-inflammatory response.[147]
- CBD significantly reduced heart-muscle dysfunction, inflammation, and heart-cell death in a mouse model of type 1 diabetes.[148]

Type 2 Diabetes

Research on the roles of the endocannabinoid system and phytocannabinoids as they relate to type 2 DM is ongoing, as it is complicated and sometimes contradictory. Yet some studies show that people who use cannabis may be at lower risk of developing type 2 DM:

- Cannabis smoking was found to possibly be protective, due to its anti-inflammatory properties, against the development of diabetes in a review of eight studies.[149]

- In a study sample of 579 cannabis users and 1,975 nonusers, cannabis use was associated with lower levels of fasting insulin, lower insulin resistance, and smaller waist size.[150]
- Cannabis users were found to have lower risk of diabetes than nonusers in a study of 10,896 adults.[151]

When obesity is present, however, the endocannabinoid system has been shown to be overactive with increased levels of endocannabinoids. Increased endocannabinoids lead to increased hunger, which worsens obesity, leading to more endocannabinoid release, triggering more hunger, creating a vicious cycle. This was the idea behind the drug rimonabant (mentioned in chapter 2), which works to block the CB_1 receptor, turning off hunger. This drug had intolerable side effects, but many researchers are still working on the idea of blocking the CB_1 receptor to not only reduce appetite but also halt the vicious cycle of endocannabinoid system overactivity.

The phytocannabinoid THCV, acting as a CB_1 receptor neutral antagonist (meaning it blocks the receptor, reducing the binding of endocannabinoids or THC), improved glucose tolerance and increased insulin sensitivity in dietary-influenced and genetically obese mice. It also helped insulin to work better in certain cells.[152]

Some of my patients with type 1 diabetes anecdotally report better control of their glucose levels when they use cannabis. Some prefer a regimen containing THC only, and some prefer a combination CBD+THC in varying ratios. None have reported a worsening of blood-glucose levels with cannabis use. Given the promising benefits of CBD in the studies on mice with type 1 DM, clinical trials in newly diagnosed humans is certainly warranted.

Some patients with type 2 DM report using cannabis for other conditions, such as chronic pain, sleep issues, anxiety, or arthritis. They state they have greater control of their glucose levels, less pain, and better sleep, allowing them to exercise more, which helps their diabetes. This outcome from cannabis use—reduced stress and better choices leading to a healthier lifestyle—is one that I hear over and over in my medical practice. I encourage all of my patients to include CBD in their medication regimen if possible, as its anti-inflammatory and antioxidant effects are potentially very important in prevention of complications from diabetes. THCV is newly available to patients, and my hope is that it will help those with obesity and/or type 2 DM to lose weight and restore a healthier metabolism.

Epilepsy

Epilepsy is a broad term for a group of conditions characterized by seizures. There are over forty different types of epilepsy and many different types of seizures. The mainstay of treatment is antiepileptic drugs (AEDs). Other treatments include a restrictive high-fat diet (called the ketogenic diet), a vagal nerve stimulator (a pacemaker-like device implanted in the chest that sends a signal to disrupt the firing of the vagus nerve), and brain surgery to remove the brain tissue that may be causing the seizures.

Approximately 47 to 50 percent of patients with epilepsy will respond to the first AED that is prescribed. Of those who do not respond to the first AED, only 13 percent will respond to the second AED, and fewer than 4 percent will respond to the third AED. This means that despite numerous new antiepileptic medications hitting the market every year, approximately 33 percent of these patients still do not achieve seizure control.[153]

A seizure is defined as "clinical manifestation of a hyperexcitable neuronal network, in which the electrical balance underlying normal neuronal activity is pathologically altered—excitation predominates over inhibition."[154] The goal of AEDs is to stop seizures by enhancing inhibition or by opposing excitation of the neuronal activity. Unfortunately for a significant portion of the population suffering from seizures, these medications may not be effective and often have severe adverse side effects. The diagnosis of intractable epilepsy is made if disabling seizures continue despite appropriate trials of two antiseizure drugs, either alone or in combination. Other terms used for this condition are refractory epilepsy, pharmacoresistant epilepsy, and treatment-resistant epilepsy (TRE).

As you have learned, the endocannabinoid system works by sending messages to maintain or restore homeostasis. In simple terms, it balances cells by regulating the neurotransmitters, specifically sending messages to neurons to decrease excitation and promote inhibition. There is compelling scientific evidence to suggest that dysfunction of the endocannabinoid system plays a critical role in the development of seizures:

- In a 2003 study, THC completely aborted seizures in a rat model of epilepsy. When the CB_1 receptor was blocked, it resulted in increased seizure duration and frequency. Researchers concluded that the endocannabinoid system modulated seizure activity.[155]
- In another study, blocking CB_1 receptors in a laboratory epilepsy model resulted in status epilepticus (continuous long-lasting difficult-to-stop seizures).[156]
- Evaluation of surgically removed epileptic human brain tissue showed a 60 percent reduction of one of the enzymes required to make the endocannabinoid 2-AG and downregulation of the cannabinoid receptor mRNA; the authors concluded that the "neuroprotective machinery involving endocannabinoids is impaired in epileptic human hippocampus."[157]
- Cerebrospinal fluid levels of endocannabinoids were found to be reduced in patients with untreated, newly diagnosed temporal-lobe epilepsy.[158]

THC as an Antiepileptic

In a review of thirty-one animal studies investigating the antiepileptic effects of different doses of THC, THC was anticonvulsant in 61 percent of the subjects, had no effect in 29 percent of the subjects, and was a proconvulsant (caused seizures) in 10 percent of the subjects.[159] The proconvulsant outcome was often due to very high doses, which medical cannabis patients do not (and should not) take. Many adults with epilepsy report that inhaled THC controls their seizures. Some are on AEDs and some are not. It is difficult to make any generalizations from these patients' experiences since they may have different types of seizures, different EEG results, and different AED regimens. However, use of THC on a daily basis for seizure control can be quite difficult for those who dislike the intoxicating effects. Another issue is the potential development of THC tolerance to the anticonvulsant effects, not ideal when trying to control a serious seizure disorder. Of note, in two separate instances two of my adult patients who had never had seizures before reported to me they experienced seizures after inadvertently overdosing on THC-rich cannabis edibles. Both patients, who were experienced users of THC, ate an entire THC-rich candy bar that, unbeknownst to them, contained high amounts of THC (approximately 180 milligrams). Each patient reported having a grand mal seizure they had never experienced before nor had experienced since. Both patients recovered quickly but were rightfully frightened by the experience. Although the amount of THC these patients ingested clearly represents a THC overdose, and is certainly not recommended dosing, this shows that THC may have proconvulsant effects in humans at high doses. Despite these concerns, some of my pediatric patients using CBD or THCA whole-plant products have benefited from the addition of low-dose THC to their cannabis regimen, with the added reduction of seizures. Doses are kept quite low, well under the patients' "ceiling dose," where intoxication can occur.

CBD as an Antiepileptic

Scientific studies documenting the antiepileptic action of cannabis in humans are limited. Importantly, CBD has been found to show anticonvulsant activity in almost all animal research. With the recent barrage of media attention on medical cannabis, and specifically on CBD use in pediatric epilepsy, researchers have focused on CBD-rich treatment as a viable option for patients with intractable epilepsy. Here is a review of the published studies, listed chronologically. As you can see, interest in CBD treatment for epilepsy in humans has spiked in the last decade:

- In 1978, nine patients with intractable epilepsy were randomized to treatment with CBD vs. placebo. Two of four patients receiving CBD achieved seizure freedom, and none of the five placebo patients reported improvement; no adverse side effects were reported.[160]

- In 1980, sixteen patients with refractory seizures were randomized to receive CBD vs. placebo. Three of the CBD patients were seizure-free, with four reporting improvement; of the placebo group, one reported improvement and seven reported no change.[161]

- In 1986, twelve adults with intractable seizures received either CBD or placebo; no benefits were reported.[162]

- In 1990, twelve adults with intractable seizures received either CBD or placebo; some reduction of seizures with CBD was seen but it was not statistically significant, and no side effects were reported.[163]

- In 2005, there was an open study of eighteen pediatric patients with refractory epilepsy treated with CBD. "[I]n most of the treated children an improvement of the crises was obtained equal to or higher than 25% in spite of the low CBD doses administered." There was clear improvement of consciousness and spasticity; no side effects were reported.[164]

- In 2013, Stanford researchers surveyed the parents of nineteen children with intractable epilepsy who used CBD-rich whole-plant extract. Results showed 11 percent became seizure-free, 42 percent reported a greater than 80 percent reduction in seizure frequency, and 32 percent reported a 25 to 60 percent seizure reduction, with beneficial side effects of better sleep, improved alertness, and better mood, and the only adverse side effect of drowsiness.[165]

- In 2013, two Colorado neurologists presented a survey of eleven patients using CBD-rich oil in which all patients reported a reduction in seizures, with 73 percent reporting a 98 to 100 percent reduction; at three months of treatment, 45 percent were seizure-free. The oil was well tolerated by all patients.[166]

- In 2015, pediatric neurologists at UCLA Medical Center performed a survey of 117 parents of children with severe refractory epilepsy who were using CBD-rich oil. Of those parents, 85 percent reported the frequency of seizures had been decreased and 14 percent had achieved seizure freedom. The only adverse side effect reported was increased appetite, but beneficial side effects were improved sleep, mood, and alertness.[167]

- In 2016, Israeli researchers reported on CBD use in seventy-four children with intractable epilepsy: 89 percent had a reduction in seizure frequency, with 52 percent having more than a 50 percent reduction; one patient became seizure-free. Benefits included improvements in behavior, alertness, language, communication, motor skills, and sleep. Adverse effects included somnolence, fatigue, gastrointestinal disturbance, and irritability.[168]

- In 2017, I co-authored an article with cannabis specialist Dustin Sulak, DO, from Maine and pediatric neurologist Russell Saneto, MD, from Washington State, documenting results of our combined experiences treating children with epilepsy with CBD-rich whole-plant oil. Overall, we saw that 86 percent had a seizure reduction, with 10 percent reporting seizure freedom.[169]

- In 2018, researchers at Vanderbilt University compared 108 patients receiving CBD without clobazam (seizure medication), CBD with clobazam, and clobazam without CBD. They reported that the addition of CBD to clobazam resulted in 39 percent of patients having a more than 50 percent reduction in seizures, with 10 percent reporting seizure freedom.[170]

In 2018, the FDA for the first time approved a cannabis-plant-derived medication, called Epidiolex, for Dravet syndrome and Lennox-Gastaut syndrome (LGS), two devastating pediatric epilepsies. It is 99 percent CBD with less than 1 percent THC, mixed in sesame oil, dehydrated alcohol, sucralose, and strawberry flavoring. It was subsequently categorized as a Schedule V controlled substance despite the fact that all other plant-derived CBD is still in the Schedule I category. Studies on Epidiolex reported children with LGS had a median percent reduction in drop seizures of 41.9 percent in those taking 20 milligrams per kilogram daily and 37.2 percent in those taking 10 milligrams per kilogram daily.[171] For those with Dravet syndrome, 43 percent of patients had at least a 50 percent reduction of convulsive seizures compared to 27 percent with placebo.[172] Epidiolex appears to have more side effects than whole-plant oil, likely because higher doses are needed (since it is 99 percent CBD, it lacks the entourage effect, which allows for lower CBD dosing). One of the side effects seen in Epidiolex that I have not seen in any of my patients on whole-plant oil is reversible elevation of liver enzymes when there is concurrent use of a drug called valproic acid. This too may be due to the higher dosing often required when CBD is used as a single compound.

How CBD Reduces Seizures

The mechanisms by which CBD reduces or prevents seizures is not fully understood. Research on this continues in many parts of the world. Remember that CBD targets many different receptors, ion channels, enzymes, and chemical transporters, so there are likely multiple sites in the brain contributing to the antiseizure effects. The following list is what scientists know so far about CBD's antiseizure mechanisms of action (discussed in detail in chapter 4):

- CBD increases our endocannabinoid levels, which in turn decreases excitatory neurotransmitters and increases inhibitory (calming) neurotransmitters, leading to a calmer brain and helping to restore homeostasis in endocannabinoid deficiency states.
- CBD modulates the flow of ions (such as calcium and potassium) in neurons, which reduces the excitability of neurons, thereby calming the brain.
- CBD blocks the GPR55 receptor, which results in fewer excitatory neurotransmitters and more of the inhibitory, or calming, neurotransmitters.
- CBD decreases neuroinflammation and is neuroprotective.

Inflammation of the brain, called "neuroinflammation," has been extensively researched over the last two decades, as both a cause of and a result of recurrent seizure activity.[173] The presence of neuroinflammation predisposes the brain to more seizures. Seizure-related inflammation may contribute to cell death. CBD is a unique compound in that it provides both anticonvulsant and anti-inflammatory effects. This dual action may be why many epilepsy patients appear to have cognitive improvement in addition to an antiepileptic effect. Moreover, many of the CBD-rich chemovars available on the market also contain the terpenoid beta-caryophyllene, which has potent anti-inflammatory properties and is synergistic with CBD in its anti-inflammatory effects.[174]

CBD as a Neuroprotectant and Stimulator of New Brain Cell Growth

CBD acts as a neuroprotective agent.[175] "Neuroprotection" refers to the preservation of nerve cells, either by mechanisms that prevent cell damage or by slowing the progression of damage or disease. The mechanism by which CBD protects the brain is not completely understood, but it is thought to be due to CBD's effect on maintaining homeostasis of the flow of calcium in brain cells.[176]

CBD also stimulates neurogenesis, the growth of new brain cells, especially in the part of the brain called the hippocampus.[177] The hippocampus is responsible for memory, spatial navigation, and emotional response, and this area of the brain is often where seizures originate. It can sustain severe damage from repeated seizures, but CBD appears to play a protective and restorative role here. More research is needed; however, these properties of CBD make it a unique compound with a preponderance of promising medicinal effects.

CBD Interactions with AEDs

It is crucial that patients who take AEDs understand the possible drug–drug interactions with CBD. **Patients on AEDs should be medically**

supervised when adding cannabis to their medication regimen. CBD is metabolized in the liver by the enzyme system cytochrome P450 (discussed in chapter 5). Because many AEDs are also metabolized in this system, drug–drug interactions may occur if both CBD and certain AEDs are present in the body at the same time. Since Epidiolex went through the process of FDA approval, we are able to use the data on drug–drug interactions from these human clinical trials to understand how CBD and AEDs interact.

- Thirty-four children with Dravet syndrome underwent laboratory testing of AED levels before beginning CBD as well as after four weeks on CBD. Results revealed an increase in the clobazam metabolite N-desmethylclobazam (which can cause sedation). There were no changes in levels of valproate (brand name Depakote), levetiracetam (brand name Keppra), topiramate (brand name Topamax), or stiripentol (brand name Diacomit). Additionally, six patients on both CBD and valproate had elevated liver enzymes normalized after valproate dosing was adjusted.[178]
- Another investigation of drug–drug interactions from the Epidiolex trials reported on thirty-nine adults and forty-two children who had AED drug levels tested before and after adding CBD to their medication regimen. As CBD dosing increased, increases in topiramate, rufinamide (brand name Banzel), and N-desmethylclobazam were seen. In adults, zonisamide (brand name Zonegran) and eslicarbazepine acetate (brand name Aptiom) were increased with increasing doses of CBD. Importantly, all changes were within the therapeutic range. Liver enzymes were significantly elevated in those taking both Epidiolex and valproate. The study's authors noted that four children who discontinued both valproate and CBD due to elevated liver enzymes and then tried CBD a second time without the concurrent use of valproate did not have any repeat abnormalities in these blood tests.[179]

In my medical practice, hundreds of pediatric patients who have intractable epilepsy have experienced benefits with whole-plant tested CBD-rich oil, taken either sublingually, orally, or via a feeding tube. Parents and patients report a reduction of seizures, improved alertness, improved memory, better mood, better sleep, better appetite, improved motor skills, improved social interaction, and less use of AEDs. Unfortunately, only about 10 percent of these patients achieve seizure freedom, but there is still a significant portion who obtain a life-changing reduction of seizures. Despite all of these therapeutic benefits, it is important to acknowledge that the addition of CBD to a medication regimen containing other AEDs can be challenging and should be medically supervised. **I cannot supply dosing information for the treatment of epilepsy since it must be customized to the patient's specific situation and should be medically supervised.**

Olivia's Story

Little Olivia came to see me in early 2014. She had been born with a brain malformation, thought to be due to a stroke that occurred while in utero. She started having seizures at a very young age and was eventually diagnosed with infantile spasms, a serious seizure disorder that occurs in babies and young children. She struggled with as many as forty seizures daily despite trials of multiple antiseizure medications. This condition has a poor prognosis, with 60 percent of children with infantile spasms going on to have other serious seizure disorders later in life.

Concerned about Olivia's quality of life, her parents had heard about CBD and were desperate to try it since nothing else was helping her. At the time of Olivia's first appointment, there were only two CBD-rich products available in California. I started her on a low dose and instructed the parents to email me every two weeks with an update, which her father did like clockwork. We slowly increased the CBD dosing, and within two months, she was having only one seizure every five days. With the neurologist's permission, she began weaning off one of the two antiseizure pharmaceuticals. We continued to increase her CBD dosing, and six months into CBD treatment, she was averaging one seizure every twenty days. Her parents reported she was also starting to be more alert and aware of her surroundings.

Olivia stopped having seizures in early 2015, was weaned off both seizure medications, and continues to have improvements in development. She has remained on the same CBD oil, albeit with dosing adjustments to keep up with her growth, from the beginning of her cannabis journey. Her parents report she loves school, is more interactive, and has a quality of life that has surpassed the terrible prognosis they were given when she was just a baby.

Fibromyalgia

Fibromyalgia is a chronic debilitating condition that includes symptoms of diffuse pain, sleep disturbance, migraine headaches, fatigue, joint pain, and irritable-bowel-type symptoms. Patients may have all or just some of these symptoms, but it appears that all patients with this condition suffer a heightened perception of pain, thought to be due to abnormal processing of pain signals in the central nervous system. This is called "central sensitization," in which the nervous system is in a state of high reactivity. Overlap with other chronic pain conditions has been observed that include chronic fatigue, irritable bowel syndrome, chronic pelvic pain, and daily headaches. Anxiety, depression, and disturbed sleep often accompany these painful symptoms. The mainstay of treatment is medication, primarily pain relievers, such as NSAIDs and opiates, antidepressants, antiepileptics, and often muscle relaxants and sleep aids.

As discussed in chapter 2, an endocannabinoid deficiency/dysregulation has been hypothesized as a possible underlying cause of fibromyalgia. Studies have not proven this theory, but research shows abnormal endocannabinoid levels, specifically higher levels of anandamide, in patients with fibromyalgia.[180] There is also evidence that fibromyalgia patients have increased levels of glutamate, an excitatory neurotransmitter that can cause inflammation and damage when it accumulates.[181] The endocannabinoid system helps to regulate glutamate and reduces its build up. Fibromyalgia patients have been found to have higher blood levels of pro-inflammatory compounds, which indicates abnormal inflammation may also play a role.[182] Remember that the endocannabinoid system is deeply involved in controlling inflammation in the brain and body.

Several studies have investigated the efficacy of cannabinoid treatment in fibromyalgia patients:

- In a small study of fibromyalgia patients who received daily doses of synthetic THC and no other pain medications, a subset of patients reported a significant reduction in daily pain.[183]
- The synthetic cannabinoid nabilone improved symptoms in forty patients with fibromyalgia in a randomized, double-blind, placebo-controlled trial.[184]
- A recent study from Spain reported that fibromyalgia patients who used cannabis had a statistically significant reduction in pain and stiffness, enhancement of relaxation, and improved sleep, with an increased feeling of well-being.[185]

I have evaluated many patients with fibromyalgia, most sharing that conventional medications are not effective and often cause side effects that make them feel worse. These patients report cannabis reduces pain and inflammation, improves mood, and promotes sleep.

I recently asked a number of my patients with fibromyalgia to list their cannabis medication regimens in an effort to see what they were finding to be helpful for their fibromyalgia. As you can see in the following list, some are on low doses, some are on high doses, some are using only one or two cannabinoids, and some are combining them. Each patient went through the "Rule it in or rule it out" method, starting with a low dose of one product, increasing the dose, looking for efficacy, and keeping it in the regimen if it helped, discontinuing if it didn't. They then tried a second cannabinoid or product, following the same process. Here are some of their reports:

- "I take 50 milligrams of CBD in the morning and afternoon, and take a 5-milligram THC gummy at night."
- "I take a tincture that contains CBD, THC, CBDA, and THCA twice a day. The total CBD is about 5 milligrams, the THC is 1 milligram, and the CBDA and THCA are both also 5 milligrams. I also rub topical 1:1 CBD:THC onto painful areas as needed. If I have trouble sleeping, I take THC through a vaporizer."
- "I only use THC, low dose in the morning (2.5 milligrams mint) that doesn't make me high, and then I smoke THC before sleep."
- "I had been using a tincture with a 4:1 ratio for the last two years, but then I added in a CBG tincture. I think it is helping with my mood and inflammation."
- "I am taking CBD oil, 100 milligrams, just at night. It has helped with pain and sleep."

Karen's Story

Karen started having what she called "strange pains" ten years ago. She consulted her family practitioner, who told her it was early arthritis and recommended over-the-counter anti-inflammatory medications. She followed this advice, but the pain relief was incomplete and short-lived. Visiting her physician again, she was referred to a rheumatologist, who diagnosed her with fibromyalgia and gave her a prescription for pregabalin (brand name Lyrica). Despite her reluctance to take prescription medication, she decided to give it a try. After experiencing severe dizziness that caused her to have to lie down for hours after only two doses, she stopped taking it.

When we met for the first time, Karen shared with me her nervousness about medical cannabis. She was worried that people might find out and think she was a "pothead," especially since she was a licensed realtor. She also told me that it was becoming more and more difficult to maintain the pace of her busy life. She said some days she would get her teenage girls off to school, and rather than go to her office, she would go back to bed. This was making her depressed and anxious, and she worried that her future would be filled with overwhelming pain and disability. She admitted to feeling desperate to find something that would help. I educated her about the endocannabinoid system and the theory that fibromyalgia may be due to a dysfunction in this system, possibly the underlying cause of her pain. Once she heard this, she was eager to try cannabis.

Karen started with high-ratio CBD:THC sublingual oil. She found only slight relief, so we added THC in a separate tincture, with the goal of customizing the CBD:THC ratio. After a few weeks of dosing adjustments, she found the combination of 50 milligrams CBD and 6 milligrams THC taken together in the morning helped reduce pain with no unwanted side effects. This works out to a CBD:THC ratio of about 8:1. She sometimes takes 5 milligrams of the THC tincture by itself at night to help with sleep and pain.

During a recent visit, we discussed using the raw cannabinoids THCA and CBDA to help reduce inflammation further. She added them to her regimen and reported back to me that she felt the combination of the various cannabinoids has reduced her pain even more, noticing that she has fewer days when pain bothers her. She also reported that her mood is better and her energy is back. She said she no longer has to go back to bed after taking her girls to school. She recently wrote in an email to me, "Although I still have fibro, I am managing it. I still haven't told anyone that I am taking these oils, but my friends and even my girls notice I am better. I guess one day I will have to let them know."

It is unfortunate that patients still worry about the stigma of cannabis use. Undoing years of propaganda is difficult, but I am hopeful that recent scientific investigations documenting endocannabinoid-related illnesses will finally help to reverse the idea that medical cannabis patients are "potheads."

Gastrointestinal Disorders

Gastrointestinal (GI) illnesses are a frequent reason for using medical cannabis. These conditions include gastroesophageal reflux disease (GERD), two inflammatory bowel diseases—Crohn's disease and ulcerative colitis—and irritable bowel syndrome (IBS).

The gut has two main functions, namely digestion of food and host defense, protecting us from foreign invaders like bacteria and viruses.[186] The endocannabinoid system, which is widely distributed throughout the gastrointestinal system, is a key player in keeping these two important functions regulated. It is found in the gut's nerves and in the cells of the immune system, working to maintain homeostasis of gastric motility (the muscular contractions that work to move food through the bowel), intestinal pain signaling, intestinal inflammation, and maintenance of the barrier of the gut lining.

The nerves in the gut are called the enteric nervous system, sometimes called the "second brain." CB_1 and CB_2 receptors are found throughout these nerves. All disorders of the gut are thought to involve the enteric nervous system, making these receptors an attractive target for treatment when illness is present. Scientists have found that the number of cannabinoid receptors can increase (upregulate) in certain intestinal illnesses, indicating that the endocannabinoid system is mounting a response to try to restore balance.[187] In addition to cannabinoid receptors, other receptors, such as PPARs, GPR55, and TRPV1, are found throughout the gut and are involved in intestinal inflammation and pain. Since cannabinoids interact with these receptors, they too are therapeutic targets for treatment by anyone using cannabis medicine for gastrointestinal disorders.

Almost 80 percent of your immune system resides in the gut. The endocannabinoid system, including the CB_2 receptors, is also present in these immune cells, ready to go into action to decrease inflammation when needed. However, if your endocannabinoid system is not working properly, it may not be able to mount the appropriate response to these triggers, leading to chronic intestinal symptoms.

Interestingly, people who have a mutation in the gene coding for one of the endocannabinoid system components are more likely to have IBS and chronic abdominal pain, evidence that endocannabinoid dysfunction may be one of the root causes of gut disorders.[188]

Gastroesophageal Reflux

GERD is very common, affecting 20 percent of all adults. GERD occurs when the stomach contents flow backward into the esophagus, causing symptoms of heartburn, chest pain, difficulty swallowing, and/or a sensation of a lump in the throat. GERD is often treated with medications; however, there are reports of possible increased risk of dementia and cancer from some of these drugs. Other interventions include altering the diet, remaining upright after meals, losing weight, and stopping tobacco use.

Animal studies showed that cannabinoid stimulation of the CB_1 receptor inhibited acid secretion and decreased damage and inflammation in the lining of the stomach.[189] Another animal study showed that cannabinoid activation of the CB_1 receptor kept the lower esophageal sphincter (the "gate" between the esophagus and stomach that works to keep stomach contents from flowing back into the esophagus) from relaxing, thereby decreasing reflux.[190] In one human study, synthetic THC given to healthy volunteers was shown to decrease the reflux rate (although there were issues in the study since the dose was very high and caused side effects).[191] It is clear that more research is needed to understand the role of cannabis in the treatment of GERD.

Clinically, some medical cannabis patients with GERD report benefits, although some do not. (As with all conditions, it is unclear as to exactly why some patients respond to cannabis and others do not.) Anecdotal reports from positive responders state they have fewer episodes of heartburn, and if they have an episode, taking cannabis decreases their discomfort. Most patients finding benefits are including some THC in their cannabis regimen, as this seems to be the cannabinoid most helpful for GERD, at least anecdotally. Some patients report a low-ratio CBD:THC product (such as 1:1, 2:1, or 4:1) helps decrease GERD symptoms with less intoxicating effects compared to THC-only products. Two terpenes, limonene and terpinolene, may also be beneficial for GERD symptoms.

Inflammatory Bowel Disease

IBD is a general term that refers to chronic inflammation of the bowel. The two main IBD conditions are Crohn's disease and ulcerative colitis. The Centers for Disease Control reports approximately three million adults were diagnosed with IBD in 2015, up from two million diagnosed in 1999. The exact cause of IBD is unknown, but recent scientific investigation reports the changes in the gut are due to "uncontrolled activation of intestinal immune cells in a genetically susceptible host."[192] Remember that immune cells are regulated by the endocannabinoid system, suggesting that endocannabinoid dysfunction may be a root cause of IBD and may serve as a therapeutic target.

Crohn's disease can affect any part of the gut but most commonly the small intestine, causing inflammation, ulcers, pain, bleeding, diarrhea, and weight loss. Ulcerative colitis is a chronic inflammatory condition affecting the large intestine, causing symptoms similar to Crohn's. Both conditions are associated with an increased risk of colorectal cancer. According to a recent article, "current therapeutic options are insufficient for a successful treatment leading to a high rate of disability and intestinal surgery in IBD patients."[193]

Activation of the CB_1 and CB_2 receptors in animal models of colitis reduces inflammation.[194] In a review of fifty-one scientific studies on cannabinoid treatment of colitis (only two were in humans), twenty-four different compounds, including synthetic cannabinoids as well as THC, CBD, and CBG, were found to be effective in reducing the severity of colitis.[195]

Studies done in a number of different countries show about 10 to 12 percent of people with IBD are using cannabis to treat their symptoms.[196] Studies in humans are limited but promising:

- A 2011 survey of thirty Crohn's patients in Israel revealed twenty-one improved significantly with cannabis, finding less need for other medication and reduced need for surgery.[197]
- A 2012 study investigating eleven patients with long-standing Crohn's disease and two patients with ulcerative colitis reported that after three months of treatment, patients reported improvement in general health perception, social functioning, ability to work, physical pain, and depression. There was a statistically significant weight gain and increase in body mass index.[198]
- A 2013 survey of 292 patients receiving care for IBD revealed approximately half reported either past or current use of cannabis. Of those, 32 percent reported medical use for abdominal pain, poor appetite, nausea, and diarrhea. Most reported that cannabis either completely relieved or was very helpful for symptoms. In this study, current users noted significant improvement in abdominal pain, poor appetite, nausea, and diarrhea.[199]
- In a 2013 study of twenty-one patients with Crohn's disease who did not respond to conventional treatments, inhaled THC or inhaled placebo was given over eight weeks. Complete remission was achieved in 45 percent of the cannabis group and 10 percent of the placebo group; 90 percent of the cannabis group had lower severity scores versus 40 percent of the placebo group. Three patients using cannabis were able to wean off steroids. The cannabis patients reported better sleep and appetite with no significant side effects. Interestingly, all patients who achieved remission relapsed within two weeks of discontinuing the cannabis treatment.[200]

- In 2019, two reports were published that reviewed hospital records through the National Inpatient Sample database, allowing researchers access to thousands of medical records. The first report looked at 615 hospitalized Crohn's disease patients who used cannabis (legally or not) and compared them to Crohn's patients who did not use cannabis. Cannabis users were found to have:
  - — Less stricturing disease (scarring built up secondary to chronic intestinal inflammation)
  - — Fewer bowel obstructions
  - — Fewer fistulas and abscesses
  - — Shorter hospital stays
  - — Fewer blood transfusions
  - — Less colectomy surgery (removal of the colon)
  - — Reduced IV nutrition requirements[201]
- The second report, using the same database of medical records, included 6,002 patients with Crohn's disease (2,999 cannabis users and 3,003 nonusers) and 1,481 patients with ulcerative colitis (742 cannabis users and 739 nonusers). This review found:
  - — Crohn's patients using cannabis had statistically significant lower incidence of cancer, less need for IV nutrition, less anemia, and shorter hospital stays with lower hospitalization costs; however, this report found an increase in fistula/abscess, GI bleeding, and hypovolemia (a decrease in circulating blood in the vessels).
  - — Ulcerative colitis patients using cannabis have statistically significant lower frequency of postoperative infections and shorter hospital stays with lower hospitalization costs; however, fluid/electrolyte imbalance and hypovolemia were increased.[202]

These reports stated that "recreational" cannabis was used. There was no mention of the type of cannabinoids used (THC, CBD, or other), nor was delivery method (smoking, edibles, etc.) or duration of use reported.

Both significant benefits and risks were found, warranting further human clinical trials.

I have evaluated many patients with gastrointestinal disorders who have had successful results with cannabis treatment. Almost all patients with Crohn's disease or ulcerative colitis who have been seen in my office have exhausted conventional options prior to seeking cannabis treatment, finding that they either were nonresponders or experienced intolerable side effects. Similar to the findings already mentioned, my patients report that their symptoms, including nausea, poor appetite, abdominal pain, diarrhea, and bloating, respond to cannabis treatment. Many patients prefer to inhale THC since the onset of relief is immediate. Patients who are reluctant to use THC-rich cannabis can use lower CBD:THC ratios, such as 1:1 or 4:1, with similar benefits but less chance of intoxication. As noted in chapter 4, THCA was found to be the main phytocannabinoid helping to regulate intestinal inflammation. With the increased availability of tinctures containing THCA, and CBDA as well, patients are finding that daily use of these raw cannabinoids, sometimes combined with CBD, is effective for anti-inflammatory effects, helping to prevent flare-ups.

Irritable Bowel Syndrome

As the most common diagnosis made by gastroenterologists, IBS affects thirty-five million people in the US alone. IBS is characterized by episodes of abdominal pain, bloating, excessive gas, and altered bowel habits (constipation, diarrhea, or mixed type). No clear cause of IBS has been identified, although endocannabinoid deficiency is suspected.[203] There usually are no abnormalities on blood tests or an endoscopy, making IBS a diagnosis based solely on the patient's history and symptoms, after ruling out other causes. IBS sufferers often struggle with other conditions, such as fibromyalgia, migraine headaches, temporomandibular joint disorders, chronic fatigue, gastroesophageal reflux, anxiety/depression, or chronic pelvic pain. Chronic stress has been linked to both the development and/or the exacerbation of IBS and should also be a focus of treatment.

There are three published human studies of cannabis use for IBS, all employing synthetic THC as the study drug. Not surprisingly, one study reported all participants to have had side effects and no benefits; the study dose of 10 milligrams THC was clearly too much for the non-cannabis users who participated.[204] The second study used lower doses, 2.5 milligrams or 5 milligrams of synthetic THC compared to placebo, and found participants with IBS diarrhea or IBS mixed type had a reduction in colonic motility, meaning THC slowed down how fast food moved through the gut.[205] The third study involved giving low-dose dronabinol for two days and had no effect on IBS diarrhea.[206] As mentioned before, findings from studies using single synthetic cannabinoid compounds are difficult to translate to outcomes in patients using whole-plant preparations.

Clinically, many medical cannabis patients with IBS report benefits, most stating simply that "it helps calm the gut." Some patients report substantial efficacy from low doses of THC taken in the evenings or just as needed when their gut is acting up. Others report using CBD preparations on a daily basis to control their symptoms. Additionally, some patients have reported that either THCA or CBDA, or both in combination, has helped with IBS, often with the patient achieving improvements in symptoms with low doses. Proper diet, regular exercise, and stress management support the endocannabinoid system, and in cases of IBS, patients find these additional interventions to be quite effective when combined with cannabinoid therapy.

It is important for patients with gut disorders to understand that long-standing inflammation will take time to respond to cannabinoid treatment. It may take eight to twelve weeks to experience significant benefits, although many report symptom reduction in the first few weeks. Edibles may cause further GI upset, so you should always read product labels to be sure you are not eating an ingredient that is a trigger for your symptoms. Terpenoids that have been found to specifically help the gut include terpinolene, beta-caryophyllene, limonene, and pinene.

Robert's Story

A tall, thin teenager with a crew cut, Robert came to my office with his parents seeking help in treating ulcerative colitis. Diagnosed two years prior, he was struggling with chronic abdominal pain, bloody diarrhea, poor appetite, and weight loss. It was no surprise he expressed feeling depressed and hopeless. He had been on numerous treatments that did not help, and according to his parents, the pharmaceuticals he tried seemed to be making him sicker, not better. He had received multiple blood transfusions due to the anemia caused by loss of blood through his gut. At the most recent visit with his GI specialist, surgery to remove part of his colon was discussed, causing Robert much distress.

Prior to meeting with me, Robert's parents caught him smoking cannabis. They were not surprised, as lately they had noticed something was different about him — maybe a lighter attitude and fewer complaints of discomfort. As a family, they Googled "cannabis for ulcerative colitis" and decided to pursue this treatment with medical supervision, as they all agreed surgery would be a last resort. When I asked Robert how cannabis helped him, he reported that all of his physical symptoms were reduced, and that he felt "normal" for a few hours. He and his parents had concerns that he was buying cannabis from unknown sources and that he was at risk for getting into legal trouble. He stated maturely, "I feel like this could be my medicine, but I don't want to be a criminal for using it."

I educated Robert and his parents about the endocannabinoid system, about the different phytocannabinoids, and about the promising, yet limited, research on cannabis use for IBD. I started Robert on low doses of a CBD:THC tincture (25:1) twice daily with the plan to increase every one to two weeks, aiming for a dose of 300 milligrams twice daily. We discussed using vaporized THC as needed for acute symptoms. After four weeks, he reported less diarrhea, less abdominal pain, and better appetite. He was sleeping better too and said his mood was improving. He continued to have blood in his stools, so THCA twice daily was added to the regimen.

Robert's red blood cell count stabilized over the next six weeks. He gained weight and happily reported he had started playing basketball again, something he had not been able to do since his initial diagnosis. His lab tests revealed a decrease in the inflammatory markers, and although they were still elevated, the decrease was evidence that the inflammation in his body was starting to respond to treatment.

Robert's GI specialist is cautiously supportive of this treatment, as he too has seen Robert's condition stabilize. Most importantly, Robert has reported a significant improvement in his quality of life, and for the first time in years, he feels optimistic about his future.

Glaucoma

Glaucoma is a group of eye disorders that can damage the optic nerve. Most cases of glaucoma result from increased pressure in the eye, called "intraocular pressure." If untreated or not properly controlled, the increased pressure damages the optic nerve, resulting in a loss of peripheral vision and eventually blindness.

The mainstay of glaucoma treatment is medication in the form of eye drops or, in some cases, surgical intervention. For many people, these treatments are successful; however, some patients are treatment resistant.

The first mention of THC's ability to lower intraocular pressure was in 1971.[207] Multiple studies have shown that THC lowers intraocular pressure via the CB_1 receptor.[208] In one particular study, 5 milligrams of THC was found to transiently lower intraocular pressure, with effects lasting only four hours, while CBD and placebo did not lower the pressure.[209] In 2002, the Research Advisory Panel of California instituted the Cannabis Therapeutic Research Program to permit cannabis use on a compassionate basis while data was collected for research. Nine patients with glaucoma were enrolled to evaluate the efficacy of THC on eye pressure. No conclusive results were obtained, except that after initial lowering of eye pressure in four of the nine patients, the decreases were not sustained. All patients elected to stop treatment. The authors concluded that "development of tolerance and significant systemic toxicity appears to limit the usefulness of this potential treatment."[210]

CBD was initially thought to not affect eye pressure, but a 2006 study, investigating both THC and CBD in six patients with glaucoma, documented that although 5 milligrams THC reduced pressure for four hours and a 20-milligram dose of CBD did not affect intraocular pressure, a 40-milligram dose of CBD increased intraocular pressure.[211] Another study from 2018, investigating how topical THC and CBD affected intraocular pressure in mice, found THC substantially decreased eye pressure in male mice for eight hours but only for four hours in female mice. This difference was discovered to be due to the presence of fewer cannabinoid receptors in the eyes of female mice. Topical CBD was found to substantially increase eye pressure. The same study showed combination CBD+THC applied topically had no effect on intraocular pressure, possibly due to CBD blocking the effects of THC. These researchers also explored which receptors were involved in cannabinoid-induced reduction of eye pressure and found a combined mechanism with both CB_1 receptor and GPR18 involvement. The authors stated in the conclusion of their report that more research on topical THC was warranted.[212]

A 2019 review of the current scientific literature on the efficacy of cannabis to reduce eye pressure revealed five randomized controlled trials that compared cannabis to a placebo. (There are no studies comparing cannabis to the current conventional treatments that lower eye pressure.) The authors concluded that the use of cannabis for treatment of glaucoma was not supported at the time due to the short duration of action, the risk of side effects, the frequency of dosing, and the lack of evidence that cannabis was effective in preventing vision loss in the long term.[213] Remember that good-quality studies of real-world cannabis use for glaucoma—meaning what patients are using in legal states—are lacking, preventing us from knowing if and how cannabis, whether inhaled, ingested, or applied topically to the eyes directly, is an effective treatment for glaucoma.

I do not advocate the use of THC-rich cannabis as *single*-drug therapy for glaucoma unless all other treatments have failed. I have a number of patients in my practice who find the addition of THC-rich cannabis to their current glaucoma treatment has been beneficial in keeping pressure in their eyes low. I encourage these patients to stay on their vision-saving medications or to pursue other options if the medications fail. Now that the latest data reports a potential increase in ocular pressure with higher doses of CBD, patients with glaucoma who want to use CBD for other indications should make sure to follow up closely with their ophthalmologist in order to ensure that CBD is not elevating pressures, potentially putting their vision at risk.

Infectious Diseases

The role of the endocannabinoid system, endocannabinoids, and phytocannabinoids in the human response to infectious diseases is an active area of research. Our complex immune system works to protect us from microbial pathogens, including bacteria, viruses, and other infections. The endocannabinoid system plays a large role in immunity, as endocannabinoids are produced and released by activated immune cells (those that have been triggered by an infection).[214] After release, the endocannabinoids attract additional immune cells, such as white blood cells, "recruiting" them to attack the infecting agent.[215]

Immune cells contain a large family of compounds called cytokines, which are secreted in response to infection. They have the important role of regulating immunity and inflammation. There are both anti- and pro-inflammatory cytokines. Numerous studies show that phytocannabinoids suppress production of cytokines, which may be beneficial when anti-inflammatory effects are desired.[216] However, studies also show that phytocannabinoids can increase the production of certain cytokines in specific cases, depending on the trigger and the cannabinoid used.[217] Due to these opposite effects, phytocannabinoids are called "immune modulators," indicating they have bidirectional effects on the immune response.[218]

"Cytokine storm" is a condition whereby the immune system overreacts in response to an infection. The infected part of the body is flooded with excessive levels of cytokines, causing more immune cells to migrate to the area, which then leads to the release of more cytokines, causing a vicious cycle of hyperinflammation. This can cause severe tissue damage and even cell death. Respiratory diseases, such as COVID-19, SARS, and MERS—all caused by coronaviruses—can result in cytokine storm, which can cause acute respiratory distress syndrome (ARDS). The high fatality of other pandemics—the 1918 Spanish flu, the 2003 H5N1 "bird flu," and the 2009 H1N1 "swine flu"—was due to cytokine storm and ARDS. In 2015, knowing that phytocannabinoids can suppress the release of cytokines, researchers at the University of South Carolina investigated the use of THC as treatment for cytokine storm in mice. The mice received a bacterial toxin known to induce cytokine storm and fatal ARDS. When untreated, all of the mice died within five days. When THC was given after the toxin exposure, all of the mice survived, with evidence of less lung inflammation and decreased levels of cytokines.[219] With these promising results and lack of other effective and safe treatment for cytokine storm, further research of phytocannabinoid efficacy is warranted.

In addition to modulating the human response to infections, phytocannabinoids have antibacterial, antiviral, and antifungal effects. THC, CBD, CBG, CBC, and CBN are strongly antibacterial in laboratory investigations, demonstrating potent activity against troublesome antibiotic-resistant *Staphylococcus* strains (often called "superbugs").[220] A recent study combining CBD with antibiotics resulted in a more powerful antibacterial effect as compared to antibiotic treatment alone.[221] Unfortunately, we are still lacking definitive clinical trials of the efficacy of phytocannabinoids to treat human bacterial infections.

Studies show conflicting results of cannabinoid treatment for viral infections.

- Although older studies demonstrated laboratory animals with viral infections who were treated with THC had worse outcomes compared to those who did not receive THC, recent reports have demonstrated the beneficial effects of cannabinoid treatment, specifically in cases in which the host's inflammatory response to the infection has become overwhelming.[222]
- In a study of sixty-two patients with HIV who were randomly assigned THC cigarettes, dronabinol (synthetic THC) capsules, or a placebo, no negative effects on the status of the virus were discovered in those using THC.[223]
- In a laboratory study investigating treatment of viral hepatitis, CBD inhibited the replication of hepatitis C with comparable efficacy to and fewer side effects than interferon, an approved anti-hepatitis medication. CBD was not effective against hepatitis B.[224]

The antifungal effects of CBC and CBG have been demonstrated in laboratory studies; however, there are no human clinical trials. Anecdotally, patients report topical cannabinoids have successfully treated minor fungal infections, such as tinea pedis (athlete's foot), however lack of research leaves us with many questions about dosing and other treatment variables.

The potential for cannabinoid treatment or an adjunctive therapy in the area of infectious diseases is exciting and may provide options for improved outcomes.

Liver Disease and Hepatitis C

The term "hepatitis" refers to inflammation of the liver. Hepatitis C specifically refers to an infection with the hepatitis C virus (HCV), which may cause either a mild, short-lived illness (acute hepatitis) or, more seriously, a lifelong condition that attacks the liver (chronic hepatitis). Approximately 75 to 85 percent of people who become infected with hepatitis C virus develop chronic infection. HCV is spread primarily through contact with the blood of an infected person, most commonly through sharing of needles during drug use. Symptoms include nausea, vomiting, abdominal pain, weight loss, fatigue, joint pain, and poor appetite. Chronic HCV can progress to cirrhosis (severe scarring of the liver) or liver cancer. An estimated 3.5 million people in the United States have chronic HCV infection.

Conventional treatment of chronic HCV consists of antiviral medications. In recent years, new antiviral medications have become available with 95 percent cure rates, depending on the type of virus being treated. These medications have fewer side effects than their predecessors, although fatigue, depression, gastrointestinal upset, insomnia, and joint pain may occur. Interestingly, in 2017 CBD was found to kill HCV and inhibit the replication of the virus by 86.4 percent in a laboratory setting (test-tube findings).[225] No animal or human studies have been performed, but certainly this discovery warrants more investigation.

Animal studies of cannabis use for liver disease show promising therapeutic results, with CBD conferring liver protective effects:

- In a mouse model of hepatic encephalopathy (defined as a decline in brain function due to severe liver disease), CBD improved cognition and locomotion due to its anti-inflammatory effects.[226]
- CBD restored liver function and improved cognition and neurological function in mice with liver failure and hepatic encephalopathy.[227]
- CBD significantly reduced liver inflammation in a mouse model of ischemia-reperfusion (cutting off blood flow, then restoring it), as is often seen in liver surgery or liver transplantation.[228]
- CBD protected the livers of mice from acute alcohol-induced steatosis, a condition in which fat infiltrates the liver cells.[229]

Human studies initially reported that THC use might cause damage to the liver in the face of hepatitis, but more recent studies show this to be unlikely:

- Three studies performed between 2005 and 2008 found that patients with hepatitis C who used THC-rich cannabis daily (vs. non-daily use) were at higher risk of moderate to severe liver fibrosis (scarring).[230]
- A study from 2013 reported the opposite, finding no link between cannabis use and progression of liver fibrosis in hepatitis C patients who were also HIV-positive. The researchers reported too that previous studies showing an association between cannabis smoking and liver fibrosis may have been biased by reverse causation, as patients use more cannabis to relieve symptoms as liver disease progresses.[231]
- Hepatitis C patients who used cannabis and were on antiviral medication to treat the disease were more likely to stay on treatment than patients who didn't use cannabis.[232]
- In a 2016 study of a large cohort of HIV/HCV coinfected women, THC was not associated with progression to significant liver fibrosis. Alcohol use was independently associated with liver fibrosis.[233]
- A review of hospital discharge records of patients with nonalcoholic fatty liver disease (also called fatty liver) found that cannabis users had significantly lower prevalence of fatty liver disease compared to nonusers, suggesting that cannabis is protective against the development of this condition.[234] The same researchers also found that alcohol users who used cannabis showed significantly lower odds of developing alcoholic changes to the liver.[235]
- Another recent analysis of hospital discharge records of 4,728 cannabis users with chronic liver disease matched to 4,728 non-cannabis users with chronic liver disease revealed that cannabis users had decreased prevalence of liver cirrhosis (and its complications) and lower total healthcare costs when compared to non-

cannabis users.[236] There was no difference found in the incidence of liver cancer, in-hospital deaths, or length of hospital stay.

Patients with hepatitis C infection or liver disease may be reluctant to take pharmaceuticals for other medical conditions, as often they are concerned about further liver damage. Patients with hepatitis or liver issues from any cause may also have coexisting chronic pain conditions. They should avoid all medications that contain acetaminophen. This compound is the active ingredient in the over-the-counter brand Tylenol and also is often combined with the opiates hydrocodone and oxycodone. Acetaminophen is a leading cause of acute liver failure, even at doses that are within the recommended range. Cannabinoids are an option for these patients, allowing them to treat their pain without concern of further liver damage.

I recommend that patients with liver disease who want to use cannabis treatment include CBD in their regimens for its anti-inflammatory and liver-protective effects.

Migraine Headaches

Migraines are quite common, affecting 12 percent of the worldwide population. They often occur in response to a specific trigger, such as hormonal changes, sleep deprivation, excess stress, a bright light, hunger, or a specific food or smell. Typical migraines escalate quickly to severe pain, with throbbing or pulsing sensations. Associated symptoms include nausea, vomiting, and sensitivity to light and/or sound. Migraine sufferers may feel sensory warning symptoms, called an aura, prior to the onset of a headache.

The mainstay of treatment is a group of drugs called triptans, which work by blocking the release of pro-inflammatory compounds in the brain. They are fairly effective for aborting or reducing the severity of migraine headaches but are expensive and come with many side effects.

Another group of medicines, called ergot alkaloids, are also prescribed for migraines, but they are less effective than triptans. A new group of injectable medications, called monoclonal antibodies, was approved by the FDA in 2018 and is showing significant efficacy with minimal side effects. However, these are costly, about six hundred dollars per month.

Unfortunately, little research exists that proves the mechanism by which cannabinoids alleviate migraines, despite the overwhelming anecdotal reports from patients. The following studies I list below suggest migraine headaches may be due to endocannabinoid deficiency and an abnormal inflammatory response. Often migraine sufferers report headaches begin in response to a trigger, which should subsequently stimulate the production of endocannabinoids to fix the imbalance and maintain cellular homeostasis, but if someone is deficient in endocannabinoids, the imbalance continues, which is thought to lead to the development of a migraine. The trigger may also cause an uncontrolled inflammatory response, contributing to the pain.

Studies assessing endocannabinoid system involvement in migraine headaches are sparse, but recent interest has increased since more patients have legal access to cannabis medicine.

- Three cases were reported of chronic heavy users of cannabis developing severe migraine attacks after abrupt cessation of use, with the authors suggesting that these rebound attacks were similar to rebound headaches experienced by migraine patients when they abruptly stop other migraine treatment.[237]
- Genes that allow for increased inflammation were found in migraine patients and not found in control subjects.[238]
- Reduced levels of anandamide were found in the cerebrospinal fluid of patients with chronic migraines.[239]
- Endocannabinoid levels were decreased in patients with chronic migraine and medication-overuse headaches, suggesting that endocannabinoid dysfunction is involved in both chronic conditions.[240]

- Of 121 approved medical cannabis patients suffering from migraine headaches, there was a decrease in frequency of headaches per month from 10.4 to 4.6, with 39.7 percent reporting positive effects.[241]
- A 2017 investigation from Italy reported migraine sufferers taking different combinations of CBD and THC found 200 milligrams of combination cannabinoids decreased acute migraine pain by 55 percent. In the second part of the study, migraine patients received either combination CBD+THC or amitriptyline, finding a slightly greater reduction of migraine attacks with the cannabinoids. There was no significant benefit in adults with cluster headaches unless they had experienced migraines as a child.[242]

Cannabis has been used for thousands of years to treat headaches. Clinically, patients report relief of pain, less nausea, and better sleep. They also report less frequency and less severity of their migraine headaches with medical cannabis use. A number of well-known triggers for migraine headaches, specifically sleep deprivation and anxiety or stress, are alleviated with cannabis, thereby contributing to improvements as well. Additionally, patients report they spend less healthcare dollars on expensive migraine medications and have fewer missed school or work days.

Patients report timing of doses is very important; if they feel the migraine coming on, immediate use can help abort or lessen the severity of a migraine. Some patients report low-dose, regular use of THC-rich medicine significantly reduces frequency and severity of the headaches. Other patients report daily CBD-rich cannabis prevents migraines from occurring. Once the headache begins, a rapid delivery method, such as inhalation or sublingual tincture, is preferred by most. I have two patients who have reported complete resolution of migraines after they started taking a sublingual oil rich in THCA and CBDA on a daily basis. In a survey of 505 patients who were approved for use of cannabis for migraines, more than 42 different preferred chemovars of cannabis were reported, supporting the idea that specific chemovar choices result from trial and error.[243] There is some evidence from this report that chemovars rich in beta-caryophyllene and myrcene are preferred by migraine sufferers.

Anna's Story

Anna, a young woman in her early thirties, came to see me seeking help with her migraine headaches. Ambitious and smart, she was working as an assistant producer for a large entertainment company and had dreams of becoming a senior producer one day. She told me about her long history of headaches, with the first migraine occurring while on vacation with her family when she was only twelve years old. Everyone thought she had caught a stomach bug or food poisoning because, in addition to the headache, she had vomited all night in the hotel. This was the beginning of years of suffering, missing school and activities due to uncontrolled migraine headaches. Her mother brought her to no fewer than eight different specialists, trying numerous medications with no luck. She sought nutritional advice, trying every dietary restriction, as well as acupuncture, chiropractic adjustments, and biofeedback—all to no avail. Her typical pattern was about one migraine per week, lasting about three days. She described that she was debilitated from pain and severe nausea on the middle day, but she pushed herself to go to work, taking nausea medication and hiding her pain from her coworkers.

About five months prior to meeting with me, she was assigned a big project at her job, requiring her to work longer hours and increasing her stress. This led to sleep issues. She began having longer migraines, noting that they were lasting almost all week with only one to two days between episodes. She reported that she had missed enough days in this time period for her boss's boss to mention it. She was terrified she was going to lose her job.

Anna had tried cannabis once or twice when she was in high school, stating, "It wasn't really my thing." We talked about the endo-

cannabinoid system and the possibility of an endocannabinoid deficiency. She felt that maybe cannabis was the answer she had been searching for and was ready to get started. Her first purchase was a vaporizer and a strain called Grand Daddy Purple. The effects on sleep and stress were immediate, allowing her to fall asleep easier and wake without a headache. After two weeks of use, she emailed me, stating that although she had only one mild headache those first two weeks on cannabis, she wanted to have something that might help prevent and/or treat pain and nausea while she was at work. She decided to try a high-ratio CBD:THC pen vaporizer. After a few weeks of intermittent use, she asked for another suggestion, as she was not getting relief. A CBD:THC vaporizer with a 1:1 ratio did the trick. She explained that she takes only one inhale when she feels a headache coming on and it completely stops the headache from progressing. If she waits too long to medicate, the headache will persist, but with less severity and duration and often without nausea.

At Anna's last visit, she reported that she had only four bad migraines the prior year, usually triggered by sleep deprivation, and although she still had occasional "regular" headaches, she was thrilled with how cannabis has helped her. She has not had to change her cannabis routine, other than occasionally trying different chemovars for nighttime use.

I am always amazed that cannabis seems to be a "last resort," only considered after years of desperate searching, after experimenting with toxic and ineffective modalities has failed. Cannabis can often be the most effective medicine and, when used properly and responsibly, have few or no side effects.

Multiple Sclerosis

MS is the most common autoimmune inflammatory disease, affecting one of every thousand people worldwide. It occurs when the immune system attacks the myelin protective covering of neurons in the brain and spinal cord, thus interfering with normal nerve function. Symptoms include numbness and/or weakness of limbs, vision problems, chronic pain, fatigue, tremor, unsteady gait, bowel or bladder problems, and muscle spasticity. Symptoms can progress over time or be episodic, called relapses or flare-ups. There is no known cure for MS. Treatment is aimed at curbing acute attacks, reducing the risk of relapse, and preventing disability. Current medications for MS include steroids and a class of drugs called "disease-modifying therapies," which aim to slow down the progression of the disease. Although patients can do well on these medications, some struggle with compliance, as they have significant adverse side effects and risks, including a potentially deadly or disabling viral infection of the brain called progressive multifocal leukoencephalopathy (PML), other serious infections, cardiac arrhythmia, macular edema (swelling of a part of the retina), autoimmune thyroiditis (up to 30 percent risk with one particular medication), kidney problems, and malignant cancers.

Numerous studies have examined the use of cannabinoids to treat MS. Much of the research comes from investigations on the efficacy of nabiximols (Sativex), a patented sublingual preparation of CBD:THC in a 1:1 ratio, which was approved in 2010 and is available by prescription in twenty-five countries for treatment of spasticity from MS. Studies of Sativex show it to be effective for spasticity, intractable peripheral neuropathy, and MS-induced pain, with minimal side effects. Sativex is not yet available in the US, but with the legalization of cannabis in many states, MS patients can use similar CBD:THC ratios from whole-plant preparations instead.

A review of the scientific literature reveals hundreds of articles when the terms "cannabinoids" and "multiple sclerosis" are searched on PubMed (a free search engine focusing on scientific articles). I am including the most recent important findings here:

- An international survey of medical cannabis patients reported that MS was one of the five medical conditions for which cannabinoids were most often used.[244] Another survey, conducted through the internet, found that 66 percent of MS patients used cannabis for treatment of symptoms.[245]

- Cannabinoids help MS by exerting neuroprotective effects through CB_1 mechanisms and by suppressing neuroinflammation through CB_2 mechanisms.[246]

- In 2010, investigators at the University of California, San Diego, reported that inhaled cannabis significantly reduced objective measures of pain intensity and spasticity in patients with MS in a placebo-controlled, randomized clinical trial. Investigators concluded that "smoked cannabis was superior to placebo in reducing spasticity and pain in patients with multiple sclerosis, and provided some benefit beyond currently prescribed treatment."[247]

- In 2017, the National Academies of Sciences, Engineering, and Medicine reviewed thousands of scientific articles assessing the efficacy of cannabinoids for MS and concluded there was conclusive or substantial evidence that oral cannabinoids are effective for improving patient-reported multiple sclerosis spasticity or pain symptoms.[248]

- Italian researchers assessed 1,615 MS patients using Sativex, finding after one month of use 70 percent of patients reported a 20 or more percent improvement and 28 percent had 30 or more percent improvement. The overall discontinuation rate was about 40 percent, due to lack of efficacy or to side effects.[249]

- A review that included 426 MS patients with neurogenic bladder found cannabinoids to be effective in decreasing the number of incontinence episodes.[250]

- In a fascinating study, whole-genome testing of MS patients before and after four weeks of treatment with Sativex showed downregulation of immune-regulated pathways, especially in those who were cannabinoid responders, meaning that treatment with cannabinoids changed the gene expression, leading to decreased production of pro-inflammatory compounds.[251]

Clinically, my patients with MS report that cannabis use reduces pain, lessens spasticity, alleviates depression, reduces fatigue, and decreases incontinence. Most of my MS patients prefer using vaporizers or sublingual tinctures, as these methods have a quicker onset and are easier to dose compared to ingested products. Although many prefer THC-rich cannabis, especially at night for pain, sleep, and relaxation, they include CBD and the raw cannabinoids THCA and CBDA for added anti-inflammatory and neuroprotective effects. Important terpenes include beta-caryophyllene, myrcene, pinene, humulene, cineole, and citronellol for their anti-inflammatory effects.

It is crucial to understand, when interpreting results from clinical trials, that treatment is restricted to the design of the study, with no ability to alter or change the regimen. This significantly affects the results. In real-world use of cannabis, patients have the ability to alter their regimen—add or replace products, change the method of taking the medications, change the timing and amount of the dosing—to customize the treatment to their needs. The product Sativex contains a 1:1 CBD:THC ratio, which may be too much THC for some patients, as evidenced by the reported side effects (psychiatric, sedation, dizziness, etc.).[252] However, with natural cannabis products, if a patient struggles with these types of side effects, which are likely due to the THC, he or she can switch to a product with less THC, such as 2:1, 4:1, or higher ratios, or even use different cannabinoids entirely. As a clinician who sees many people benefit from cannabis, I can share with you that the ability to personalize cannabis to your needs is crucial to achieving positive therapeutic benefits.

Neurodegenerative Disorders

Neurodegenerative disorders refer to conditions in which there is progressive loss of structure and function of nerve cells, leading to cell death. Currently there are no known cures for the various neurodegenerative disorders, such as Lou Gehrig's, Alzheimer's, Huntington's, and Parkinson's diseases. These conditions can be devastating, causing significant loss of function and decreased quality of life for those afflicted as well as their families.

Cannabinoids have numerous properties that make them attractive medicines for central nervous system disorders, namely they provide neuroprotection, are antioxidants, and are potent anti-inflammatories. Interestingly, healthy brains do not have many CB_2 receptors; however, in the face of neuroinflammation, there is an influx of immune cells that have many CB_2 receptors, adding another therapeutic target in addition to the CB_1 receptors already present.

Amyotrophic Lateral Sclerosis

ALS—also known as Lou Gehrig's disease—is a neurodegenerative disorder characterized by progressive motor neuron loss, paralysis, and death within two to five years of diagnosis. The cause of ALS is unknown, but there is evidence of a genetic basis in a small number of cases. Theories as to the possible causes of ALS include autoimmune disease, in which the body's immune system attacks its own cells and kills them; a chemical imbalance of glutamate, a neurotransmitter that can build up and cause toxicity to brain cells; or possibly an abnormal accumulation of a protein called TDP-43, which triggers cell damage and cell death. There are four FDA-approved medications for ALS, which work by decreasing the excitatory neurotransmitter glutamate.

The neuroprotective and anti-inflammatory properties of cannabis combined with its excellent safety profile have stimulated interest in it as a treatment for all neurodegenerative disorders.

- THC delayed motor impairment and prolonged survival in mice with ALS.[253]
- A synthetic cannabinoid targeting both CB_1 and CB_2 receptors in mice with ALS significantly slowed the progression of the disease.[254]
- A synthetic cannabinoid that binds to the CB_2 receptor was given to mice with ALS, resulting in a delay in disease progression.[255]

- The same synthetic cannabinoid selective for the CB_2 receptor given to mice with ALS prolonged survival.[256]
- A small survey of ALS patients using THC-rich cannabis found efficacy for appetite stimulation, depression, pain, spasticity, and drooling. There was no improvement reported in speech, swallowing, or sexual dysfunction.[257]
- A study using dronabinol for symptoms in ALS patients reported benefits for sleep, appetite, and spasticity, as well as an acceptable safety profile.[258]
- A human clinical trial in Italy reported that nabiximols (Sativex) had a positive effect on spasticity, with an acceptable safety and tolerability profile.[259]

Many patients suffering with ALS have a poor quality of life, with pain, muscle spasms, wasting, trouble breathing, drooling, insomnia, anxiety, and depression. Cannabis can help all of these symptoms since it works as a pain reliever, a muscle relaxant, an appetite stimulant, a bronchodilator (opens up the lungs), and a sleep and mood enhancer. Because it causes drying of the mouth, it also helps with excess drooling and secretions. I have successfully treated a few patients with ALS who reported an improved quality of life with cannabis use. These patients found good results with THC-rich cannabis delivered by vaporizer, edibles, or sublingual tinctures. Some ALS patients may also choose to add CBD to their regimen to help with spasticity and mood. An upcoming human clinical trial, to be done in Australia, using high-CBD, low-THC cannabis for early onset ALS was announced in 2019.

Alzheimer's Disease

Alzheimer's disease (AD) is a chronic neurodegenerative disorder that affects millions of people worldwide. Symptoms include memory loss, problems with language, disorientation, mood swings, and difficulty managing activities of daily living. About 70 percent of cases are thought to be genetic. Researchers have found that the brains of those with AD have abnormal protein deposits called amyloid-beta plaques and tau neurofibrillary tangles. Plaques and tangles disrupt the brain cells' ability to function properly and lead to cell death, which subsequently leads to the terrible symptoms of AD. Neuroinflammation is also a big part of AD. Two kinds of immune cells, astrocytes and microglia, are activated in the brain with AD, releasing numerous pro-inflammatory chemicals. It is still unknown if neuroinflammation is a cause or consequence of AD. Researchers report both benefits and detriments from these immune cells in the brain, and the current theory is that anti-inflammatory treatment may allow for the benefits to dominate while the detrimental effects are lessened.

Cannabinoids are well-known to be potent anti-inflammatory compounds and have been shown in multiple studies to decrease neuroinflammation. Research investigating the use of cannabinoids for AD is summarized here:

- CBD reduced the formation of amyloid-beta protein.[260]
- CBD blocked the pathway leading to tau protein buildup.[261]
- THC also reduced the formation of amyloid-beta protein.[262]
- A synthetic cannabinoid, through activation of the CB_2 receptor, helped to remove amyloid-beta protein from human brain cells.[263]
- A synthetic cannabinoid, through activation of CB_1 receptors, blocked the formation of tau neurofibrillary tangles.[264]
- Mice with AD improved when given a synthetic cannabinoid that targets the CB_2 receptor, with a better result when it was given before the symptoms began. The cannabinoid blocked pro-inflammatory chemicals from being released and blocked the formation of tau protein.[265]
- Mice with AD improved when given a synthetic cannabinoid targeting CB_1 receptors.[266]
- Treatment of mice with AD using a combination of THC and CBD preserved memory and decreased learning impairment.[267]

One of the main concerns involved in deciding to treat patients with Alzheimer's disease with cannabis is that THC itself can cause memory loss, disorientation, agitation, and anxiety in some people. However, it can also do the opposite, reducing agitation, stimulating appetite, and promoting sleep. It is therefore recommended that if THC is to be used, dosing should start low, about 1 milligram, with small increases to the desired effect. Tinctures with low concentrations, such as 5 or 10 milligrams per 1 milliliter, are good for this indication, as accurate dosing can be achieved. Chemovars rich in the terpenoid myrcene are sedating and can be helpful for agitated AD patients. Pinene may be helpful as well since it can assist memory.

Research supports using THC and CBD together for patients with AD. In my practice, I encourage patients to try both high-ratio and low-ratio CBD:THC products. CBD may protect patients from memory loss and can counteract the anxiety and paranoia that can occur in some who take THC.[268] However, I have seen a few patients whose agitation became worse with CBD. Unfortunately, there are no published human trials looking at the efficacy of cannabis for the prevention of or delay of the progression of AD.

Huntington's Disease

Huntington's disease (HD) is a progressive, inherited neurodegenerative disorder that affects motor coordination. It is caused by a mutation in the huntingtin gene (*IT15*), which controls the production of a protein by the same name. Symptoms include uncontrolled movements (called chorea); changes in behavior, emotion, judgment, and cognition; and eventual progression to dementia and severe disability. There is no cure for HD, but there are medications and interventions, such as physical therapy, that can help with management of the symptoms.

Endocannabinoid system abnormalities have been found in mice with HD, with evidence that as the course of HD progresses, the endocannabinoid system becomes less functional.[269] Treatment of HD may require adjustments as the disease progresses since the changing endocannabinoid system will likely respond differently to different cannabinoid compounds. Experimentally, cannabinoids have shown some preliminary promise in delaying the progression of the disease.

- The number of CB_1 receptors in the area of the brain that controls movement, called the basal ganglia, are lower than normal in mice with HD. Those that were lacking CB_1 receptors had worse symptoms than those with CB_1 receptors. Pure THC improved motor symptoms in these mice.[270]
- Mice with HD that did not have CB_2 receptors had quicker onset and increased severity of motor deficits. Treatment with a cannabinoid that targets the CB_2 receptor extended life span, improved motor deficits, and decreased central nervous system inflammation.[271]
- Mice with HD that were given CBG had a reduction of the mutant huntingtin protein and an increase in prosurvival compounds.[272]
- Multiple mice studies reported that treatment with cannabinoids delayed the progression of the disease and showed less damage of the neurons involved in HD.[273]
- Mice with HD that were treated with nabiximols (Sativex) from a young age with the goal of preventing progression of the disease had some benefits, but efficacy was less when compared to pure THC.[274]

As you have learned, phytocannabinoids exert a protective effect on damaged nerve cells due to their neuroprotective, anti-inflammatory, antioxidant, and neuroregenerative properties. Cannabinoids have been examined in a few clinical trials in humans for relief of symptoms of chorea and behavior issues, listed here:

- The synthetic cannabinoid nabilone was found to improve symptoms in two studies of HD and worsen symptoms in another.[275]
- Fifteen patients with HD received CBD, with an average dose of 700 milligrams per day for six weeks, with no improvement or worsening of symptoms and no adverse side effects.[276]

- Twenty-four HD patients received nabiximols (Sativex) in a safety trial and found improvement of sleep and anxiety with no adverse effects or tolerability issues.[277]

Because of the ability to identify who will develop HD through genetic testing, patients may benefit from early intervention with cannabinoids prior to the onset of symptoms. Research is desperately needed to determine if cannabinoids can prevent or delay the progression of HD. If so, which cannabinoids, what dosing, and when to start treatment are all critical questions.

Patients with HD may choose to use cannabis to help improve their quality of life. Choice of cannabinoids should be based on the stage of the disease as well as individual response, but evidence so far points to benefits from the combination of CBD and THC in a low ratio.[278]

Parkinson's Disease

Parkinson's disease (PD) is a neurodegenerative disorder that primarily affects motor function and coordination. It results from the death of dopamine-producing nerve cells in the area of the brain called the substantia nigra, a part of the basal ganglia, which is responsible for movement. The cause of PD in most cases is unknown; however, 10 to 15 percent of cases are genetic. Some environmental risk factors have been associated with an increased risk of PD, including pesticide exposure and head injury. PD patients suffer with tremors, rigidity, bradykinesia (slow movement), and postural instability. Patients may also experience depression, cognitive decline, sleep disorders, and occasionally psychosis. Research shows 60 percent of PD patients suffer with pain and are prescribed more pain medications than the general population, but pain is often insufficiently treated.[279] The mainstay of treatment is medication, rehabilitation with exercise, and occupational therapy, as well as, in some cases, surgery.

There is tremendous interest in the use of cannabinoids to treat as well as delay the progress of the symptoms of Parkinson's. We know that the endocannabinoid system plays a major role in the modulation of dopamine in the basal ganglia. Researchers have found both TRPV1 and CB_2 receptors are present in this part of the brain, both targets of cannabinoid treatment.[280] As with Huntington's disease, the endocannabinoid system goes through various changes during the progression of PD, in part as a response to the onset of the disease, and then as a result of the disease.[281] It appears that certain cannabinoids may help early in the disease, which may aggravate the condition as it progresses, necessitating a change in the cannabinoid regimen.

There are a number of published studies on cannabinoid treatment of PD, almost all of which show therapeutic benefits for symptoms:

- In a randomized, double-blind, placebo-controlled crossover trial with seven patients with PD, the synthetic cannabinoid nabilone significantly reduced levodopa-induced dyskinesia (abnormal, uncontrollable, involuntary movements caused by the use of PD medication).[282]
- In a randomized, placebo-controlled crossover study with seventeen patients with PD, oral cannabis extract was given over four weeks with no subjective/objective improvements noted; however, the treatment was deemed safe and well tolerated.[283]
- In a survey of 339 patients attending a movement disorder clinic, 25 percent reported experimenting with cannabis to treat symptoms. Almost half of those using cannabis reported improvement with at least once-a-day use. Use over three months resulted in more significant alleviation of symptoms. Only four patients reported worsening symptoms with cannabis use. The researchers reported that "long-term regular use of cannabinoids is crucial" to obtaining good results with cannabis for PD.[284]
- Six patients with Parkinson's psychosis were treated with pure CBD, 150 to 600 milligrams daily over four weeks, with significant improvement in thinking and anxiety, and decreases in psychotic symptoms, with no adverse effects.[285]

- Twenty-two patients with PD were evaluated at baseline and thirty minutes after smoking cannabis flowers, with significant improvement in the Unified Parkinson's Disease Rating Scale, as well as decreases noted in tremor, rigidity, and bradykinesia. Additionally, there was improvement in sleep and pain, with no adverse side effects.[286]

- In a study of twenty-one patients with PD, treatment with a placebo, 75 milligrams CBD, or 300 milligrams CBD was given for six weeks. There were no differences in the Unified Parkinson's Disease Rating Scale; however, another PD rating scale, called PDQ-39, showed a statistical difference between the placebo and the higher CBD dose.[287]

- Four patients with PD who had REM sleep behavior disorder were treated with CBD, with three receiving 75 milligrams per day and one receiving 300 milligrams per day. Three patients reported a complete resolution of symptoms and one reported a significant reduction of symptoms. Symptoms returned when CBD was discontinued.[288]

- A survey of forty-seven men with PD using medical cannabis to treat symptoms (thirty-eight of the forty-seven inhaled via smoking) found improvement in falls, pain, depression, tremor, muscle stiffness, and sleep.[289]

- A 2020 placebo-controlled trial of twenty-four patients with PD given CBD 300 milligrams daily showed decreased anxiety and decreased tremor amplitude in an anxiety-provoking situation.[290]

An interesting animal model investigated THCV for PD, finding a decrease in motor symptoms in addition to a decrease in the loss of neurons, demonstrating not only symptomatic benefits but also potential disease-delaying effects.[291] These effects are thought to be due to its antioxidant properties and through its interaction with the CB_2 receptor. An earlier published report supports THCV in combination with CBD for use in PD as well.[292]

It is important to note that patients start cannabis treatment when they are at different stages of a disease, and certain cannabinoids may be helpful at one point in treatment but may need to be altered as the disease progresses. For instance, a person in the early stages of PD with mild symptoms may find relief from CBD; however, as time passes and their condition and symptoms change, they may need to add in THC or another cannabinoid.

Patients with PD often report significant relief from tremors, better sleep, and less anxiety with inhaled THC. Some have found relief with high doses of CBD-rich cannabis taken sublingually or in capsules. I usually recommend a combination of THC and CBD to start and then customize the cannabinoids and dosing depending on a patient's response. Starting with a low dose and titrating up is recommended to avoid unwanted side effects, particularly with THC-rich cannabis. THCV has recently become available in California, so its efficacy for Parkinson's in real-world patients will be interesting to see.

―⁓―

Mary's Story

Mary's husband, Mike, contacted my office, desperate for his wife to be evaluated quickly. A mother and grandmother, Mary had been the picture of health. She was devoted to her family and had always made time to be involved in her church and community. When she was sixty-six years old, her family noted that she began having memory issues. Her family noted more changes throughout the next year, including episodes during which she seemed agitated, lost, and disconnected, not herself. Mary's family was devastated after she was diagnosed with dementia.

Over the next three years, Mary declined rapidly, eventually requiring a caregiver to help provide home care. She had good days and bad days. Mike sought out second and third medical opinions, and Mary ended up on multiple medications, but there was no real improvement. At one point Mary became very aggressive, hitting and screaming all the time, and she was eventually hospitalized in order to safely introduce a new antipsychotic to her regimen. She worsened, becoming terribly confused, refusing to eat, and requiring help with basic activities of daily living. It was at this point that a friend of Mike's referred them to me.

Mary started taking a CBD-rich tincture once she got home from the hospital, but it caused more agitation. This was not surprising, as some patients become overstimulated by it. I advised trying a THCA tincture next, and the results were "remarkable," according to Mike. In an email after she'd been on this oil a few weeks, he wrote to me that she was doing better, had more periods of alertness, an improved appetite, and "a desire to be on her own two feet." I advised a low-dose THC tincture for times of increased agitation, and this helped as well. Over the next year, with the help of a new neurologist, Mary was weaned off three of her five pharmaceuticals, and her life improved even more.

Two years after she started cannabis, I received an email from Mike, addressed to me as well as Mary's primary care physician and neurologist, both of whom were supportive of her cannabis use. Mike had forwarded a touching article about a man who lost his life to dementia. Here is the email:

This time two years ago, Mary was hospitalized for the purpose of safely dosing her up on quetiapine to address her anxiety, agitation, and physical issues. During those twenty-eight days I watched her physical self change so dramatically that when I took her out, she could barely stand, was hunched over, could not hold her head up, and needed assistance moving. She was receiving increased doses of quetiapine and was intermittently receiving shots of haloperidol.

The man described in the article lost his life. I feared that Mary was going to as well.

So, thank you, all three of you. Your collaboration in titrating her safely from quetiapine and introducing her to cannabis therapy has helped her thrive. It has allowed me to enjoy her every day. She is in a stable state, where she is happy and joyful. Her sense of humor appears often, and she is upright, able to walk with slight assistance, and most importantly *alive*. I'm not sure I could say that if we hadn't made the changes that we did starting in 2017.

Post-Traumatic Stress Disorder

PTSD is a condition brought on by experiencing or witnessing a terrifying event. A recent study reported that PTSD has a large genetic component, which explains why only some individuals who suffer through a traumatic ordeal develop PTSD.[293] Symptoms of PTSD include reliving the traumatic event, flashbacks, nightmares, emotional numbness, disturbed sleep, irritability, anger, and severe anxiety that interferes with normal functioning.

The mainstay of treatment for PTSD is therapy and medications, such as antidepressants, antianxiety medications, and antipsychotics. These medications may cause significant side effects (especially when more than one is taken at a time) and have been shown to have limited effectiveness.[294] PTSD sufferers are desperate for effective yet nontoxic treatment and many have found that cannabis helps to quell the nightmares, promote sleep, and alleviate anxiety and irritability.

Understanding how cannabis may help patients with PTSD is a major focus of research, as the number of military veterans with this medical condition has increased significantly over the past few decades. The discovery of the endocannabinoid system and the mapping of cannabinoid receptors (reviewed in chapter 2) shows that cannabinoid receptors are expressed in high levels in the part of the brain called the amygdala, which controls anxiety, fear memory, and emotional response to stress.[295] In order to have an adaptive response to fear and to the resulting traumatic memories, a properly functioning endocannabinoid system must be present. An abnormality in the endocannabinoid system can predispose a person to PTSD. Additionally, chronic stress that results from PTSD can further impair the functioning of the endocannabinoid system, worsening the condition.

Although published research on the use of cannabis for PTSD is limited, there are some studies that show a relationship between the endocannabinoid system, PTSD, and cannabis use:

- Nabilone, a synthetic cannabinoid that binds to CB_1, was found to either eliminate or significantly reduce nightmares in 72 percent of PTSD patients who did not respond to conventional treatments. Participants reported improved quality of sleep and a reduction of daytime flashbacks. When nabilone was discontinued, nightmares returned, resolving again when the drug was restarted.[296]
- In a Canadian study, nabilone given to prison inmates with PTSD showed significant improvement in insomnia, nightmares, and other PTSD symptoms as well as on the Global Assessment of Functioning scale. A number of participants were able to discontinue antipsychotic and/or sedating/hypnotic medications, reducing unwanted side effects.[297]
- Multiple abnormalities within the endocannabinoid system were found in people with PTSD.[298]
- PTSD patients who were approved for use of medical cannabis as part of the New Mexico Medical Cannabis Program reported an over 75 percent reduction in symptoms with cannabis use.[299]
- In Israel, ten patients with chronic PTSD were given oral THC doses of 5 milligrams twice a day and showed a statistically significant improvement in global symptom severity, sleep quality, frequency of nightmares, and PTSD hyperarousal symptoms; three patients reported mild adverse side effects but did not discontinue use of the medication.[300]
- In another report from Canada, a randomized, double-blind, placebo-controlled crossover study of military veterans with treatment-resistant PTSD, nabilone administration significantly reduced the severity and frequency of nightmares, and increased general well-being.[301]

- In a 2019 retrospective study of eleven patients with PTSD who received CBD for eight weeks, 91 percent reported a decrease in symptom severity, with less anxiety, better sleep, and improved focus. CBD also relieved nightmares in a subset of patients who reported this as a symptom of their PTSD. CBD was well tolerated, and no patients discontinued treatment. Four patients continued on CBD for thirty-six weeks, and all experienced long-term, sustained decreases in the severity of their PTSD symptoms.[302]

Cannabinoid treatment is effective for many of the symptoms of PTSD, but it is critical that patients understand the concept of receptor downregulation with THC use. Remember that chronic heavy use of THC-rich cannabis can cause a decrease in cannabinoid receptor numbers that will lead to tolerance and eventually to a loss of effectiveness. **Patients with PTSD must be thoughtful about frequency and dosing of THC-rich cannabis so that tolerance can be minimized and effectiveness can be maximized.**

Some patients with PTSD report to me that using low to moderate doses of THC with intermittent breaks from use (one day a week or four to seven days every few months after they have improved symptoms) has been very effective in reducing their PTSD symptoms. I have a few patients with PTSD who reported a loss of benefits from the use of THC-rich cannabis due to overmedicating with high-potency, concentrated formulations, which created a very high tolerance and worsening anxiety. In addition to abstaining from cannabis for at least a week in order to upregulate their receptors, use of high-ratio CBD:THC (approximately 18:1 to 25:1) cannabis during the time of abstinence helped to minimize THC withdrawal symptoms in some of these patients. I encourage my patients to include some CBD in their cannabis medicine regimen since it can be quite helpful in reducing anxiety and minimizing tolerance. One particular patient has been able to conquer his PTSD symptoms with daily use of CBD and CBG tinctures and small doses of THC at night for sleep.

PTSD patients using chemovars with high THCV potency anecdotally report that this phytocannabinoid also helps to decrease anxiety and can block panic attacks without causing sedation. Chemovars with significant amounts of THCV are still somewhat rare to find at this time and often contain an equal amount of THC, which may or may not be desired. Terpenoids that may help with PTSD symptoms include myrcene for its sedating effects, linalool for its calming effects, and limonene for its antianxiety and mood-enhancing effects. Chemovars high in pinene may have unwanted effects since this terpenoid can aid and enhance memory, which is not desirable for someone who is trying to forget their traumatic experience.

Edward's Story

Edward came to see me for help with his PTSD and severe insomnia. He is a war veteran and served two difficult tours of duty in Iraq. When he came home after the second tour, he was completely drained but happy to be back with his wife and young child, eager to grow his family. He started going to school, as he had always dreamed of becoming a paramedic. It seemed like a fresh start until the nightmares began a few months after returning home. He became fearful as night fell, dreading the dark, since it meant he would relive his worst memories. Staying up late became his routine, and sometimes he didn't fall asleep until dawn. He started missing classes, fought with his wife, and began drinking alcohol, telling me when we met that he had just wanted to "stop feeling."

A friend convinced Edward to go to the VA, and after a number of visits, he was diagnosed with PTSD and prescribed medications for sleep and depression. Feeling worse, he continued to drink. The breaking point came when he was supposed to be watching his young son while his wife was at work. She came home to find the small child unsupervised, playing in the bathroom, while Edward was passed out on the couch. Knowing he could not continue like this, and hearing from his military buddies that cannabis was helping them, he decided it was time to make a change.

Edward was reluctant to talk about his experiences in Iraq and his nightmares when we met, so we talked about his family. He shared how much they meant to him, how he was terrified of losing them, afraid that he was out of control. Edward started taking a CBD-rich tincture twice a day with instructions to slowly increase the dose and to report back to me regularly. We talked about the role of THC in sleep and breakthrough anxiety, and he decided to try low-dose edibles at night, with the goal of normalizing sleep. Since many of my patients who suffered from similar nightmare episodes had found they resolved with cannabis, I reassured him that this was possible.

The first report from Edward was positive. He was falling asleep earlier and easier, and was staying asleep longer. He had one nightmare the first week of CBD treatment but none after increasing the dose from 25 to 50 milligrams twice a day. He had tried a 5-milligram THC edible product but was too drowsy in the morning, finding half that dose quite effective on nights when he felt particularly anxious. He was pleased to share with me that he had cut back on his drinking, which also had pleased his wife. Edward asked about vaping for breakthrough anxiety, and I recommended he try 1:1 CBD:THC, which he subsequently reported to be effective and not intoxicating when he took only one or two puffs.

The last time we met, Edward told me he still felt damaged by the war but proud of his success in getting his life back together. He was going to group therapy at the VA, exercising regularly, and back in school. He said cannabis was a piece of the puzzle that helped him get better and saved his family life. His face lit up when he shared a picture of his son and told me another child was on the way.

Schizophrenia

Schizophrenia is a chronic, severe, debilitating brain disorder that affects about 1 percent of the population. Symptoms are categorized into three types: positive symptoms, which include delusions, hallucinations, agitated movements, and disorganized thinking; negative symptoms, which include "flat affect" (a reduction of emotional expressiveness), social withdrawal, and a lack of pleasure in everyday life; and cognitive symptoms, which include poor attention, poor executive functioning, trouble with decision-making, and poor memory. Hyperactivity of dopamine and serotonin, two important neurotransmitters, plays an important role in the cause of schizophrenia; however, other neurotransmitters and their receptors are involved as well.[303]

Cannabinoid receptors exist in high numbers in the area of the brain implicated in schizophrenia, with accumulating evidence that endocannabinoid system dysfunction is likely to play a role in this condition.[304] Remember that if the endocannabinoid system is not functioning properly, the brain cannot balance the hyperactivity of the involved neurotransmitters, which results in an imbalance in the messages brain cells are sending to each other. Cerebrospinal fluid of schizophrenic patients reveals significantly elevated anandamide, thought to be a result of the endocannabinoid system's attempt to restore homeostasis. Interestingly, researchers found the higher the anandamide, the fewer delusions and other positive symptoms.[305] There are also numerous studies that report schizophrenia is likely an inflammatory illness, again evidence of endocannabinoid system dysfunction.

Conventional treatment for patients with schizophrenia is antipsychotic medications. These drugs have been shown to be effective in reducing the positive symptoms of schizophrenia but do not appear to help with the negative or the cognitive symptoms. Additionally, antipsychotic medications have numerous side effects that can become intolerable, causing patients to discontinue use. Approximately one-third of patients are treatment resistant, meaning they do not respond to two or more medications.

There has been some concern about cannabis, namely THC, causing schizophrenia (as mentioned in chapter 6). Many teenagers use cannabis, but only a small fraction develop schizophrenia. Researchers have found that an underlying genetic susceptibility is likely at play.[306] The adolescent who starts using THC-rich cannabis at a young age and also has a first-degree family member with mental illness, such as schizophrenia or bipolar disorder, appears to be the most vulnerable. Once the brain is fully developed, it seems there is no increased risk of schizophrenia with cannabis use.

The first case report of a patient with schizophrenia responding to CBD treatment was published in 1995.[307] Since that time, there have been a few published human trials of the benefits of CBD for psychosis, summarized here:

- In a double-blind, controlled clinical trial, CBD significantly reduced acute psychotic symptoms after two and four weeks of treatment. In this trial, CBD did not differ in efficacy from an atypical antipsychotic except for a lower incidence of side effects.[308]
- In another double-blind study of thirty-nine acutely psychotic inpatients, cannabidiol improved symptoms similarly to another antipsychotic medication; however, CBD had fewer unwanted side effects.[309]
- In a randomized, placebo-controlled study, forty-five patients with schizophrenia who received 1,000 milligrams of CBD per day had lower levels of positive psychotic symptoms and were more likely to have been rated as improved and as not severely unwell by the treating physician. There were no adverse effects.[310]
- A case report of a fifty-seven-year-old female with treatment-resistant schizophrenia added CBD, up to 1,500 milligrams per day, to the existing pharmaceutical regimen of clozapine and lamotrigine, resulting in significant improvement.[311]
- Two studies did not show improvement. The first gave only a single dose of either 300 or 600 milligrams of CBD and found no difference when compared to a placebo.[312] The other study looked at stable patients, meaning not acutely psychotic, and found no difference with 600-milligram daily dosing.[313]

Although there is concern about patients with schizophrenia using THC, I have a small number of patients with this condition using THC-rich cannabis with excellent results, mostly to treat breakthrough anxiety. They have been educated about the important terpenes that target anxiety—namely myrcene, limonene, and linalool—and are choosing chemovars that give antianxiety and calming effects. Others are using CBD-rich cannabis with reports that they experience fewer hallucinations and delusions, with improved mood and much less anxiety. Almost all of these patients are combining cannabis with conventional antipsychotic medications with good results, as indicated by fewer hospitalizations and reports of improved interpersonal relationships and better functioning. The biggest issue with CBD for use in schizophrenia is the cost of high daily doses, which can range from 300 to 800 milligrams per day, costing three hundred dollars or more per month, a large out-of-pocket expense for someone who may be unable to work due to their illness.

Skin Disorders

The skin is the human body's largest organ and serves as a most important barrier, protecting us from the external world. Both CB_1 and CB_2 receptors are found throughout human skin tissue. The role of the endocannabinoid system in skin is thought to regulate cell growth, both promoting wound healing and blocking skin cell growth in certain conditions. It is also responsible for controlling the immune function of skin, regulating what is called "cutaneous homeostasis." Our understanding of the endocannabinoid system and its role in skin conditions is still in its infancy. The following are the main research findings.

Acne

As one of the most common skin disorders, acne can cause psychological distress and negatively impact quality of life. Acne is considered a multifactorial condition—that is, many factors contribute to its development and course. Experts studying the effects of cannabinoids on this condition have found that CBD, CBDV, and THCV exert potent anti-acne effects, with THCV having the most potency in a test-tube study.[314] There are no human clinical trials using phytocannabinoids for acne; however, a number of companies are investigating patented synthetic cannabinoids for this indication.

Allergic Contact Dermatitis

Allergic contact dermatitis is a red, itchy rash that occurs due to direct contact with a substance causing an allergic reaction. Often caused by soaps, jewelry, plants, or cosmetics, the rash can be quite uncomfortable. In one study, topical THC applied to allergic contact dermatitis in mice decreased allergic swelling as well as inflammatory cells and compounds found in the skin.[315]

Atopic Dermatitis/Eczema

Atopic dermatitis, also called eczema, is a chronic skin condition characterized by dry, itchy, scaly skin. It is thought to be caused by allergies. Eczema flare-ups are when the skin becomes inflamed with large red patches. There is no known cure for this condition, but topical medications, including steroids, are often prescribed. Animal studies have found the endocannabinoid system to play a large role in regulating skin inflammation.

- Mice bred without an endocannabinoid system developed severe skin inflammation and, on skin biopsy, had significantly more inflammatory cells throughout the layers of their skin.[316]
- Mice bred to have no FAAH, the enzyme that breaks down anandamide (meaning anandamide stayed around longer), had fewer allergic responses. Additionally, compounds that blocked the cannabinoid receptors aggravated allergic inflammation.[317]
- In mice with chemically induced atopic dermatitis, topical application of CB_1 receptor activators reduced inflammatory compounds

in the skin, including histamine, a compound that causes inflammation after it is released in response to an allergic trigger.[318]

- In a study of 2,456 patients with allergic eczema, treatment with a topical cream containing the endocannabinoid N-palmitoylethanolamide (PEA) significantly improved dryness, scaling, and redness in 70 percent of patients, with 56 percent reporting they were able to eliminate topical steroid creams.[319] (A quick note about PEA: this endocannabinoid does not bind to CB_1 or CB_2 receptors; rather, it blocks the breakdown of anandamide, enhancing its effects.)

Collectively these studies show the skin's inflammatory response is likely under the control of the endocannabinoid system.

Pruritis/Itching

Pruritis is the medical term for the unpleasant sensation of itchiness that leads to excessive scratching. Pruritis is present in many common skin conditions and is notoriously difficult to treat.

Animal studies documented that cannabinoids are effective at reducing pruritis.[320] Additionally, human trials using topical preparations containing cannabinoids reduced itching significantly.[321]

In the aforementioned study of 2,456 patients with allergic eczema, which causes uncomfortable pruritis, treatment with a topical cream containing the endocannabinoid PEA significantly decreased itchiness without side effects.[322] Patients also reported better sleep. Three other studies using creams containing PEA as well as additional cannabinoids found similar findings, with either resolution or a significant reduction of itching without any adverse side effects.[323]

Psoriasis

Psoriasis is a skin disorder in which skin cells, called keratinocytes, multiply faster than normal, building up and forming scales and itchy, dry patches. There are a few different types of psoriasis, with plaque psoriasis being most common. Sometimes joints are inflamed as well, indicating the type of psoriasis called psoriatic arthritis. Psoriasis is considered to be an autoimmune disorder. Many factors can trigger it, including hormonal changes, stress, smoking, alcohol, certain medications, and infections. Treatment consists of topical medications, light therapy, and systemic medications.

There is some evidence that psoriasis may be due to endocannabinoid system dysfunction, with multiple abnormalities of endocannabinoid system components. For instance, blood tests on patients with psoriasis revealed their endocannabinoid levels were elevated, as were the enzymes that break them down, along with upregulation of CB_1 and CB_2 receptors.[324]

A 2007 article investigated a number of phytocannabinoids, specifically THC, CBD, CBG, and CBN, for their ability to inhibit hyperproliferating keratinocytes, the cells that build up in psoriasis. All four compounds were found to inhibit the skin cells from multiplying, with CBG being the most potent and CBD the second most potent. The researchers found that these effects were not due to interaction with the cannabinoid receptors.[325]

I have successfully treated a number of patients with psoriasis. Most use daily topical cannabinoid preparations with CBD, CBG, and/or THC. Patients report inhaled, sublingual, or oral THC-rich or CBD:THC preparations to be helpful with anti-inflammatory effects, improving sleep, reducing anxiety, and reducing itching. CBDA and THCA, with their potent anti-inflammatory effects, may be beneficial for this condition as well.

Skin Cancer

There are three types of skin cancer: basal cell carcinoma, squamous cell carcinoma, and melanoma. Basal cell and squamous cell carcinoma are for the most part not life-threatening and commonly result from prolonged exposure to UV radiation from the sun. Melanoma, the most serious of skin cancers, starts in melanocytes, cells that make the skin pigment melanin. Melanoma is more dangerous because it is more likely to metastasize.

In a multipart study investigating cannabinoids as a treatment for skin cancer, researchers found that CB_1 and CB_2 receptors were expressed not only in healthy skin cells but also in all skin cancer cells, including melanoma.[326] Cannabinoids caused apoptosis (cell suicide) of skin cancer cells implanted into mice, inhibited tumor growth, and inhibited angiogenesis (the growth of blood vessels feeding the cancer cells). Cannabinoids also decreased epidermal growth factor receptor (EGFR), a chemical that encourages the cancer to grow. Multiple studies report the use of cannabinoids decreased the number of viable melanoma cells in the laboratory and in mice.[327] Unfortunately, there are no human studies.

Clinically, there are many anecdotal reports of patients using topical preparations of cannabinoids for various skin rashes and skin cancers. Preparations can be of any of the available cannabinoids, and often patients will apply different combinations to find what works best. Skin itchiness may respond to topical preparations, but often patients have reported taking THC-rich cannabis and/or combination CBD+THC preparations in order to sleep. There are anecdotal reports of less serious skin cancers responding to a topical application of cannabinoids.

Sleep Disorders

Sleep disturbance is one of the most common reasons patients come to my office. Poor sleep is associated with increased risk of inflammation and "all cause mortality"—meaning sleep is crucially important to living and to living healthfully.[328] Significant conditions that have a negative impact on your life—such as anxiety, depression, poor memory, anger, increased risk of accidents, and increased risk of cardiovascular diseases—are all increased when you are not getting good sleep. Even the Centers for Disease Control has called insufficient sleep a public health crisis.[329]

Those suffering from sleep difficulty will often try over-the-counter sleep aids or prescription sleep medications, both of which fall into a group of medications called hypnotics. In addition to the well-known and unwanted side effects of morning grogginess and potential sleep behaviors (for instance, waking and eating in the middle of the night with no memory of doing so), research shows that taking hypnotics is associated with a greater than threefold increased risk of death as well as an increased risk of cancer.[330]

Numerous studies on the effects of cannabinoids and cannabis for sleep have been published. Unfortunately, the overall quality of most of the reports is considered low, as confounding factors such as age of participants, type of cannabis or cannabinoids, cannabinoid dosing, and duration of use were not controlled and varied greatly from study to study. It is quite difficult to draw any useful conclusions since the findings from these studies are often conflicting.

A 2014 review of the literature documents the findings from thirty-nine studies, summarized here:

- With recreational use (the focus of eleven studies with 203 participants), the results varied tremendously, some showing better sleep and some not, making it difficult to determine the true effects on sleep.
- With medicinal cannabis use (the focus of twenty-eight studies with 3,658 participants), the studies included sleep as a treatment outcome while primarily concerned with the efficacy of medicinal cannabis for other conditions, such as pain, MS, and cancer. Approximately 65 percent of the studies used synthetic cannabinoids, with the rest using nabiximols (CBD:THC 1:1, Sativex). Although there was no objective measure of sleep, twenty of the twenty-eight studies showed a significant and positive impact on sleep.[331]

Additionally, some patients, especially those with PTSD, report that cannabis helps prevent nightmares. A few studies have shown that it reduces the frequency and intensity of nightmares and improves sleep.[332]

We still have a long way to go in sorting out how cannabis and cannabinoids affect sleep. That being stated, many of the patients I have evaluated for use of cannabis report better sleep. Most struggle primarily with pain, chronic illness, anxiety, and other conditions in which sleep has been negatively affected. Cannabis serves multiple purposes, often replacing both pain medications and sleep aids. I have also successfully treated patients with primary insomnia, sleep apnea, restless leg syndrome, nightmares, and bruxism (grinding of the teeth). Patients who report better sleep with cannabis use tell me they have a quicker onset of sleep and are able to stay asleep through the night. They also feel well rested upon awakening and, for the most part, do not experience morning grogginess. Those who feel tired the next morning can easily resolve this issue with a change of dosing, product, or timing of dosing.

THC and the terpenes myrcene and linalool are sedating for most people. Pinene, through its interaction with GABA, has been shown to enhance non-REM sleep and help the onset of sleep in mice.[333] Patients are using various methods to achieve better sleep. Inhalation or sublingual use of THC-rich cannabis helps with the onset of sleep. Ingestion of cannabis edibles often will prevent waking in the middle of the night due to their longer-lasting effects; however, they can take about two hours to be effective, so they should be ingested at least a few hours before the desired bedtime. It is always best for anyone new to cannabis to start with a very low dose of edibles, such as 1 to 2.5 milligrams, because higher doses may be too stimulating at first. Almost all patients using cannabis to help with sleep have to experiment with different doses and methods, adjusting to fit their individual needs.

Some patients who are using sleeping pills on a regular basis may have rebound insomnia when switching to cannabis. Poor sleep is likely due to the brain adjusting to the lack of sleeping pills, and in time, better sleep will be restored. I have witnessed many patients discontinue use of sleeping pills by adding cannabis and get through the transition period with the result of improved quality of sleep and no adverse side effects.

Just a reminder that CBD in low doses can be alerting (but not for everyone) and in higher doses can be sedating. These effects vary from person to person. Some patients report not feeling either alert or sedated with CBD. If you are using CBD for another condition, you may want to avoid taking it right before bedtime, as it can interfere with sleep in some patients. Once you see how it affects you, you can adjust the timing so that it does not adversely interfere with sleep.

Sleep Apnea

Sleep apnea is a disorder in which breathing is repeatedly interrupted during sleep, leaving the affected individual tired in the daytime. It can be obstructive (airway blockage from relaxation of soft tissue in the throat), called OSA, or central (the brain fails to signal breathing). It is associated with obesity, older age, a large tongue, a large neck, or large tonsils, and it can increase the risk of health problems such as heart attack, high blood pressure, depression, ADHD, and headache. Treatment of OSA is with a device called a continuous positive airway pressure (CPAP) machine, which is highly effective but often associated with poor compliance due to discomfort or a sense of claustrophobia with the mask, the loud noise of the machine, or intolerance to the forced air from the mask.

A 2002 study of mice, looking at the effects of an endocannabinoid and THC, showed that both suppressed sleep apnea.[334] Three human studies assessed the use of dronabinol ranging in doses from 2.5 milligrams up to 10 milligrams to treat OSA. All three found the cannabinoid to reduce the apnea episodes, although some side effects were reported (which may be due to the use of a synthetic cannabinoid, as clinically, patients using whole-plant products do not report similar side effects).[335]

Many of my patients with sleep apnea report that a low dose of THC at night helps them to stay compliant with the use of the CPAP because they have less discomfort from the device and are able to fall asleep easier.

Spinal Cord Injury

Spinal cord injury refers to any injury to the spinal cord or to the nerves at the bottom of the cord, causing permanent changes in strength, sensation, and other body functions below the site of the injury. People with spinal cord injuries suffer loss of movement and sensation, chronic pain, bowel and bladder problems, and extremity contractures (permanent tightening of the skin, muscles, tendons), as well as anxiety, depression, and sleep issues. Unfortunately, there is no way to reverse spinal cord damage.

Damage results from not only the initial spinal cord injury but also a secondary injury, brought on by the body's reaction to the insult. A massive inflammatory response descends on the area involved, creating more long-term tissue damage, swelling, cell death, and spinal cord dysfunction. Cannabis research, although scarce, has focused on prevention of this secondary response as well as symptomatic relief for patients. Both animal and human studies are listed here, showing promising therapeutic benefits, including pain relief and a decrease in spasticity:

- Mice with spinal cord injuries given a synthetic compound that binds to the CB_2 receptor had improved motor function and improved bladder function, and seven days after the injury, there was a significant reduction of the cells causing inflammation as well as pro-inflammatory compounds.[336]
- Mice with pain from spinal cord injuries given a synthetic cannabinoid showed improvement in pain response.[337]
- A survey of forty-three people with spinal cord injuries reported decreased spasticity with cannabis use.[338]
- Of 117 patients with spinal cord injuries and chronic pain who were surveyed, 32 percent reported significant pain relief from cannabis; additionally, it was rated the most effective of all treatments reviewed by participants.[339]

- In a 2007 study, twenty-five patients with spinal cord injury received either oral THC or rectal THC-hemisuccinate, resulting in a significant decrease in spasticity scores. The researchers concluded, "THC is an effective and safe drug in the treatment of spasticity."[340]
- A report of eleven patients with spinal cord injury given the synthetic cannabinoid nabilone found significant reduction of spasticity.[341]
- In 2016, in a placebo-controlled trial, forty-two patients with neuropathic pain from spinal cord injury vaporized placebo, low-dose THC, or high-dose THC. Both doses of THC provided highly statistically significant pain relief.[342]

Patients with spinal cord injury often find relief with either THC-rich cannabis or combination CBD+THC products based on personal preference and response. Some prefer to inhale since the rapid onset provides quicker relief of spasticity and pain. A few of my patients report that sublingual tinctures and/or edibles give a longer, more even effect. THCA, CBDA, and CBG may also be used for pain and decreased inflammation. I encourage patients with cervical or thoracic injuries who want to inhale to use vaporizers rather than smoking to reduce any risk of pulmonary infection. Terpenoids that are relaxing and sedating, such as linalool and myrcene, can be helpful for spasticity, anxiety, and sleep.

—⁓—

Andrew's Story

Andrew has been my patient for many years, and I wrote about him in my previous book. An update is included at the end of the original story.

Andrew initially injured himself while working with shipping containers on the docks in Long Beach. He had to undergo surgery on his back to fuse two vertebrae and was declared disabled, suffering near-constant pain. He was prescribed opiates, but they made him anxious, and worried they were only a Band-Aid, he got used to living with pain. He underwent months of physical therapy, which restored some mobility and allowed him to function better.

Andrew is a single father of four children and loved tinkering and riding ATVs with them. Two years after his back surgery, while traveling on a country fire road in canyon country with his kids, his vehicle hit a rut, wobbled, and then hit a cow fence. The ATV stopped, but he kept going. He was airlifted from the site and learned soon after that he was paralyzed from the nipples down.

"I'm not dead," Andrew stated, despite the paralysis. His arms still worked, so he went back to work as a clerk. The hours it took to get ready to go to work on the docks were often filled with pain. He had developed digestive problems because of the paralysis, and he experienced a considerable amount of nausea, pain, and anxiety daily. Some days his stomach hurt so much that he had to leave work early. He could barely eat. His back constantly seized up and contracted. If someone touched his skin, he might feel nothing, but internally he could feel it as it deflected to his stomach. His kids noticed, winced at his pain, but learned to live with it just as he did. The doctors prescribed many different medications, but these made him even more depressed and increased his anxiety. He continued to try various prescriptions, determined to be present and a good father for his kids, but the ten medications he was prescribed, along with many OTC medicines, only made him feel worse.

Andrew knew nothing about the medicinal value of cannabis and had even tried Marinol (synthetic THC available with a prescription) with no effect. He was dubious that medical cannabis would do anything for his constant pain and nausea, but he decided to try it. It has changed his life. Both inhaling it and taking cannabis edibles have helped to lessen the stomach issues and the anxiety. He reports that he is able to eat, his back spasms have improved, and his anxiety has diminished considerably. Cannabis even helps ease the severe and debilitating pain he's had in his left hip ever since the accident.

Andrew uses his cannabis medicine before work, later at his lunch break, and when he gets home. Far more independent, he is able to stretch every day and perform a series of exercises to keep himself strong. Getting up in the dark hours before dawn, Andrew is determined to be as hardworking and independent as he's ever been. He has had great results and has overcome many obstacles.

His children have witnessed his pain and problems and seen how much the cannabis helps him. Andrew and his kids have a mission-like intensity about educating the public on the medicinal value of cannabis. Andrew wants to change the stigma around it and share how it has improved the quality of his and his family's life.

Update: *I recently spoke with Andrew, who continues to struggle with issues related to his paralysis. He still relies on cannabis as his medicine to treat his chronic pain. Although the pain is never really gone, cannabis makes it tolerable. He was recently hospitalized after breaking a bone, and since the hospital forbids cannabis use, he was forced to take pharmaceuticals for his medical issues. He told me the experience made him reflect on just how much cannabis has helped him, sharing that he could not imagine his life without it.*

Tourette Syndrome

Tourette syndrome (TS) is a neurological disorder manifested by repetitive, involuntary movements and vocalizations called tics. The disorder is named for Dr. Georges Gilles de la Tourette, the French neurologist who first described the condition in an eighty-six-year-old French noblewoman in 1885.

The cause of TS is still unknown. Recent research points to a genetic cause, with about a 50 percent chance of parents passing the gene on to their children. Abnormalities in certain brain regions, including the basal ganglia, cortex, and frontal lobes, and in the neurotransmitters dopamine, serotonin, and norepinephrine, have been found in persons suffering from TS and are a focus of current research.

Many patients with TS are finding relief from their symptoms with cannabis. A large percentage of people who have been diagnosed with TS also suffer from other significant conditions, such as OCD, ADHD, mood disorders, and anxiety. The conventional medications used to treat these conditions are not always helpful and often cause a wide array of unwanted side effects.

Research on the use of cannabis for TS has been led by neurologist and psychiatrist Kirsten Müller-Vahl, MD, and her group at Germany's Hannover Medical School. Here is a summary of her research, along with other results on human use of cannabis for Tourette syndrome:

- Of the TS patients who reported prior use of cannabis, 82 percent experienced a "reduction or complete remission of motor and vocal tics and amelioration of premonitory urges and OCD symptoms."[343]
- A 1999 report documented the successful treatment of a twenty-five-year-old male with Tourette syndrome who received a single dose of 10 milligrams of THC, with reduction of his tic severity score from 41 pre-THC to 7 post-THC treatment.[344]
- A case study of a twenty-four-year-old female with TS and extreme tics showed that she improved with a combination of THC and an antipsychotic medication called amisulpride.[345]
- A 2002 report found a significant improvement of tics and obsessive-compulsive behavior after treatment with THC compared to placebo in twelve adult patients with TS who also had other psychiatric disorders.[346]
- In a randomized, double-blind, placebo-controlled study, twenty-four patients with TS treated over a six-week period with up to 10 milligrams per day of THC showed statistically significant improvement in symptoms.[347]
- In the first of a two-part study, twelve patients with TS found that THC significantly reduced motor and vocal tics compared to treatment with a placebo. The second part included twenty-four patients who were treated with THC or a placebo for six weeks. The authors concluded, "THC reduces tics in TS patients without any serious

adverse side effects and no impairment on neuropsychological performance."[348]

- A case report of a forty-two-year-old man with treatment-resistant TS showed a significant reduction of tics with THC, with improvement in concentration and visual perception.[349]

- In another case report, two teenage males suffering with incapacitating stuttering caused by vocal-blocking tics received medical cannabis or dronabinol and had significant improvement of speech and a reduction of tics.[350]

- A 2018 survey conducted in Israel reported that thirty-eight of forty-two patients who used medical cannabis for TS had reduced tic severity, better sleep, and improved mood.[351]

- A case report of a seven-year-old boy with severe TS and ADHD — who, after becoming depressed, suicidal, and socially isolated, did not respond to conventional medication — showed that oral THC drops significantly decreased his tics and improved his focus, social interaction, and overall quality of life, with no adverse effects.[352]

- A case report of a twelve-year-old with TS, who was treated by parents with vaporized and oral THC, showed immediate and nearly complete remission of tics with no adverse side effects.[353]

- In 2019, German researchers surveyed patients who used cannabinoids for TS, with the majority reporting a subjective improvement in tics, sleep, OCD, ADHD, and tolerable side effects. Whole-plant THC-rich strains were preferred over a CBD+THC combination and synthetic cannabinoids (dronabinol).[354]

- A case report of a female with TS showed a rapid and highly significant improvement with 20 milligrams CBD plus 10 milligrams THC.[355]

All of the patients with TS who have come to my office seeking help have tried numerous pharmaceuticals and found them to cause intolerable side effects and/or to be ineffective. The adult patients in my practice are using mainly THC-rich cannabis products to help decrease the number of tics and other symptoms of TS and its related conditions, and they report improved quality of life and no adverse side effects. Tolerance has been an issue for a few, who now take a short break in treatment as part of their routine, usually one to three days off THC every few months, with a return of efficacy at lower doses. In the pediatric population, a number of patients have responded to both high-ratio and low-ratio CBD:THC preparations, with a wide range of effective dosing. Recently I treated a teenage boy with TS who had increased anxiety with THC and no efficacy of high-ratio CBD:THC, but he responded with a reduction of tics and anxiety on a combination of THCA and CBG.

Traumatic Brain Injury

Traumatic brain injury (TBI) occurs when an external force delivers a violent blow to the head, resulting in brain dysfunction. Blunt-force trauma, penetrating injury, and/or a severe skull fracture can be the cause. TBI may be mild, with temporary brain damage, or quite serious, causing permanent and long-term complications and death. The symptoms of TBI vary widely and can include headache, nausea or vomiting, fatigue, difficulty sleeping, loss of balance, sensitivity to light or sound, seizures, communication problems, memory or concentration problems, mood swings, depression and/or anxiety, slurred speech, agitation, and/or combativeness. It also has been linked to dementia and chronic neurodegenerative changes in the brain. TBI interferes with the quality of life for both the patient and their family.

A concussion is considered a mild traumatic brain injury that may cause temporary symptoms before a full recovery is made; however, 15 to 30 percent of people with a concussion will go on to have post-concussion syndrome. This is a complex condition that affects memory, attention, energy level, sleep, and mood. There are no pharmacological treatments for post-concussion syndrome.

Chronic traumatic encephalopathy (CTE) is a neurodegenerative disease that has been associated with repetitive mild TBI, and is common in football players and other athletes.

After initial treatment and stabilization of any of these head injuries, many patients go through rehabilitation to relearn basic life functions and how to perform daily activities. They often end up on multiple medications, such as sleeping pills, antidepressants, antianxiety medications, mood stabilizers, anticonvulsants, pain relievers, and antipsychotics.

When the brain sustains an injury, there is immediate damage to brain cells. This is followed by a secondary response from the immune system, which descends upon the brain to help repair the affected brain cells. However, this response from the immune system includes a release of pro-inflammatory compounds known to contribute to more brain cell injury. Scientists have been searching for a way to improve the beneficial "repairing" immune response and minimize the unwanted "damaging" secondary response. Currently there are no adequate conventional treatments to do this.[356] The endocannabinoid system and phytocannabinoids may be the answer.

Phytocannabinoids are proven neuroprotective agents with potent anti-inflammatory properties, and thus the use of cannabis is a major focus of investigation for TBI and related neurodegenerative conditions by researchers all over the world. Animal studies are promising and summarized here:

- Immediately after a brain injury, endocannabinoids are significantly increased, providing neuroprotection.[357]
- Endocannabinoids decrease the intensity and duration of toxicity to brain cells after induced chemical damage.[358]
- After a brain injury, endocannabinoids lessen the inflammatory process and enhance brain cell survival.[359]
- Synthetic cannabinoids given to animals with brain injury protected against brain cell death and injury in multiple studies.[360]
- CBD given immediately after both oxygen and blood-flow deprivation reduced brain cell injury, cerebral hemodynamic impairment,

brain swelling, and seizures. Motor function and behavioral performance were restored within seventy-two hours after the insult.[361]

- A synthetic compound that selectively binds to CB_2 receptors (with no interaction at the CB_1 receptors) decreased inflammation, reduced swelling, enhanced blood flow to the brain, and improved behavior (less anxiety, better motor skills) after TBI.[362]

- Mice that underwent TBI and developed chronic pain, anxiety, and aggression were improved with oral CBD given during the first two weeks after the injury and again for ten days starting on day 50 after the injury, corresponding to times when symptoms from the injury were observed. CBD normalized the neurotransmitters glutamate and GABA after a TBI. CBD decreased aggression and depression and improved sociability.[363]

Human clinical trials have not been done, but two reports on patients with TBI who used cannabis reveal some benefits:

- A three-year retrospective review revealed that a positive THC screen was associated with decreased mortality in adult patients sustaining TBI; mortality of patients was 2.4 percent with a positive THC test and 11.5 percent with a negative THC test.[364]

- Cannabis users who sustained concussions had significantly fewer symptoms during week 3 and week 4 after the injury when compared to tobacco and alcohol users.[365]

In my clinical experience, patients with TBI benefit from cannabis. They report a relief from pain, enhanced sleep, less agitation, and mood stabilization. They also report no adverse side effects from cannabis use and are able to discontinue most, if not all, pharmaceuticals. Depending on personal preference, some are using high-ratio CBD:THC and others prefer low-ratio products. I encourage all of my patients with TBI to include CBD-rich cannabis in their regimen for its added anti-inflammatory and neuroprotective properties. Additionally, CBG or the raw cannabinoids THCA and CBDA may help enhance anti-inflammatory effects.

～ww～

Patrick's Story

Patrick is a fifty-two-year-old firefighter who, after thirty years on the job, still loved his work but wanted to spend more time with his family. He figured he would retire at fifty-five and still be young enough to pursue his other interest, restoring old cars. "I made plans, but God decided to change them," he said when we met.

Patrick's firehouse was called to a large warehouse fire. They responded and got to work putting out the fire. Patrick doesn't remember the injury but says that his fellow firefighters reported he was hit in the head when a ladder accidentally fell over, striking his helmet and causing him to fall to the ground, where he hit his head again on the concrete. Losing consciousness, he reportedly was out for only one minute. He was checked out by the paramedics on the scene, who told him he should go to the ER for an evaluation of the head injury. Despite his protests that he was fine, his colleagues told him that he seemed dazed and slow to respond.

After the fire was extinguished and the firefighters were back at the firehouse, Patrick started experiencing nausea and vomiting, accompanied by a terrible headache. He went to the ER, and after a number of tests, he was diagnosed with a grade 4 concussion. He stayed home for the next two weeks, and although he initially felt better, he started to have more headaches and dizziness. His primary care physician diagnosed him with post-concussion syndrome, stressing the need for further rest.

After two months of what Patrick called "being a bum," he returned to work despite continuing to experience headaches, irritability, and occasional dizziness, as well as having difficulty focusing. He also struggled to work on the hot rod he was restoring, and after another few months of continued symptoms, Patrick started to feel depressed and anxious that he would never fully recover. He was prescribed antianxiety medications and antidepressants, which he was reluctant to take. He tried some other interventions, including acupuncture and physical therapy, but nothing seemed to help. After almost one year of struggling with symptoms, Patrick considered suicide, as he could no longer work, enjoy his family, or enjoy his beloved car hobby.

One of Patrick's friends mentioned cannabis to him, but after having a bad experience in high school, he was reluctant to try it. When his wife asked him to reconsider, stating he had nothing to lose, he did some research and read about others who had had positive responses to CBD. When I met Patrick, he seemed nervous. But it was obvious to me that he was suffering. His eyes welled up with tears when he told me he loved being a firefighter and was devastated to think he would no longer be able to work as one.

Patrick began with low doses of an 18:1 CBD:THC tincture, working up over a few weeks to higher doses of about 150 milligrams twice a day. He noted in the first week that he felt better, and by about six weeks of treatment, he reported his headaches had resolved, his mood was better, and he was no longer depressed and anxious. He also noted, though, that he still felt dizzy during and after exercising. He tried a higher dose of CBD (200 milligrams twice a day), and after a number of weeks, these symptoms were almost completely resolved. Patrick has not experienced any unwanted side effects from CBD and has continued taking it for the last few years, reporting he feels like his old self. He wrote in an email to me:

It seems crazy that no one had anything to help me get better and the one thing that is helping me is still illegal. This seems so unfair for those that are suffering.

Acknowledgments

I am so fortunate to have tremendous support from many wonderful people, allowing me to realize my childhood dream of helping people heal from illness.

To Bonnie Solow, for your invaluable guidance, expertise, and kindness. I am so lucky to have found you.

Thank you to everyone at Hachette Book Group; Little, Brown Spark; and Headline Publishing Group for making this book possible: Marisa Vigilante, for seeking me out and serving as the editorial light of this book; Tracy Behar, for believing in my work; Ian Straus, for supporting me throughout the publishing process; and Alyssa Persons, Massey Barner, Craig Young, Laura Mamelock, Karen Landry, Jessica Chun, Kirin Diemont, Dianna Stirpe, Anna Steadman, Antonia Whitton, and Georgina Polhill, for your expert advice and dedicated support.

To Doug and Becky Francis, your friendship and unconditional support of my work leaves me speechless. Thank you from the bottom of my heart.

To Chris Beals, Carl Fillichio, and everyone at Weedmaps, thank you for fighting for cannabis freedom.

To Fred Gardner, Martin Lee, Jeff Raber, and Dustin Sulak, thank you for answering my endless questions and for doing all that you do for cannabis patients. To the scientists and physicians who paved the way — Raphael Mechoulam, Ethan Russo, Jeffrey Hergenrather, Tod Mikuriya — and the multitude of devoted cannabinoid researchers around the world, thank you for your dedication to the truth in the face of so much doubt. You have helped me help others.

To Margot Gonzalez, thank you for controlling my chaos on a daily basis with a smile on your face. I am indebted to you forever.

To Michael Levinsohn, thank you for your sage advice and for always having my back.

Last but not least...

To my parents, Fran and Murray, I hit the parent lottery for sure. You guys are the best.

To my sisters and their families, I love you all for always supporting me. (Or should that be putting up with me?)

And to my husband, Jim, and son, Jake, the loves of my life, no words can express how much you both mean to me.

Appendix A

The History of Cannabis

The history of cannabis and its path to illegality is fascinating. The plant was cultivated in Asia over ten thousand years ago, and its use as a medicine has been well documented. Here is a time line that highlights important dates:

2700 BCE: Legendary Chinese emperor Shen Nung writes about herbal remedies in *Shen-nung Pen Ts'ao Ching,* in which cannabis is recorded as a treatment for pain associated with gout and arthritis.

2350 BCE: A description of cannabis is entered in the Pyramid Texts of Egypt.

1700 BCE: Cannabis is described in the medical papyri in ancient Egypt and Mesopotamia (*Ramesseum III Papyrus* and *Eber's Papyrus*) as a treatment for eye conditions, female disorders, migraine headaches, and toenail conditions.

1350 BCE: Traces of hashish (concentrated cannabis resin) are placed with the remains of a young woman who died in childbirth; it is thought to have been used to ease the labor of childbirth.

1200 BCE: The Atharva Veda, a collection of Hindu texts, lists cannabis as one of the five sacred plants.

440 BCE: Herodotus writes about Scythians using cannabis during funeral rites.

1542: *Cannabis sativa* is named by German physician and botanist Leonhart Fuchs in his book *De Historia Stirpium Commentarii Insignes*.

1600s: Cannabis is used for sleep, dysentery, appetite, headaches, and digestive problems in India.

1798: Napoleon's soldiers bring hashish from Egypt back to France, where it becomes a focus of study by scientists for its pain-relieving and sedating properties.

1833: Irish physician Dr. William O'Shaughnessy travels to India, where he witnesses cannabis being used for arthritis, rabies, cholera, and convulsions.

1840s: A tincture of cannabis (cannabis in alcohol) becomes available as a medicine in Europe and in the United States.

1842: Dr. O'Shaughnessy brings cannabis back to Europe, where it becomes popular for treatment of depression, asthma, migraine headaches, female disorders, nerve pain, and muscle spasms.

1840–1900: Numerous reports of the therapeutic and medicinal benefits of cannabis are published in medical literature. In 1894, the *Report of the Indian Hemp Drugs Commission* is published, concluding that "moderate use practically produces no ill effects."[1]

1911: Massachusetts passes a law making it illegal to sell or possess cannabis and other "hypnotic" drugs without a prescription; New York and Maine follow suit in 1914. Between 1915 and 1927, eight more states pass anti-cannabis laws.

1936: The film *Reefer Madness* is released to warn parents about the dangers of cannabis use, brainwashing an entire generation with misinformation.

1937: Harry Anslinger, the first commissioner of the US Treasury Department's Federal Bureau of Narcotics, gets the Marihuana Tax Act of 1937 passed. Taxes are placed on anyone who wants to use hemp industrially or cannabis medically, and those who do not comply are fined heavily or jailed for tax evasion.

1938: New York's mayor Fiorello La Guardia appoints a committee of scientists to assess the medical, sociological, and psychological aspects of cannabis use in New York City.

1941: Cannabis is removed from the National Formulary and is no longer available for medical use in the US.

1944: Mayor La Guardia's study of cannabis reports no proof of major crime associated with cannabis, no association with aggression or antisocial behavior, and no evidence of personality change or sexual overstimulation. The study is denounced and ignored.

1951: Congress passes the Boggs Act, which sets harsh mandatory sentences for violations of the Marihuana Tax Act of 1937.

1964: Israeli researchers isolate and identify delta-9-tetrahydrocannabinol as the psychoactive compound in the cannabis plant.

1970: Congress and President Nixon pass the Controlled Substances Act into law, which places cannabis into the most restrictive category, Schedule I, defined as having no medicinal value, a high potential for abuse, and a high potential for addiction.

1972: The National Organization for the Reform of Marijuana Laws (NORML) launches the first petition to reschedule marijuana from Schedule I to Schedule II. The petition was eventually given a hearing in 1986 and was ultimately denied.

1973: Researchers led by UCLA pulmonologist Dr. Donald Tashkin find that both smoked cannabis and oral THC cause an opening of the pulmonary airways, not a constriction of the lungs as was previously presumed. Oregon is the first state to decriminalize cannabis.

1975: Researchers report in the *Journal of the National Cancer Institute* that some cannabinoids have the ability to shrink tumors in a dose-dependent manner.

1976: Glaucoma patient Robert Randall files a lawsuit against the Food and Drug Administration (FDA), the Drug Enforcement Administration (DEA), the National Institute on Drug Abuse (NIDA), the

Department of Justice (DOJ), and the Department of Health, Education and Welfare (HEW), claiming that cultivation of marijuana, for which he is being prosecuted, is a medical necessity. The charges against him are dropped, and federal agencies begin providing him with FDA-approved medical marijuana. Although he wins this case, the government tries to prevent him from gaining legal access to marijuana, and after filing another lawsuit in 1978, he gains access to medical marijuana through a federal pharmacy.

Mid-1980s: Randall's case leads to the FDA's Investigational New Drug (IND) program, which under a "compassionate use" designation allows thirty patients to receive medical marijuana from the government. The program stops accepting patients in 1992 after President George H. W. Bush's administration decides to "get tough on drugs."

1988: The DEA's own administrative law judge, Francis L. Young, states that marijuana "is one of the safest therapeutically active substances known to man" and recommends that it be reclassified as a Schedule II drug. The DEA responds by setting new criteria for accepted medical use of a drug and refuses to reclassify cannabis.

1988: Researchers discover that rats have endogenous cannabinoid receptors, which leads to the mapping of the locations of a cannabinoid receptor system in a human in 1990 and the discovery of naturally occurring cannabis-like compounds, endocannabinoids, in the human brain in 1992.

1991: The federal program that was providing free cannabis to those approved under the FDA IND program is suspended after the number of applicants surges due to the AIDS epidemic. The first medical cannabis initiative, called Proposition P, passes in San Francisco with 79 percent of the vote as the AIDS epidemic surges.

1994: The DEA issues a final rejection of all pending requests to reclassify cannabis.

1995: NORML files another petition to change the Schedule I status of cannabis.

1996: California becomes the first state to pass a medical marijuana law with voter initiative Proposition 215, the Compassionate Use Act of 1996, getting 55.6 percent of the vote.

1998: Alaska, Oregon, and Washington pass medical cannabis laws.

1999: Maine passes a medical cannabis law.

2000: Colorado, Hawaii, and Nevada pass medical cannabis laws.

2002: Patients and patient advocates petition the DEA to reschedule cannabis. This is ultimately rejected nine years later in 2011.

2004: Montana and Vermont pass medical cannabis laws.

2006: Rhode Island passes a medical cannabis law.

2007: New Mexico passes a medical cannabis law.

2008: Michigan passes a medical cannabis law.

2009: US attorney general Eric Holder states the Obama administration will end federal raids of cannabis dispensaries in states with medical cannabis laws.

2010: Arizona, New Jersey, and Washington, DC, all pass medical cannabis laws. Oregon reclassifies cannabis at the state level as a Schedule II drug.

2011: Delaware and Arizona pass medical cannabis laws.

2012: Colorado and Washington voters pass adult-use cannabis laws. The country of Uruguay legalizes cannabis for adult use. Washington, DC, decriminalizes personal use and possession of cannabis for anyone over twenty-one years of age. Connecticut and Massachusetts pass laws legalizing medical use of cannabis.

2013: A federal appeals court rejects a petition from three medical cannabis advocacy groups that seek to reclassify cannabis. Illinois and New Hampshire pass medical cannabis laws. The US Department of Justice issues the Cole Memorandum, stating it will not enforce federal cannabis prohibition in states that have legalized cannabis in some form.

2014: The federal Farm Bill passes, otherwise known as the Agricultural Act of 2014, which states that hemp is defined as containing 0.3 or less percent THC and allows for industrial hemp to be grown in state-sanctioned research programs. This opens the door for industrial hemp entrepreneurs to start selling hemp-derived CBD. The Rohrabacher-Farr Amendment is signed into federal law, prohibiting the Justice Department from spending funds to interfere with the implementation of state medical cannabis laws. Maryland, Minnesota, and New York all pass laws legalizing medical use of cannabis. Alaska, Oregon, and Washington, DC, all pass laws allowing for adult use of cannabis. Florida, Alabama, Iowa, Kentucky, Mississippi, Missouri, North Carolina, South Carolina, Tennessee, Utah, and Wisconsin all pass CBD-only laws.

2015: The FDA sends cease and desist letters to numerous companies making medical claims about hemp-derived CBD products after tests reveal that the majority of products do not contain CBD. The country of Jamaica decriminalizes cannabis. Puerto Rico passes a medical cannabis law. Texas, Wyoming, Georgia, Oklahoma, and Virginia all pass CBD-only laws.

2016: California, Nevada, Maine, Vermont, and Massachusetts all pass adult-use cannabis laws. Arkansas, Florida, North Dakota, Ohio, Louisiana, West Virginia, and Pennsylvania all pass laws legalizing medical use of cannabis.

2017: The country of Argentina begins to provide free cannabis for medical conditions. Indiana passes a CBD-only law.

2018: US attorney general Jeff Sessions rescinds the Cole Memorandum and other Obama administration policies, effectively removing all assurances that cannabis companies and patients in states with cannabis laws will be protected from federal arrest and prosecution. Oklahoma passes a medical cannabis law. Vermont passes an adult-use cannabis law. Canada becomes the first major world economy to legalize adult-use cannabis. South Korea and Thailand pass medical cannabis laws. Oklahoma, Utah, and Missouri expand their medical cannabis laws.

2019: The US House of Representatives passes a bill that would protect financial institutions offering banking services to cannabis-related businesses; however, the bill stalls in the US Senate. Kansas passes a CBD-only law. Hawaii decriminalizes cannabis. Illinois legalizes recreational sales through an act of the state legislature and begins the expungement of 700,000 cannabis-related police records and court convictions.

2020: Virginia decriminalizes cannabis.

Appendix B

The Pharmacokinetics of Phytocannabinoids

Pharmacokinetics is the branch of pharmacology concerned with the movement of drugs within the human body. The pharmacokinetics of cannabis refers to the absorption, distribution, and metabolism of cannabinoids. Since cannabis can be taken in many ways, the method of delivery influences how much is absorbed and metabolized. Delivery methods include inhalation (smoking and vaporizing), ingestion, sublingual tinctures, topical application, rectal suppositories, and transdermal patches, discussed in detail in chapter 5. The information included here reviews the scientific literature exploring how cannabis acts in the body once it is taken internally.

The Different Delivery Methods

Inhalation

When inhaled, the absorption of THC and CBD through the lungs is rapid and levels of both in plasma can be detected within seconds, peaking within three to ten minutes.[1] Maximum concentrations are higher compared to ingestion.[2] The bioavailability (how much of the compound is actually used by the body) of inhaled THC varies from 10 to 35 percent due to variables such as the dose inhaled, the depth of inhalation, and the length of time the breath is held.[3] Bioavailability of inhaled CBD has been measured at approximately 31 percent.[4] Inhaling cannabis is the most efficient method of delivery, and experienced users have been shown to exhibit increased efficiency compared to occasional users.[5]

Ingestion

Oral absorption of THC and CBD is poor and unpredictable, with absorption rates based on numerous variables, such as the person's stomach contents, including gastric acid, the dose ingested, the carrier medium, and the presence of other drugs.[6] Bioavailability is low with oral ingestion and has been documented at 4 to 20 percent.[7] Oral THC undergoes extensive metabolism in the liver (called the first pass effect).[8] Peak plasma levels of THC have been reported between two and six hours after ingestion.[9] CBD has similar low bioavailability when orally ingested.[10] A recent study showed that taking cannabinoids with fatty food slightly delays the onset of action but increases the overall cannabinoid exposure, with female subjects having a greater peak plasma concentration.[11]

Sublingual Tinctures

Sublingual administration of THC and CBD has highly variable rates of absorption and is difficult to measure, as some of the product may be swallowed, which can affect bioavailability. Studies of nabiximols (Sativex) report excellent bioavailability if the oil is held sublingually and allowed to absorb.[12] These studies also report resulting plasma concentrations of THC from sublingual administration to be higher than from oral ingestion but lower when compared to inhaled THC. The bioavailability of sublingual THC is higher than the bioavailability of sublingual CBD.[13]

Topical Application

Topical application of cannabinoids is difficult because they are lipophilic (fat loving) and do not penetrate the deeper layers of the aqueous skin efficiently; however, if they are prepared properly, they can have effects at the local application site. Bioavailability studies in humans on topical use of cannabis have not been performed, but the permeability of

CBD was found to be ten times higher than that of both delta-9-THC and delta-8-THC, consistent with CBD being less lipophilic.[14]

Rectal Suppositories

The pharmacokinetics of rectal administration based on limited studies report that THC by itself is not absorbed rectally.[15] When THC was combined with a chemical compound called hemisuccinate, which was performed in a laboratory and is not currently available to patients, the bioavailability from rectal suppositories was double that of the oral route. To date, the only study looking at rectal bioavailability of CBD reported improved colitis symptoms in mice if rectal CBD was given prior to the insult causing the colitis; in this report, rectal CBD was more effective than oral CBD at reducing the changes in the gut due to colitis.[16]

Transdermal Patches

Transdermal differs from topical in that transdermal application is meant to penetrate deeper through the skin with the potential for penetration into the bloodstream, whereas topical application can be expected to work locally where it is applied. The pharmacokinetics of cannabinoid delivery with this method is limited. Likely the hydrophobic (not soluble in water) cannabinoids require the addition of a chemical "permeation enhancer" so the compounds can penetrate the aqueous layer of the skin to reach the bloodstream. In one report, delta-8-THC delivered by transdermal patch in both animals and humans achieved a steady-state level in plasma in 1.4 hours and maintained this level for 48 hours.[17] This study also reported that the permeability of CBD and CBN was greater than that of delta-8-THC.

THC Distribution and Metabolism

Since THC is highly lipophilic (fat loving and not water soluble), after absorption it is initially distributed and taken up by tissues that are highly perfused, such as the heart, lung, brain, and liver. Over time, THC redistributes into fatty tissue and may be retained there for weeks.[18] THC is broken down in the liver into numerous compounds. The primary breakdown products are 11-hydroxy-THC (11-OH-THC) and 11-carboxy-THC (11-COOH-THC). The amount of 11-hydroxy-THC formed after inhalation is relatively small, but quite large after oral ingestion of THC, as blood containing absorbed THC from the intestines passes through the liver. Whereas 11-hydroxy-THC is intoxicating and sedating, 11-carboxy-THC is not.[19]

THC and its metabolites are excreted mainly in feces and urine.[20] The elimination of one dose of THC from the body takes approximately three to five days. THC and its metabolites are stored in the body's fat tissues. When the metabolites move out of the fat, they bind to a sugar compound and become slightly soluble in water, and are then eliminated in feces and urine. The presence of THC metabolites in the body's fat tissues causes no intoxicating effects. If THC is used regularly, its metabolites will accumulate in the body and continue to be excreted for months after use. Studies show that there is extreme variation in excretion patterns for different individuals.[21]

CBD Distribution and Metabolism

CBD is taken up by the brain and adipose tissue. It is highly protein bound, and about 10 percent of the absorbed CBD in the body is bound to circulating red blood cells. CBD is metabolized in the liver, where it is hydroxylated to 7-hydroxy-CBD by the cytochrome P450 system. This breakdown product is then broken down further in the liver and excreted primarily in feces with some excretion in urine.[22] CBD is reported to have a long elimination half-life of approximately two to five days.[23]

Appendix C

Phytocannabinoids and Their Effects

Phytocannabinoid	Acronym	Medicinal effects	Helpful facts
Cannabichromene	CBC	Anti-acne	Not intoxicating
		Antibacterial	Allows endocannabinoids to last longer
		Anticancer	
		Antidepressant	
		Antifungal	
		Anti-inflammatory	
		Relieves pain	
Cannabidiol	CBD	Antibacterial	Not intoxicating
		Anticancer	No tolerance or withdrawal
		Anticonvulsant	Alerting effect in lower doses; sedating effect in higher doses
		Anti-inflammatory	Can be used to treat THC withdrawal
		Antioxidant	
		Antipsychotic	Allows brain-produced endocannabinoids to last longer by inhibiting the enzyme called fatty acid amide hydroxylase (FAAH), which breaks down the endocannabinoid
		Neuroprotectant	
		Promotes bone growth	
		Reduces anxiety and depression	
		Reduces/eliminates nausea and vomiting	
		Reduces intraocular pressure	
		Reduces spasticity and muscle spasms	
		Relieves chronic pain	
		Stimulates appetite	

Phytocannabinoid	Acronym	Medicinal effects	Helpful facts
Cannabidiolic acid	CBDA	Antianxiety Antidepressant Anti-inflammatory Potential anticonvulsant Reduces/eliminates nausea and vomiting Relieves pain	Not intoxicating Found in raw cannabis flowers Converts to CBD with heat More potent than CBD for antinausea effects Pain relief may be enhanced in combination with THC
Cannabidivarin	CBDV	Anticonvulsant Relieves neuropathic pain	Not intoxicating May help in Rett syndrome
Cannabigerol	CBG	Antibacterial/anti-MRSA Anticancer Antidepressant Anti-inflammatory Antioxidant Anti-psoriasis Neuroprotectant Promotes bone growth Reduces bladder spasms Reduces bowel inflammation Reduces intraocular pressure Reduces/eliminates nausea and vomiting Stimulates appetite	Not intoxicating Found in higher amounts in hemp May block antinausea effects of CBD May enhance anti-inflammatory effects of CBD

Phytocannabinoid	Acronym	Medicinal effects	Helpful facts
Cannabinol	CBN	Antibacterial Anticonvulsant Promotes bone growth Reduces intraocular pressure Relieves pain Stimulates appetite	A breakdown product of THC CBN content increases as THC degrades over time May enhance the intoxicating effects of THC Not present in freshly cut flowers
Delta-8-tetrahydrocannabinol	Δ^8-THC	Antianxiety Anticancer Neuroprotectant Reduces intraocular pressure Reduces nausea and vomiting Relieves pain Stimulates appetite	Not intoxicating
Delta-9-tetrahydrocannabinol	Δ^9-THC	Anticancer Anti-inflammatory Antioxidant Improves sleep/sedating Neuroprotectant Reduces anxiety and depression Reduces/eliminates nausea and vomiting Reduces intraocular pressure Reduces spasticity and muscle spasms Relieves chronic pain Stimulates appetite	The most prominent phytocannabinoid Results from the heating of THCA Intoxicating Mimics brain-produced endocannabinoids by binding to cannabinoid receptors Tolerance can develop with chronic use Withdrawal can occur with cessation of chronic heavy use

Phytocannabinoid	Acronym	Medicinal effects	Helpful facts
Tetrahydrocannabinolic acid	THCA	Anticancer	Not intoxicating
		Anticonvulsant	The main compound in raw cannabis flowers
		Anti-inflammatory	Converts to THC with heat
		Antispasmodic	Found to be the main phytocannabinoid influencing anti-inflammatory effects in the colon
		Blocks anticipatory nausea	
		Neuroprotectant	
		Potential antidepressant	
Delta-9-tetrahydrocannabivarin	THCV	Anticancer	Not intoxicating in low doses
		Anticonvulsant	May be beneficial for Parkinson's disease when combined with CBD
		Anti-inflammatory	
		Antioxidant	
		Antipsychotic	
		Appetite suppressant	
		Neuroprotectant	
		Potentially improves glucose tolerance and increases insulin sensitivity	
		Relieves pain	

Appendix D

Terpenoids and Their Effects[1]

Terpenoid	Also found in	Medicinal effects	Aroma	Synergistic with
Alpha-bisabolol	Chamomile	Anticancer[†] Anti-inflammatory Neuroprotectant	Floral	Unknown
Alpha-pinene *The most common terpene in all plants	Basil Dill Eucalyptus Parsley Pine trees Rosemary Sage	Analgesic Anti-inflammatory Bronchodilator Increases focus and alertness Increases permeability of blood–brain barrier Reduces THC-induced memory loss	Pine "Skunky"	CBD—enhances anti-inflammatory effect THC—enhances bronchodilatory effect
Beta-caryophyllene *Often found in CBD-rich chemovars *Activates the CB₂ receptor	Basil Black pepper Cinnamon Cloves Hops Lavender Oregano Rosemary	Analgesic Antibacterial Anticancer[†] Antifungal Anti-inflammatory Anti-itching Antimalarial Antioxidant Gastrointestinal relief May reduce alcohol intake	Spicy Woodsy	THC—enhances gastric cell protection CBD—enhances anti-inflammatory effect

*Activates the CB_2 receptor

Terpenoid	Also found in	Medicinal effects	Aroma	Synergistic with
Borneol	Camphor Cinnamon Mint Rosemary Wormwood	Analgesic Antibacterial Bronchodilator Sedating	Camphor	Unknown
Caryophyllene oxide	Basil Cloves Eucalyptus Hops Lavender Lemon balm Oregano Pepper Rosemary Salvia	Analgesic Anticancer[+] Antifungal Anti-inflammatory Antioxidant Antiviral	Woodsy	Unknown
Cineole	Basil Eucalyptus Mugwort Rosemary Tea tree Wormwood	Analgesic Antibacterial/antifungal Anticancer[+] Antidepressant Anti-inflammatory Antioxidant Stimulating due to increased cerebral blood flow, enhancing memory and cognitive learning	Camphor Minty	Unknown

Terpenoid	Also found in	Medicinal effects	Aroma	Synergistic with
Citronellol	Basil Chamomile Geraniums Lavender Lemongrass Roses Sandalwood	Analgesic Antibacterial/antifungal Anticancer[+] Anti-inflammatory Antioxidant Promotes wound healing Sedating	Citrus Floral Fruity Rose	Unknown
Geraniol	Geraniums Lemons Roses	Antibacterial/antifungal Anticancer[+] Anti-inflammatory Antioxidant	Rose	Unknown
Guaiol	Cypress trees Guaiacum	Anti-inflammatory Antimicrobial	Pine Rose Woodsy	Unknown
Humulene ***Isomer** **of beta-caryophyllene**	Basil Coriander Ginger Ginseng Hops Sage Spearmint	Analgesic Anticancer[+] Antibacterial Anti-inflammatory Appetite suppressant	Earthy Herbaceous	Unknown

Terpenoid	Also found in	Medicinal effects	Aroma	Synergistic with
Limonene ***The second most common terpenoid in cannabis**	Caraway seeds Citrus rinds Dill seeds Juniper berries Peppermint Rosemary	Analgesic Antianxiety Anticancer* Antidepressant Anti-inflammatory Antioxidant Bronchodilator GERD suppressant	Citrus Orange Spicy	CBD—enhances antidepressant and antianxiety effects CBD and CBG—enhances anticancer† effect THC—enhances anti-GERD effect
Linalool ***A precursor ingredient in the formation of vitamin E** ***The most powerful sedative of all terpenoids**	Birch trees Citrus Coriander Lavender Rosewood	Active against acne bacteria Analgesic Antianxiety Antibacterial/antifungal Anticonvulsant Antidepressant Anti-inflammatory Antimalarial	Citrus Floral Spicy	CBD—enhances antianxiety and analgesic effects CBD/THCV/CBDV—enhances anticonvulsant effect THC—enhances sedation and analgesic effects
Myrcene ***The most common terpenoid found in cannabis** ***Not found in hemp**	Bay leaves Eucalyptus Hops Lemongrass Mangoes Parsley Wild thyme	Analgesic Antianxiety Antibacterial Anticancer† Antidepressant Anti-inflammatory Antioxidant Muscle relaxant Sedating/hypnotic	Clove Earthy Fruity	CBD—enhances anti-inflammatory effect CBG—enhances anti-inflammatory effect THC—may enhance effects of THC

Terpenoid	Also found in	Medicinal effects	Aroma	Synergistic with
Nerolidol	Ginger Jasmine Lavender Lemongrass Oranges Tea tree	Antifungal Antimalarial Sedating	Earthy Fruity Woodsy	THC/CBN—enhances sedation
Ocimene	Basil Hops Lavender Mangoes Mint Oregano Parsley Pepper	Antibacterial/antifungal Anti-inflammatory Antiviral Decongestant	Citrus Clove Thyme Woodsy	Unknown
Phytol ***A breakdown product of chlorophyll**	Green tea Wild lettuce	Antifungal Immunosuppressant Sedating	Balsamic Floral	Unknown
Terpineol ***Often found in chemovars high in pinene**	Eucalyptus Lilac blossoms Lime blossoms Pine trees	Analgesic Antianxiety Antibacterial/antifungal Anticancer† Anti-inflammatory Antioxidant Antiviral Sedating	Citrus Floral Lilac	Unknown

Terpenoid	Also found in	Medicinal effects	Aroma	Synergistic with
Terpinolene	Apples	Analgesic	Earthy	Unknown
	Coriander	Antibacterial/antifungal	Pine	
	Cumin	Anticancer[†]	Woodsy	
	Lilac blossoms	Antioxidant		
	Nutmeg	Gastrointestinal relief		
	Tea tree	Sedating		
Valencene	Grapefruits	Antiallergy	Citrus	Unknown
	Oranges	Anti-inflammatory	Spicy	
	Tangerines			

[†] Note that the anticancer effects of terpenes are likely to require much higher doses than occur naturally in cannabis (J. K. Booth et al., "Terpenes in *Cannabis Sativa*: From Plant Genome to Humans," *Plant Science* [20˙9]: 67–72).

Notes

Part I: The Science of Cannabis

Chapter 1: The Cannabis Plant

1. M. A. ElSohly et al., "Phytochemistry of *Cannabis Sativa L.*," in *Progress in the Chemistry of Organic Natural Products* 103 (2017): 1–36.
2. S. Chandra, "New Trends in Cannabis Potency in USA and Europe During the Last Decade (2008–2017)," *European Archives of Psychiatry and Clinical Neuroscience* 269, no. 1 (2019): 5–15.
3. E. B. Russo, "Taming THC: Potential Cannabis Synergy and Phytocannabinoid–Terpenoid Entourage Effects," *British Journal of Pharmacology* 163, no. 7 (2011): 1344–64.
4. E. B. Russo et al., "A Tale of Two Cannabinoids: The Therapeutic Rationale for Combining Tetrahydrocannabinol and Cannabidiol," *Medical Hypotheses* 66, no. 2 (2006): 234–46.
5. R. Brenneisen, "Chemistry and Analysis of Phytocannabinoids and Other *Cannabis* Constituents," in *Forensic Science and Medicine: Marijuana and the Cannabinoid,* ed. M. A. ElSohly (Totowa, NJ: Humana Press, 2007), 17–49.
6. B. Singh et al., "Plant Terpenes: Defense Responses, Phylogenetic Analysis, Regulation, and Clinical Applications," *3 Biotech* 5, no. 2 (2015): 129–51.
7. L. M. Lopes Campêlo et al., "Sedative, Anxiolytic, and Antidepressant Activities of Citrus Limon (Burn) Essential Oil in Mice," *Die Pharmazie—An International Journal of Pharmaceutical Sciences* 66, no. 8 (2011): 623–27.
8. K. H. C. Baser et al., eds., *Handbook of Essential Oils: Science, Technology and Application* (Boca Raton, FL; London; New York: CRC Press/Taylor and Francis Group, 2010), 1021.
9. M.-H. Pan et al., "Anti-inflammatory Activity of Natural Dietary Flavonoids," *Food and Function* 1, no. 1 (2010): 15–31.
10. H. D. Woo et al., "Dietary Flavonoids and Gastric Cancer Risk in a Korean Population," *Nutrients* 6, no. 11 (2014): 4961–73.
11. M. L. Neuhouser, "Dietary Flavonoids and Cancer Risk: Evidence from Human Population Studies," *Nutrition and Cancer* 50, no. 1 (2004): 1–7.
12. Y.-J. Liu et al., "Dietary Flavonoids Intake and Risk of Type 2 Diabetes: A Meta-Analysis of Prospective Cohort Studies," *Clinical Nutrition* (Edinburgh, Scotland) 33, no. 1 (2014): 59–63.
13. F. Comelli et al., "Antihyperalgesic Effect of a *Cannabis Sativa* Extract in a Rat Model of Neuropathic Pain: Mechanisms Involved," *Phytotherapy Research* 22, no. 8 (2008): 1017–24.
14. A. Pollio, "The Name of *Cannabis:* A Short Guide for Nonbotanists," *Cannabis and Cannabinoid Research* 1, no. 1 (2016): 234–38.

15. M. A. Lee, "Marijuana, Industrial Hemp, and the Vagaries of Federal Law," Project CBD, accessed February 2020, https://www.projectcbd.org/article/sourcing-cbd-marijuana-industrial-hemp-vagaries -federal-law.

Chapter 2: The Endocannabinoid System

1. Y. Gaoni et al., "Isolation, Structure, and Partial Synthesis of an Active Constituent of Hashish," *Journal of the American Chemical Society* 86, no. 8 (1964): 1646–47.
2. W. A. Devane et al., "Determination and Characterization of a Cannabinoid Receptor in Rat Brain," *Molecular Pharmacology* 34, no. 5 (1988): 605–13.
3. W. A. Devane et al., "Isolation and Structure of a Brain Constituent That Binds to the Cannabinoid Receptor," *Science* (New York) 258, no. 5090 (1992): 1946–49.
4. S. Munro et al., "Molecular Characterization of a Peripheral Receptor for Cannabinoids," *Nature* 365, no. 6441 (1993): 61–65.
5. R. Mechoulam et al., "Identification of an Endogenous 2-Monoglyceride, Present in Canine Gut, That Binds to Cannabinoid Receptors," *Biochemical Pharmacology* 50, no. 1 (1995): 83–90.
6. V. Di Marzo et al., "Endocannabinoids: Endogenous Cannabinoid Receptor Ligands with Neuro-modulatory Action," *Trends in Neurosciences* 21, no. 12 (1998): 521–28.
7. P. B. Sparling et al., "Exercise Activates the Endocannabinoid System," *Neuroreport* 14, no. 17 (2003): 2209–11; and C. J. Fowler, "The Cannabinoid System and Its Pharmacological Manipulation—a Review, with Emphasis upon the Uptake and Hydrolysis of Anandamide," *Fundamental and Clinical Pharmacology* 20, no. 6 (2006): 549–62.
8. V. Di Marzo, "'Endocannabinoids' and Other Fatty Acid Derivatives with Cannabimimetic Properties: Biochemistry and Possible Physiopathological Relevance," *Biochimica et Biophysica Acta* 1392, nos. 2–3 (1998): 153–75.
9. O. Aizpurua-Olaizola et al., "Targeting the Endocannabinoid System: Future Therapeutic Strategies," *Drug Discovery Today* 22, no. 1 (2017): 105–10.
10. R. Mechoulam, "Plant Cannabinoids: A Neglected Pharmacological Treasure Trove," *British Journal of Pharmacology* 146, no. 7 (2005): 913–15.
11. P. Strohbeck-Kuehner et al., "Cannabis Improves Symptoms of ADHD," *Cannabinoids* 3, no. 1 (2008): 1–3.
12. D. Centonze et al., "Altered Anandamide Degradation in Attention-Deficit/Hyperactivity Disorder," *Neurology* 72, no. 17 (2009): 1526–27.
13. M. Herkenham et al., "Cannabinoid Receptor Localization in Brain," *PNAS* 87, no. 5 (1990): 1932–36; G. Ferguson et al., "Review Article: Sleep, Pain, and Cannabis," *Journal of Sleep Disorders and Therapy* 4, no. 2 (2015): 191; and I. Svíženská et al., "Cannabinoid Receptors 1 and 2 (CB_1 and CB_2), Their Distribution, Ligands, and Functional Involvement in Nervous System Structures—a Short Review," *Pharmacology Biochemistry and Behavior* 90, no. 4 (2008): 501–11.
14. E. B. Russo, "Clinical Endocannabinoid Deficiency Reconsidered: Current Research Supports the Theory in Migraine, Fibromyalgia, Irritable Bowel, and Other Treatment-Resistant Syndromes," *Cannabis and Cannabinoid Research* 1, no. 1 (2016): 154–65; P. Sarchielli et al., "Endocannabinoids in Chronic Migraine: CSF Findings Suggest a System Failure," *Neuropsychopharmacology* 32, no. 6 (2007): 1384–90; M. N. Hill et al., "Reductions in Circulating Endocannabinoid Levels in Individuals with Post-traumatic Stress Disorder Following Exposure to the World Trade Center Attacks," *Psychoneuroendocrinology* 38, no. 12 (2013): 2952–61; M. N. Hill et al., "Is There a Role for the Endocannabinoid System in the Etiology and Treatment of Melancholic Depression?," *Behavioural Pharmacology* 16, nos. 5–6 (2005): 333–52; A. F. Giuffrida et al., "Cerebrospinal Anan-

Notes

damide Levels Are Elevated in Acute Schizophrenia and Are Inversely Correlated with Psychotic Symptoms," *Neuropsychopharmacology* 29, no. 11 (2004): 2108–14; and S. C. Smith et al., "Clinical Endocannabinoid Deficiency (CECD) Revisited," *Neuroendocrinology Letters* 35, no. 3 (2014): 198–201.

15. C. H. Ashton et al., "Endocannabinoid System Dysfunction in Mood and Related Disorders," *Acta Psychiatrica Scandinavica* 124, no. 4 (2011): 250–61; A.-Q. Yin et al., "Integrating Endocannabinoid Signaling in the Regulation of Anxiety and Depression," *Acta Pharmacologica Sinica* 40, no. 3 (2019): 336–41; J. Lazary et al., "Genetic Analysis of the Endocannabinoid Signalling in Association with Anxious and Depressive Phenotype," in *European Neuropsychopharmacology* 27, no. 4 (2017): S600; B. L. Hungund et al., "Upregulation of CB_1 Receptors and Agonist-Stimulated [^{35}S] GTPYS Binding in the Prefrontal Cortex of Depressed Suicide Victims," *Molecular Psychiatry* 9, no. 2 (2004): 184–90; and C. J. Hillard et al., "Contributions of Endocannabinoid Signaling to Psychiatric Disorders in Humans: Genetic and Biochemical Evidence," *Neuroscience* 204 (2012): 207–29.

16. D. Centonze et al., "The Endocannabinoid System Is Dysregulated in Multiple Sclerosis and in Experimental Autoimmune Encephalomyelitis," *Brain* 130, pt. 10 (2007): 2543–53; J. C. Sipe et al., "Reduced Endocannabinoid Immune Modulation by a Common Cannabinoid 2 (CB2) Receptor Gene Polymorphism: Possible Risk for Autoimmune Disorders," *Journal of Leukocyte Biology* 78, no. 1 (2005): 231–38; and G. A. Cabral et al., "Emerging Role of the Cannabinoid Receptor CB_2 in Immune Regulation: Therapeutic Prospects for Neuroinflammation," *Expert Reviews in Molecular Medicine* 11 (2009): e3.

17. F. Montecucco et al., "At the Heart of the Matter: The Endocannabinoid System in Cardiovascular Function and Dysfunction," *Trends in Pharmacological Sciences* 33, no. 6 (2012): 331–40; P. Pacher et al., "Modulation of the Endocannabinoid System in Cardiovascular Disease: Therapeutic Potential and Limitations," *Hypertension* 52, no. 4 (2008): 601–7; and P. Pacher et al., "The Emerging Role of the Endocannabinoid System in Cardiovascular Disease," *Seminars in Immunopathology* 31, no. 1 (2009): 63–77.

18. I. Kaufmann et al., "Enhanced Anandamide Plasma Levels in Patients with Complex Regional Pain Syndrome Following Traumatic Injury: A Preliminary Report," *European Surgical Research* 43, no. 4 (2009): 325–29.

19. P. Monteleone et al., "Blood Levels of the Endocannabinoid Anandamide Are Increased in Anorexia Nervosa and in Binge-Eating Disorder, but Not in Bulimia Nervosa," *Neuropsychopharmacology* 30, no. 6 (2005): 1216–21.

20. M. J. Wallace et al., "The Endogenous Cannabinoid System Regulates Seizure Frequency and Duration in a Model of Temporal Lobe Epilepsy," *Journal of Pharmacology and Experimental Therapeutics* 307, no. 1 (2003): 129–37; and A. Ludányi et al., "Downregulation of the CB_1 Cannabinoid Receptor and Related Molecular Elements of the Endocannabinoid System in Epileptic Human Hippocampus," *Journal of Neuroscience* 28, no. 12 (2008): 2976–90.

21. E. Fride et al., "Endocannabinoids and Food Intake: Newborn Suckling and Appetite Regulation in Adulthood," *Experimental Biology and Medicine* (Maywood, NJ) 230, no. 4 (2005): 225–34.

22. I. Kaufmann et al., "Anandamide and Neutrophil Function in Patients with Fibromyalgia," *Psychoneuroendocrinology* 33, no. 5 (2008): 676–85; and C. Fede et al., "Expression of the Endocannabinoid Receptors in Human Fascial Tissue," *European Journal of Histochemistry* 60, no. 2 (2016): 2643.

23. M. D. Sepers et al., "Endocannabinoid-Specific Impairment in Synaptic Plasticity in Striatum of Huntington's Disease Mouse Model," *Journal of Neuroscience* 38, no. 3 (2018): 544–54.

24. M. A. Storr et al., "The Role of the Endocannabinoid System in the Pathophysiology and Treatment of Irritable Bowel Syndrome," *Neurogastroenterology and Motility* 20, no. 8 (2008): 857–68; and M. Pesce et al., "Endocannabinoid-Related Compounds in Gastrointestinal Diseases," *Journal of Cellular and Molecular Medicine* 22, no. 2 (2018): 706–15.

25. Sarchielli et al., "Endocannabinoids in Chronic Migraine," 1384–90; and Z. Volfe et al., "Cannabinoids Block Release of Serotonin from Platelets Induced by Plasma from Migraine Patients," *International Journal of Clinical Pharmacology Research* 5, no. 4 (1985): 243–46.

26. V. Chiurchiù et al., "The Endocannabinoid System and Its Therapeutic Exploitation in Multiple Sclerosis: Clues for Other Neuroinflammatory Diseases," *Progress in Neurobiology* 160 (2018): 82–100; and M. Di Filippo et al., "Abnormalities in the Cerebrospinal Fluid Levels of Endocannabinoids in Multiple Sclerosis," *Journal of Neurology, Neurosurgery, and Psychiatry* 79, no. 11 (2008): 1224–29.

27. M. A. Sticht et al., "Endocannabinoid Mechanisms Influencing Nausea," *International Review of Neurobiology* 125 (2015): 127–62; and A. Choukèr et al., "Motion Sickness, Stress, and the Endocannabinoid System," *PLoS One* 5, no. 5 (2010): e10752.

28. A. Giuffrida et al., "The Endocannabinoid System and Parkinson Disease," in *The Endocannabinoid System*, ed. E. Murillo-Rodriguez (Cambridge, MA: Academic Press, 2017), 63–81.

29. D. Koethe et al., "Familial Abnormalities of Endocannabinoid Signaling in Schizophrenia," *World Journal of Biological Psychiatry* 20, no. 2 (2019): 117–25; and F. M. Leweke et al., "Role of the Endocannabinoid System in the Pathophysiology of Schizophrenia: Implications for Pharmacological Intervention," *CNS Drugs* 32, no. 7 (2018): 605–19.

30. V. Di Marzo, "The Endocannabinoid System in Obesity and Type 2 Diabetes," *Diabetologia* 51, no. 8 (2008): 1356–67.

31. I. Matias et al., "Regulation, Function, and Dysregulation of Endocannabinoids in Models of Adipose and Beta-Pancreatic Cells and in Obesity and Hyperglycemia," *Journal of Clinical Endocrinology and Metabolism* 91, no. 8 (2006): 3171–80.

32. V. Di Marzo et al., "Changes in Plasma Endocannabinoid Levels in Viscerally Obese Men Following a 1 Year Lifestyle Modification Programme and Waist Circumference Reduction: Associations with Changes in Metabolic Risk Factors," *Diabetologia* 52, no. 2 (2009): 213–17.

33. A. H. Sam et al., "Rimonabant: From RIO to Ban," *Journal of Obesity* 2011 (2011): 432607.

34. L. K. Miller et al., "The Highs and Lows of Cannabinoid Receptor Expression in Disease: Mechanisms and Their Therapeutic Implications," *Pharmacological Reviews* 63, no. 3 (2011): 461–70.

35. M. R. Karlócai et al., "Redistribution of CB$_1$ Cannabinoid Receptors in the Acute and Chronic Phases of Pilocarpine-Induced Epilepsy," *PLoS One* 6, no. 11 (2011): e27196.

36. A. A. Izzo et al., "Cannabinoid CB$_1$-Receptor-Mediated Regulation of Gastrointestinal Motility in Mice in a Model of Intestinal Inflammation," *British Journal of Pharmacology* 134, no. 3 (2001): 563–70.

37. A. Siegling et al., "Cannabinoid CB$_1$ Receptor Upregulation in a Rat Model of Chronic Neuropathic Pain," *European Journal of Pharmacology* 415, no. 1 (2001): R5–7.

38. L. Navarro et al., "Potential Role of the Cannabinoid Receptor CB$_1$ in Rapid Eye Movement Sleep Rebound," *Neuroscience* 120, no. 3 (2003): 855–59

39. D. Siniscalco et al., "Cannabinoid Receptor Type 2, but Not Type 1, Is Up-Regulated in Peripheral Blood Mononuclear Cells of Children Affected by Autistic Disorders," *Journal of Autism and Developmental Disorders* 43, no. 11 (2013): 2686–95.

40. Hungund et al., "Upregulation of CB$_1$ Receptors and Agonist-Stimulated [^{35}S]GTPγS Binding," 184–90.

41. F. Rodriguez de Fonseca et al., "Downregulation of Rat Brain Cannabinoid Binding Sites After Chronic Delta-9-Tetrahydrocannabinol Treatment," *Pharmacology, Biochemistry, and Behavior* 47, no. 1 (1994): 33–40; and J. Hirvonen et al., "Reversible and Regionally Selective Downregulation of Brain Cannabinoid CB$_1$ Receptors in Chronic Daily Cannabis Smokers," *Molecular Psychiatry* 17, no. 6 (2012): 642.

42. Hirvonen et al., "Reversible and Regionally Selective Downregulation of Brain Cannabinoid CB$_1$ Receptors," 642.

Notes

Chapter 3: The Safety Profile of Cannabis

1. "New DEA Leader Suspects Marijuana Is Not as Bad as Heroin," *Cannabis News Report,* July 30, 2015, http://cannabisnewsreport.com/news/new-dea-leader-suspects-marijuana-is-not-as-bad-as-heroin-0045068/.

2. T. H. Mikuriya, "Physical, Mental, and Moral Effects of Marijuana: The Indian Hemp Drugs Commission Report," Schaffer Library of Drug Policy website, accessed May 14, 2020, http://www.druglibrary.org/schaffer/library/effects.htm.

3. Mayor's Committee on Marihuana, by the New York Academy of Medicine, *The Laguardia Committee Report New York, USA (1944): The Marihuana Problem in the City of New York* (City of New York, 1944).

4. D. L. Farnsworth, "Summary of the Report from the National Commission on Marihuana and Drug Abuse: Marihuana: A Signal of Misunderstanding," *Psychiatric Annals* 2, no. 5 (1972): 8–9.

5. Drug Enforcement Administration, Diversion Control Division, "Controlled Substance Schedules: Definition of Controlled Substance Schedules," https://www.deadiversion.usdoj.gov/schedules/#define.

6. US Department of Justice, Drug Enforcement Administration, "In the Matter of Marijuana Rescheduling Petition, Docket No. 86-22, Opinion and Recommended Ruling, Findings of Fact, Conclusions of Law, and Decision of Administrative Law Judge Francis L. Young," September 6, 1988, 58–59.

7. J. E. Joy et al., eds. *Marijuana and Medicine: Assessing the Science Base* (Washington, DC: National Academies Press, 1999).

8. "New Surgeon General Dr. Vivek Murthy: Measles Vaccine Is Safe and Effective," *CBS This Morning,* video, February 3, 2015, https://www.cbsnews.com/video/new-surgeon-general-dr-vivek-murthy-measles-vaccine-is-safe-and-effective/.

9. National Academies of Sciences, Engineering, and Medicine, *The Health Effects of Cannabis and Cannabinoids: The Current State of Evidence and Recommendations for Research* (Washington, DC: National Academies Press, 2017).

10. G. R. Thompson et al., "Comparison of Acute Oral Toxicity of Cannabinoids in Rats, Dogs, and Monkeys," *Toxicology and Applied Pharmacology* 25, no. 3 (1973): 363–72.

11. K. Kochanek et al., Centers for Disease Control and Prevention, "Deaths: Final Data for 2017," National Vital Statistics Reports, 68, no. 9 (June 24, 2019), accessed January 2020, https://www.cdc.gov/nchs/data/nvsr/nvsr68/nvsr68_09-508.pdf.

12. M. H. Meier et al., "Associations Between Cannabis Use and Physical Health Problems in Early Midlife," *JAMA Psychiatry* 73, no. 7 (2016): 731–40.

13. H. G. Pope et al., "Neuropsychological Performance in Long-Term Cannabis Users," *Archives of General Psychiatry* 58, no. 10 (2001): 909–15.

14. M. A. Ware et al., "Cannabis for the Management of Pain: Assessment of Safety Study (COMPASS)," *Journal of Pain* 16, no. 12 (2015): 1233–42.

15. S. A. Gruber et al., "Splendor in the Grass? A Pilot Study Assessing the Impact of Medical Marijuana on Executive Function," *Frontiers in Pharmacology* 7 (2016): 355.

16. S. A. Gruber et al., "The Grass Might Be Greener: Medical Marijuana Patients Exhibit Altered Brain Activity and Improved Executive Function After 3 Months of Treatment," *Frontiers in Pharmacology* 8 (2018): 983.

17. R. Abuhasira et al., "Epidemiological Characteristics, Safety, and Efficacy of Medical Cannabis in the Elderly," *European Journal of Internal Medicine* 49 (2018): 44–50.

18. S. Jafari et al., "Diagnosis and Treatment of Marijuana Dependence," *BCMJ* 58, no. 6 (2016): 315–17.

19. C. Lopez-Quintero et al., "Probability and Predictors of Transition from First Use to Dependence on Nicotine, Alcohol, Cannabis, and Cocaine: Results of the National Epidemiologic Survey on Alcohol and Related Conditions (NESARC)," *Drug and Alcohol Dependence* 115, nos. 1–2 (2011): 120–30.

20. A. Zehra et al., "Cannabis Addiction and the Brain: A Review," *Focus (American Psychiatric Publishing)* 17, no. 2 (2019): 169–82.

21. G. Katz et al., "Cannabis Withdrawal: A New Diagnostic Category in DSM-5," *Israel Journal of Psychiatry and Related Sciences* 51, no. 4 (2014): 270–75.

Chapter 4: The Medicinal Effects of Phytocannabinoids

1. Y. Gaoni et al., "Isolation, Structure, and Partial Synthesis of an Active Constituent of Hashish," *Journal of the American Chemical Society* 86, no. 8 (1964): 1646–47.

2. E. B. Russo, "Clinical Endocannabinoid Deficiency Reconsidered: Current Research Supports the Theory in Migraine, Fibromyalgia, Irritable Bowel, and Other Treatment-Resistant Syndromes," *Cannabis and Cannabinoid Research* 1, no. 1 (2016): 154–65; and F. A. Iannotti et al., "Endocannabinoids and Endocannabinoid-Related Mediators: Targets, Metabolism, and Role in Neurological Disorders," *Progress in Lipid Research* 62 (2016): 107–28.

3. C. Muller et al., "Cannabinoid Ligands Targeting TRP Channels," *Frontiers in Molecular Neuroscience* 11 (2019): 487.

4. W. Xiong et al., "Cannabinoid Potentiation of Glycine Receptors Contributes to Cannabis-Induced Analgesia," *Nature Chemical Biology* 7, no. 5 (2011): 296–303; and C. F. Burgos et al., "Structure and Pharmacologic Modulation of Inhibitory Glycine Receptors," *Molecular Pharmacology* 90, no. 3 (2016): 318–25.

5. S. Haj-Dahmane et al., "Modulation of the Serotonin System by Endocannabinoid Signaling," *Neuropharmacology* 61, no. 3 (2011): 414–20.

6. S. E. O'Sullivan, "An Update on PPAR Activation by Cannabinoids," *British Journal of Pharmacology* 173, no. 12 (2016): 1899–910.

7. N. Sotudeh et al., "Towards a Molecular Understanding of the Cannabinoid Related Orphan Receptor GPR18: A Focus on Its Constitutive Activity," *International Journal of Molecular Sciences* 20, no. 9 (2019): E2300.

8. E. Tudurí et al., "GPR55: A New Promising Target for Metabolism?," *Journal of Molecular Endocrinology* 58, no. 3 (2017): R191–202.

9. M. Kathmann et al., "Cannabidiol Is an Allosteric Modulator at Mu- and Delta-Opioid Receptors," *Naunyn-Schmiedeberg's Archives of Pharmacology* 372, no. 5 (2006): 354–61; and P. J. Vaysse et al., "Modulation of Rat Brain Opioid Receptors by Cannabinoids," *Journal of Pharmacology and Experimental Therapeutics* 241, no. 2 (1987): 534–39.

10. R. Mechoulam et al., "Hashish. I: The Structure of Cannabidiol," *Tetrahedron* 19, no. 12 (1963): 2073–78.

11. C. Ibeas Bih et al., "Molecular Targets of Cannabidiol in Neurological Disorders," *Neurotherapeutics* 12, no. 4 (2015): 699–730.

12. R. B. Laprairie et al., "Cannabidiol Is a Negative Allosteric Modulator of the Cannabinoid CB_1 Receptor," *British Journal of Pharmacology* 172, no. 20 (2015): 4790–805.

13. W. Xiong et al., "Cannabinoids Suppress Inflammatory and Neuropathic Pain by Targeting α3 Glycine Receptors," *Journal of Experimental Medicine* 209, no. 6 (2012): 1121–34.

14. T. Bakas et al., "The Direct Actions of Cannabidiol and 2-Arachidonoyl Glycerol at $GABA_A$ Receptors," *Pharmacological Research* 119 (2017): 358–70.

Notes

15. E. B. Russo et al., "Agonistic Properties of Cannabidiol at 5-HT1a Receptors," *Neurochemical Research* 30, no. 8 (2005): 1037–43.

16. R. Ramer et al., "COX-2 and PPAR-γ Confer Cannabidiol-Induced Apoptosis of Human Lung Cancer Cells," *Molecular Cancer Therapeutics* 12, no. 1 (2013): 69–82.

17. Ibeas Bih et al., "Molecular Targets of Cannabidiol in Neurological Disorders," 699–730.

18. M. Bazelot et al., "Investigating the Involvement of GPR55 Signaling in the Antiepileptic Effects of Cannabidiol," *Neurology* 86, suppl. 16 (2016): P5.244.

19. D. McHugh et al., "Delta-9-Tetrahydrocannabinol and N-Arachidonyl Glycine Are Full Agonists at GPR18 Receptors and Induce Migration in Human Endometrial HEC-1B Cells," *British Journal of Pharmacology* 165, no. 8 (2012): 2414–24.

20. A. S. Laun et al., "GPR3, GPR6, and GPR12 as Novel Molecular Targets: Their Biological Functions and Interaction with Cannabidiol," *Acta Pharmacologica Sinica* 40, no. 3 (2019): 300–8.

21. Kathmann et al., "Cannabidiol Is an Allosteric Modulator at Mu- and Delta-Opioid Receptors," 354–61; and Vaysse et al., "Modulation of Rat Brain Opioid Receptors by Cannabinoids," 534–39.

22. Ibeas Bih et al., "Molecular Targets of Cannabidiol in Neurological Disorders," 699–730.

23. Ibid.

24. C. J. Morgan et al., "Impact of Cannabidiol on the Acute Memory and Psychotomimetic Effects of Smoked Cannabis: Naturalistic Study," *British Journal of Psychiatry* 197, no. 4 (2010): 285–90; and A. Englund et al., "Cannabidiol Inhibits THC-Elicited Paranoid Symptoms and Hippocampal-Dependent Memory Impairment," *Journal of Psychopharmacology* 27, no. 1 (2013): 19–27.

25. R. Gallily et al., "Overcoming the Bell-Shaped Dose-Response of Cannabidiol by Using Cannabis Extract Enriched in Cannabidiol," *Pharmacology and Pharmacy* 6, no. 2 (2015): 75–85.

26. L. M. Bornheim et al., "Characterization of Cytochrome P450 3A Inactivation by Cannabidiol: Possible Involvement of Cannabidiol-Hydroxyquinone as a P450 Inactivator," *Chemical Research in Toxicology* 11, no. 10 (1998): 1209–16.

27. T. Etges et al., "An Observational Postmarketing Safety Registry of Patients in the UK, Germany, and Switzerland Who Have Been Prescribed Sativex® (THC:CBD, Nabiximols) Oromucosal Spray," *Therapeutics and Clinical Risk Management* 12 (2016): 1667.

28. R. G. Pertwee, "Cannabinoid Pharmacology: The First 66 Years," *British Journal of Pharmacology* 147, suppl. 1 (2006): S163–71.

29. R. G. Pertwee, "The Diverse CB_1 and CB_2 Receptor Pharmacology of Three Plant Cannabinoids: Delta-9-Tetrahydrocannabinol, Cannabidiol, and Delta-9-Tetrahydrocannabivarin," *British Journal of Pharmacology* 153, no. 2 (2008): 199–215.

30. L. De Petrocellis et al., "Effects of Cannabinoids and Cannabinoid–Enriched *Cannabis* Extracts on TRP Channels and Endocannabinoid Metabolic Enzymes," *British Journal of Pharmacology* 163, no. 7 (2011): 1479–94.

31. Pertwee, "The Diverse CB_1 and CB_2 Receptor Pharmacology," 199–215; L. E. Hollister, "Cannabidiol and Cannabinol in Man," *Experientia* 29, no. 7 (1973): 825–26; I. G. Karniol et al., "Effects of Delta-9-Tetrahydrocannabinol and Cannabinol in Man," *Pharmacology* 13, no. 6 (1975): 502–12; and K. D. Bird et al., "Interactions Among the Cannabinoids (THC, CBD, and CBN) Alone and When Combined with Ethanol: Effects on Human Performance," in *Proceedings of the 8th International Conference on Alcohol, Drugs, and Traffic Safety Held 15–19 June 1980*, vol. 3, ed. L. Goldberg (Stockholm, Sweden: Almqvist and Wiksell, 1981), 1111–25.

32. G. Appendino et al., "Antibacterial Cannabinoids from *Cannabis Sativa:* A Structure-Activity Study," *Journal of Natural Products* 71, no. 8 (2008): 1427–30.

33. P. Consroe et al., "Cannabidiol—Antiepileptic Drug Comparisons and Interactions in Experimentally Induced Seizures in Rats," *Journal of Pharmacology and Experimental Therapeutics* 201, no. 1 (1977): 26–32.

Notes

34. A. Scutt et al., "Cannabinoids Stimulate Fibroblastic Colony Formation by Bone Marrow Cells Indirectly via CB_2 Receptors," *Calcified Tissue International* 80, no. 1 (2007): 50–59.

35. B. K. Colasanti et al., "Intraocular Pressure, Ocular Toxicity, and Neurotoxicity After Administration of Cannabinol or Cannabigerol," *Experimental Eye Research* 39, no. 3 (1984): 251–59.

36. P. M. Zygmunt et al., "Delta-9-Tetrahydrocannabinol and Cannabinol Activate Capsaicin-Sensitive Sensory Nerves via a CB_1 and CB_2 Cannabinoid Receptor-Independent Mechanism," *Journal of Neuroscience* 22, no. 11 (2002): 4720–27; and H. Wong et al., "Cannabidiol, Cannabinol, and Their Combinations Act as Peripheral Analgesics in a Rat Model of Myofascial Pain," *Archives of Oral Biology* 104 (2019): 33–39.

37. J. A. Farrimond et al., "Cannabinol and Cannabidiol Exert Opposing Effects on Rat Feeding Patterns," *Psychopharmacology* (Berlin) 223, no. 1 (2012): 117–29.

38. D. Schubert et al., "Efficacy of Cannabinoids in a Pre-Clinical Drug-Screening Platform for Alzheimer's Disease," *Molecular Neurobiology* 56, no. 11 (2019): 7719–30.

39. Wong et al., "Cannabidiol, Cannabinol, and Their Combinations," 33–39.

40. R. E. Musty et al., "Interactions of Delta-9-Tetrahydrocannabinol and Cannabinol in Man," in *The Pharmacology of Marihuana*, vol. 2, ed. M. C. Braude et al. (New York: Raven Press, 1976), 559–63.

41. F. Korte et al., "Tetrahydrocannabinolcarboxylic Acid, a Component of Hashish," *Angewandte Chemie International Edition* 4, no. 10 (1965): 872.

42. R. Mechoulam et al., "A New Tetrahydrocannabinolic Acid," *Tetrahedron Letters* 10, no. 28 (1969): 2339–41.

43. S. Sirikantaramas et al., "Tetrahydrocannabinolic Acid Synthase, the Enzyme Controlling Marijuana Psychoactivity, Is Secreted into the Storage Cavity of the Glandular Trichomes," *Plant and Cell Physiology* 46, no. 9 (2005): 1578–82.

44. G. Moreno-Sanz, "Can You Pass the Acid Test? Critical Review and Novel Therapeutic Perspectives of Delta-9-Tetrahydrocannabinolic Acid A," *Cannabis and Cannabinoid Research* 1, no. 1 (2016): 124–30.

45. R. Karler et al., "The Cannabinoids as Potential Antiepileptics," *Journal of Clinical Pharmacology* 21, no. S1 (1981): 437–44S.

46. A. Varatharaj et al., "The Blood–Brain Barrier in Systemic Inflammation," *Brain, Behavior, and Immunity* 60 (2017): 1–12; E. Severance et al., "8.4 Gut Dysbiosis and Autoimmune Features in Schizophrenia Fuel Broken Barrier Hypotheses," *Schizophrenia Bulletin* 45, suppl. 2 (2019): S101; D. Shlosberg et al., "Blood–Brain Barrier Breakdown as a Therapeutic Target in Traumatic Brain Injury," *Nature Reviews Neurology* 6, no. 7 (2010): 393–403; and B. Obermeier et al., "Development, Maintenance, and Disruption of the Blood–Brain Barrier," *Nature Medicine* 19, no. 12 (2013): 1584–96.

47. X. Nadal et al., "Tetrahydrocannabinolic Acid Is a Potent PPARγ Agonist with Neuroprotective Activity," *British Journal of Pharmacology* 174, no. 23 (2017): 4263–76.

48. R. Nallathambi et al., "Anti-inflammatory Activity in Colon Models Is Derived from Delta-9-Tetrahydrocannabinolic Acid That Interacts with Additional Compounds in *Cannabis* Extracts," *Cannabis and Cannabinoid Research* 2, no. 1 (2017): 167–82.

49. L. R. Ruhaak et al., "Evaluation of the Cyclooxygenase Inhibiting Effects of Six Major Cannabinoids Isolated from *Cannabis Sativa*," *Biological and Pharmaceutical Bulletin* 34, no. 5 (2011): 774–78.

50. L. De Petrocellis et al., "Non-THC Cannabinoids Inhibit Prostate Carcinoma Growth In Vitro and In Vivo: Pro-Apoptotic Effects and Underlying Mechanisms," *British Journal of Pharmacology* 168, no. 1 (2013): 79–102.

51. Y. Shen et al., "Peroxisome Proliferator-Activated Receptor-γ and Its Ligands in the Treatment of Tumors in the Nervous System," *Current Stem Cell Research and Therapy* 11, no. 3 (2016): 208–15; and A. Ligresti et al., "Antitumor Activity of Plant Cannabinoids with Emphasis on the Effect of

Notes

Cannabidiol on Human Breast Carcinoma," *Journal of Pharmacology and Experimental Therapeutics* 318, no. 3 (2006): 1375–87.

52. R. Karler et al., "Cannabis and Epilepsy," in *Marihuana Biological Effects,* ed. G. G. Nahas et al. (Oxford, England: Pergamon, 1979), 619–41.

53. K. C. M. Verhoeckx et al., "Unheated *Cannabis Sativa* Extracts and Its Major Compound THC-Acid Have Potential Immuno-Modulating Properties Not Mediated by CB_1 and CB_2 Receptor Coupled Pathways," *International Immunopharmacology* 6, no. 4 (2006): 656–65.

54. C. E. Turner et al., "Constituents of *Cannabis Sativa* L. XVII. A Review of the Natural Constituents," *Journal of Natural Products* 43, no. 2 (1980): 169–234.

55. E. M. Rock et al., "Effect of Phytocannabinoids on Nausea and Vomiting," in *Handbook of Cannabis,* ed. R. G. Pertwee (Oxford, England: Oxford University Press, 2014), 435–54.

56. Nadal et al., "Tetrahydrocannabinolic Acid Is a Potent PPARɣ Agonist with Neuroprotective Activity," 4263–76; and R. Moldzio et al., "Effects of Cannabinoids Delta-9-Tetrahydrocannabinol, Delta-9-Tetrahydrocannabinolic Acid, and Cannabidiol in MPP+ Affected Murine Mesencephalic Cultures," *Phytomedicine* 19, nos. 8–9 (2012): 819–24.

57. R. Colle et al., "PPAR-ɣ Agonists for the Treatment of Major Depression: A Review," *Pharmacopsychiatry* 50, no. 2 (2017): 49–55.

58. Pertwee, "Cannabinoid Pharmacology: The First 66 Years," S163–71.

59. D. Bolognini et al., "Cannabidiolic Acid Prevents Vomiting in *Suncus Murinus* and Nausea-Induced Behaviour in Rats by Enhancing 5-HT1A Receptor Activation," *British Journal of Pharmacology* 168, no. 6 (2013): 1456–70.

60. E. M. Rock et al., "Effect of Combined Doses of Delta-9-Tetrahydrocannabinol (THC) and Cannabidiolic Acid (CBDA) on Acute and Anticipatory Nausea Using Rat (Sprague-Dawley) Models of Conditioned Gaping," *Psychopharmacology* (Berlin) 232, no. 24 (2015): 4445–54.

61. E. M. Rock et al., "Synergy Between Cannabidiol, Cannabidiolic Acid, and Delta-9-Tetrahydrocannabinol in the Regulation of Emesis in the *Suncus Murinus* (House Musk Shrew)," *Behavioral Neuroscience* 129, no. 3 (2015): 368–70.

62. E. M. Rock et al., "Effect of Prior Foot Shock Stress and Delta-9-Tetrahydrocannabinol, Cannabidiolic Acid, and Cannabidiol on Anxiety-Like Responding in the Light-Dark Emergence Test in Rats," *Psychopharmacology* (Berlin) 234, no. 14 (2017): 2207–17.

63. De Petrocellis et al., "Effects of Cannabinoids and Cannabinoid-Enriched *Cannabis* Extracts," 1479–94.

64. Ibid.

65. Ibid.

66. Ruhaak et al., "Evaluation of the Cyclooxygenase Inhibiting Effects of Six Major Cannabinoids," 774–78.

67. S. Takeda et al., "Down-Regulation of Cyclooxygenase-2 (COX-2) by Cannabidiolic Acid in Human Breast Cancer Cells," *Journal of Toxicological Sciences* 39, no. 5 (2014): 711–16; S. Takeda et al., "Cannabidiolic Acid, a Major Cannabinoid in Fiber-Type Cannabis, Is an Inhibitor of MDA-MB-231 Breast Cancer Cell Migration," *Toxicology Letters* 214, no. 3 (2012): 314–19; S. Takeda et al., "Cannabidiolic Acid-Mediated Selective Down-Regulation of C-Fos in Highly Aggressive Breast Cancer MDA-MB-231 Cells: Possible Involvement of Its Down-Regulation in the Abrogation of Aggressiveness," *Journal of Natural Medicines* 71, no. 1 (2017): 286–91; and S. Takeda et al., "DNA Microarray Analysis of Genes in Highly Metastatic 4T1E/M3 Murine Breast Cancer Cells Following Exposure to Cannabidiolic Acid," *Fundamental Toxicological Sciences* 2, no. 2 (2015): 89–94.

68. D. Hen-Shoval et al., "Acute Oral Cannabidiolic Acid Methyl Ester Reduces Depression-Like Behavior in Two Genetic Animal Models of Depression," *Behavioural Brain Research* 351 (2018): 1–3.

69. C. Stott et al., "Use of Canabinoids in the Treatment of Epilepsy," World Intellectual Property Organization (Patent Cooperation Treaty) publication WO2017025712A1 (2017), https://patents.google.com/patent/WO2017025712A1/en#patentCitations.

70. L. L. Anderson et al., "Pharmacokinetics of Phytocannabinoid Acids and Anticonvulsant Effect of Cannabidiolic Acid in a Mouse Model of Dravet Syndrome," *Journal of Natural Products* 82, no. 11 (2019): 3047–55.

71. E. Murillo-Rodríguez et al., "Sleep and Neurochemical Modulation by Cannabidiolic Acid Methyl Ester in Rats," *Brain Research Bulletin* 155 (2020): 166–73.

72. M. G. Cascio et al., "Evidence That the Plant Cannabinoid Cannabigerol Is a Highly Potent Alpha-2-Adrenoceptor Agonist and Moderately Potent 5HT1A Receptor Antagonist," *British Journal of Pharmacology* 159, no. 1 (2010): 129–41.

73. Ligresti et al., "Antitumor Activity of Plant Cannabinoids," 1375–87.

74. De Petrocellis et al., "Effects of Cannabinoids and Cannabinoid-Enriched *Cannabis* Extracts," 1479–94.

75. Ibid.; and L. De Petrocellis et al., "Plant-Derived Cannabinoids Modulate the Activity of Transient Receptor Potential Channels of Ankyrin Type-1 and Melastatin Type-8," *Journal of Pharmacology and Experimental Therapeutics* 325, no. 3 (2008): 1007–15.

76. S. P. Banerjee et al., "Cannabinoids: Influence on Neurotransmitter Uptake in Rat Brain Synaptosomes," *Journal of Pharmacology and Experimental Therapeutics* 194, no. 1 (1975): 74–81.

77. Cascio et al., "Evidence That the Plant Cannabinoid Cannabigerol," 129–41.

78. A. G. Granja et al., "A Cannabigerol Quinone Alleviates Neuroinflammation in a Chronic Model of Multiple Sclerosis," *Journal of Neuroimmune Pharmacology* 7, no. 4 (2012): 1002–16.

79. Cascio et al., "Evidence That the Plant Cannabinoid Cannabigerol," 129–41.

80. E. M. Rock et al., "Interaction Between Non-Psychotropic Cannabinoids in Marihuana: Effect of Cannabigerol (CBG) on the Anti-nausea or Anti-emetic Effects of Cannabidiol (CBD) in Rats and Shrews," *Psychopharmacology* (Berlin) 215, no. 3 (2011): 505–12.

81. S. Mammana et al., "Could the Combination of Two Non-Psychotropic Cannabinoids Counteract Neuroinflammation? Effectiveness of Cannabidiol Associated with Cannabigerol," *Medicina* (Kaunas) 55, no. 11 (2019): E747.

82. D. I. Brierley et al., "Chemotherapy-Induced Cachexia Dysregulates Hypothalamic and Systemic Lipoamines and Is Attenuated by Cannabigerol," *Journal of Cachexia, Sarcopenia and Muscle* 10, no. 4 (2019): 844–59.

83. Appendino et al., "Antibacterial Cannabinoids from *Cannabis Sativa*," 1427–30.

84. Ligresti et al., "Antitumor Activity of Plant Cannabinoids," 1375–87; K. A. Scott et al., "Enhancing the Activity of Cannabidiol and Other Cannabinoids In Vitro Through Modifications to Drug Combinations and Treatment Schedules," *Anticancer Research* 33, no. 10 (2013): 4373–80; S. H. Baek et al., "Boron Trifluoride Etherate on Silica-A Modified Lewis Acid Reagent (VII). Antitumor Activity of Cannabigerol Against Human Oral Epitheloid Carcinoma Cells," *Archives of Pharmacal Research* 21, no. 3 (1998): 353–56; and F. Borrelli et al., "Colon Carcinogenesis Is Inhibited by the TRPM8 Antagonist Cannabigerol, a Cannabis-Derived Non-Psychotropic Cannabinoid," *Carcinogenesis* 35, no. 12 (2014): 2787–97.

85. R. Musty et al., "A Cannabigerol Extract Alters Behavioral Despair in an Animal Model of Depression," in *16th Annual Symposium on the Cannabinoids, Tihany, Hungary, June 24–28, 2006, Program and Abstracts* (Burlington, VT: International Cannabinoid Research Society, 2006), 32.

86. A. Gugliandolo et al., "In Vitro Model of Neuroinflammation: Efficacy of Cannabigerol, a Non-Psychoactive Cannabinoid," *International Journal of Molecular Sciences* 19, no. 7 (2018): E1992.

87. A. A. Izzo et al., "Non-Psychotropic Plant Cannabinoids: New Therapeutic Opportunities from an Ancient Herb," *Trends in Pharmacological Sciences* 30, no. 10 (2009): 515–27; and A. J. Hill et al.,

Notes

"Phytocannabinoids as Novel Therapeutic Agents in CNS Disorders," *Pharmacology and Therapeutics* 133, no. 1 (2012): 79–97.

88. "Cannabinoids Inhibit Human Keratinocyte Proliferation Through a Non-CB_1/CB_2 Mechanism and Have a Potential Therapeutic Value in the Treatment of Psoriasis," *Journal of Dermatological Science* 45, no. 2 (2007): 87–92.

89. S. Valdeolivas et al., "Neuroprotective Properties of Cannabigerol in Huntington's Disease: Studies in R6/2 Mice and 3-Nitropropionate-Lesioned Mice," *Neurotherapeutics* 12, no. 1 (2015): 185–99; and Gugliandolo et al., "In Vitro Model of Neuroinflammation," E1992.

90. Scutt et al., "Cannabinoids Stimulate Fibroblastic Colony Formation," 50–59.

91. E. Pagano et al., "Effect of Non-Psychotropic Plant-Derived Cannabinoids on Bladder Contractility: Focus on Cannabigerol," *Natural Product Communications* 10, no. 6 (2015): 1009–12.

92. F. Borrelli et al., "Beneficial Effect of the Non-Psychotropic Plant Cannabinoid Cannabigerol on Experimental Inflammatory Bowel Disease," *Biochemical Pharmacology* 85, no. 9 (2013): 1306–16.

93. Colasanti et al., "Intraocular Pressure, Ocular Toxicity, and Neurotoxicity After Administration of Cannabinol or Cannabigerol," 251–59.

94. Rock et al., "Interaction Between Non-Psychotropic Cannabinoids in Marihuana," 505–12.

95. D. I. Brierley et al., "Cannabigerol Is a Novel, Well-Tolerated Appetite Stimulant in Pre-Satiated Rats," *Psychopharmacology* (Berlin) 233, nos. 19–20 (2016): 3603–13; and D. I. Brierley et al., "A Cannabigerol-Rich *Cannabis Sativa* Extract, Devoid of Delta-9-Tetrahydrocannabinol, Elicits Hyperphagia in Rats," *Behavioural Pharmacology* 28, no. 4 (2017): 280–84.

96. E. W. Gill et al., "Preliminary Experiments on the Chemistry and Pharmacology of Cannabis," *Nature* 228, no. 5267 (1970): 134–36; and F. W. H. M. Merkus, "Cannabivarin and Tetrahydrocannabivarin, Two New Constituents of Hashish," *Nature* 232, no. 5312 (1971): 579–80.

97. A. Abioye et al., "Delta-9-Tetrahydrocannabivarin (THCV): A Commentary on Potential Therapeutic Benefit for the Management of Obesity and Diabetes," *Journal of Cannabis Research* 2, no. 1 (2020): 1–6.

98. D. Bolognini et al., "The Plant Cannabinoid Delta-9-Tetrahydrocannabivarin Can Decrease Signs of Inflammation and Inflammatory Pain in Mice," *British Journal of Pharmacology* 160, no. 3 (2010): 677–87.

99. De Petrocellis et al., "Effects of Cannabinoids and Cannabinoid-Enriched *Cannabis* Extracts," 1479–94; and Abioye et al., "Delta-9-Tetrahydrocannabivarin (THCV)," 1–6.

100. M. G. Cascio et al., "The Phytocannabinoid, Delta-9-Tetrahydrocannabivarin, Can Act Through 5-HT_{1A} Receptors to Produce Antipsychotic Effects," *British Journal of Pharmacology* 172, no. 5 (2015): 1305–18.

101. S. Anavi-Goffer et al., "Modulation of l-Alpha-Lysophosphatidylinositol/GPR55 Mitogen-Activated Protein Kinase (MAPK) Signaling by Cannabinoids," *Journal of Biological Chemistry* 287, no. 1 (2012): 91–104.

102. A. J. Hill et al., "Delta-9-Tetrahydrocannabivarin Suppresses In Vitro Epileptiform and In Vivo Seizure Activity in Adult Rats," *Epilepsia* 51, no. 8 (2010): 1522–32.

103. G. Riedel et al., "Synthetic and Plant-Derived Cannabinoid Receptor Antagonists Show Hypophagic Properties in Fasted and Non-Fasted Mice," *British Journal of Pharmacology* 156, no. 7 (2009): 1154–66.

104. De Petrocellis et al., "Effects of Cannabinoids and Cannabinoid-Enriched *Cannabis* Extracts," 1479–94.

105. GW Research, "GWMD1092 - GWP42003 : GWP42004 Together Plus Alone in Type II Diabetes," ClinicalTrials.gov, last modified September 18, 2104, accessed January 2020, https://clinicaltrials.gov/ct2/show/NCT01217112.

106. GW Research, "A Randomised, Double Blind, Placebo Controlled, Parallel Group, Dose Ranging Study of GWP42004 as Add On to Metformin in the Treatment of Participants with Type 2 Diabetes,"

ClinicalTrials.gov, last modified September 23, 2018, accessed January 2020, https://www
.clinicaltrialsregister.eu/ctr-search/trial/2013-001140-61/results.

107. C. García et al., "Symptom-Relieving and Neuroprotective Effects of the Phytocannabinoid Delta-9-THCV in Animal Models of Parkinson's Disease," *British Journal of Pharmacology* 163, no. 7 (2011): 1495–506.

108. S. Maione et al., "Cannabidivarin for Use in the Treatment of Neuropathic Pain," patent EP2709604B1, accessed January 2020, https://patents.google.com/patent/EP2709604B1/en.

109. A. Englund et al., "The Effect of Five Day Dosing with THCV on THC-Induced Cognitive, Psychological, and Physiological Effects in Healthy Male Human Volunteers: A Placebo-Controlled, Double-Blind, Crossover Pilot Trial," *Journal of Psychopharmacology* 30, no. 2 (2016): 140–51.

110. L. Vollner et al., "Hashish. XX. Cannabidivarin, a New Hashish Constituent" [in German], *Tetrahedron Letters* 3 (1969): 145–47.

111. A. Hill et al., "Cannabidivarin Is Anticonvulsant in Mouse and Rat," *British Journal of Pharmacology* 167, no. 8 (2012): 1629–42; F. A. Iannotti et al., "Nonpsychotropic Plant Cannabinoids, Cannabidivarin (CBDV) and Cannabidiol (CBD), Activate and Desensitize Transient Receptor Potential Vanilloid 1 (TRPV1) Channels In Vitro: Potential for the Treatment of Neuronal Hyperexcitability," *ACS Chemical Neuroscience* 5, no. 11 (2014): 1131–41; A. Capasso, "Do Cannabinoids Confer Neuroprotection Against Epilepsy? An Overview," *Open Neurology Journal* 11 (2017): 61–73; and A. Morano et al., "Cannabis in Epilepsy: From Clinical Practice to Basic Research Focusing on the Possible Role of Cannabidivarin," *Epilepsia Open* 1, nos. 3–4 (2016): 145–51.

112. S. Rosenthaler et al., "Differences in Receptor Binding Affinity of Several Phytocannabinoids Do Not Explain Their Effects on Neural Cell Cultures," *Neurotoxicology and Teratology* 46 (2014): 49–56.

113. De Petrocellis et al., "Effects of Cannabinoids and Cannabinoid-Enriched *Cannabis* Extracts," 1479–94.

114. Iannotti et al., "Nonpsychotropic Plant Cannabinoids, Cannabidivarin (CBDV) and Cannabidiol (CBD)," 1131–41; and E. M. Rock et al., "Evaluation of the Potential of the Phytocannabinoids, Cannabidivarin (CBDV), and Delta-9-Tetrahydrocannabivarin (THCV), to Produce CB_1 Receptor Inverse Agonism Symptoms of Nausea in Rats," *British Journal of Pharmacology* 170, no. 3 (2013): 671–78.

115. Anavi-Goffer et al., "Modulation of L-Alpha-Lysophosphatidylinositol/GPR55 Mitogen-Activated Protein Kinase (MAPK)," 91–104.

116. A. Morano et al., "Cannabis in Epilepsy: From Clinical Practice to Basic Research Focusing on the Possible Role of Cannabidivarin," *Epilepsia Open* 1, nos. 3–4 (2016): 145–51.

117. D. Vigli et al., "Chronic Treatment with the Phytocannabinoid Cannabidivarin (CBDV) Rescues Behavioural Alterations and Brain Atrophy in a Mouse Model of Rett Syndrome," *Neuropharmacology* 140 (2018): 121–29.

118. Maione et al., "Cannabidivarin for Use in the Treatment of Neuropathic Pain," https://patents .google.com/patent/EP2709604B1/en.

119. Morano et al., "Cannabis in Epilepsy," 145–51.

120. New Cannabis Ventures Newswire, "GW Phrame Phase 2 Trial Using CBDV to Treat Adults with Focal Seizures Misses Primary Endpoint," February 21, 2018, accessed January 2020, https://www .newcannabisventures.com/gw-pharma-phase-2-trial-using-cbdv-to-treat-adults-with-focal-seizures -misses-primary-endpoint/.

121. King's College London, "Shifting Brain Excitation-Inhibition Balance in Autism Spectrum Disorder," ClinicalTrials.gov, last modified May 25, 2018, accessed January 2020, https://clinicaltrials .gov/ct2/show/NCT03537950; and E. Hollander et al., "Cannabidivarin (CBDV) vs. Placebo in Children with Autism Spectrum Disorder (ASD)," ClinicalTrials.gov, last modified October 18, 2019, accessed January 2020, https://clinicaltrials.gov/ct2/show/record/NCT03202303.

122. L. E. Hollister et al., "Delta-8- and Delta-9-Tetrahydrocannabinol; Comparison in Man by Oral and Intravenous Administration," *Clinical Pharmacology and Therapeutics* 14, no. 3 (1973): 353–57; and B. R. Martin, "Cellular Effects of Cannabinoids," *Pharmacological Reviews* 38, no. 1 (1986): 45–74.

123. Y. Avraham et al., "Very Low Doses of Delta-8-THC Increase Food Consumption and Alter Neurotransmitter Levels Following Weight Loss," *Pharmacology Biochemistry and Behavior* 77, no. 4 (2004): 675–84.

124. H. L. Tripathi et al., "Effects of Cannabinoids on Levels of Acetylcholine and Choline and on Turnover Rate of Acetylcholine in Various Regions of the Mouse Brain," *Alcohol and Drug Research* 7, nos. 5–6 (1987): 525–32.

125. A. E. Munson et al., "Antineoplastic Activity of Cannabinoids," *Journal of the National Cancer Institute* 55, no. 3 (1975): 597–602.

126. S. Muchtar et al., "A Submicron Emulsion as Ocular Vehicle for Delta-8-Tetrahydrocannabinol: Effect on Intraocular Pressure in Rabbits," *Ophthalmic Research* 24, no. 3 (1992): 142–49; J. Merritt et al., "Topical Delta-8-Tetrahydrocannabinol as a Potential Glaucoma Agent," *Glaucoma* 4 (1982): 253–55; and N. S. Punyamurthula et al., "Ocular Disposition of Delta-8-Tetrahydrocannabinol from Various Topical Ophthalmic Formulations," *AAPS PharmSciTech* 18, no. 6 (2017): 1936–45.

127. A. Abrahamov et al., "An Efficient New Cannabinoid Antiemetic in Pediatric Oncology," *Life Sciences* 56, nos. 23–24 (1995): 2097–102.

128. B. W. Sandage Jr., "Anti-emetic Uses of (3R, 4R)-Delta-8-Tetrahydrocannabinol-11-OIC Acids," patent application 20070099988, Indevus Pharmaceuticals, May 3, 2007, http://appft.uspto.gov/netacgi/nph-Parser?p=1&u=%2Fnetahtml%2FPTO%2Fsearch-adv.html&r=1&f=G&l=50&d=PG01&s1=20070099988.PN.&OS=PN/20070099988&RS=PN/20070099988.

129. Y. Gaoni et al., "Cannabichromene, a New Active Principle in Hashish," *Chemical Communications* (London) 1 (1966): 20–21.

130. L. Booker et al., "Evaluation of Prevalent Phytocannabinoids in the Acetic Acid Model of Visceral Nociception," *Drug and Alcohol Dependence* 105, nos. 1–2 (2009): 42–47.

131. De Petrocellis et al., "Plant-Derived Cannabinoids Modulate the Activity of Transient Receptor Potential Channels," 1007–15.

132. Ibid.

133. A. Oláh et al., "Differential Effectiveness of Selected Non-Psychotropic Phytocannabinoids on Human Sebocyte Functions Implicates Their Introduction in Dry/Seborrhoeic Skin and Acne Treatment," *Experimental Dermatology* 25, no. 9 (2016): 701–7.

134. Ligresti et al., "Antitumor Activity of Plant Cannabinoids," 1375–87.

135. R. Deyo et al., "A Cannabichromene (CBC) Extract Alters Behavioral Despair on the Mouse Tail Suspension Test of Depression," in *13th Symposium on the Cannabinoids, Cornwall, Ontario, June 24–29, 2003* (Winston-Salem, NC: International Cannabinoid Research Society, 2003), 146; and A. T. El-Alfy et al., "Antidepressant-Like Effect of Delta-9-Tetrahydrocannabinol and Other Cannabinoids Isolated from *Cannabis Sativa L.*," *Pharmacology Biochemistry and Behavior* 95, no. 4 (2010): 434–42.

136. W. Davis et al., "Neurobehavioral Actions of Cannabichromene and Interactions with Delta-9-Tetrahydrocannabinol," *General Pharmacology* 14, no. 2 (1983): 247–52.

137. G. T. DeLong et al., "Pharmacological Evaluation of the Natural Constituent of *Cannabis Sativa*, Cannabichromene, and Its Modulation by Delta-9-Tetrahydrocannabinol," *Drug and Alcohol Dependence* 112, nos. 1–2 (2010): 126–33.

138. C. E. Turner et al., "Biological Activity of Cannabichromene, Its Homologs and Isomers," *Journal of Clinical Pharmacology* 21, no. S1 (1981): 283S–291S.

139. N. S. Hatoum et al., "Cannabichromene and Delta-9-Tetrahydrocannabinol: Interactions Relative to Lethality, Hypothermia, and Hexobarbital Hypnosis," *General Pharmacology* 12, no. 5 (1981): 357–62.

140. N. Shinjyo et al., "The Effect of Cannabichromene on Adult Neural Stem/Progenitor Cells," *Neurochemistry International* 63, no. 5 (2013): 432–37.

Notes

Chapter 5: How to Use Cannabis as Medicine

1. K.-H. Kim et al., "Exposure to Pesticides and the Associated Human Health Effects," *Science of the Total Environment* 575 (2017): 525–35; and P. Nicolopoulou-Stamati et al., "Chemical Pesticides and Human Health: The Urgent Need for a New Concept in Agriculture," *Frontiers in Public Health* 4 (2016): 148.

2. D. Gieringer, "The California NORML/MAPS Smoking Device Study," originally printed in MAPS Newsletter 1996, last modified November 1999, https://www.420magazine.com/community/threads/the-california-norml-maps-smoking-device-study.77173/.

3. L. Navon et al., "Risk Factors for E-Cigarette, or Vaping, Product Use-Associated Lung Injury (EVALI) Among Adults Who Use E-Cigarette, or Vaping, Products—Illinois, July–October 2019," *Morbidity and Mortality Weekly Report* 68, no. 45 (2019): 1034–39.

4. Z. Eisenberg et al., "Contaminant Analysis of Illicit vs. Regulated Market Extracts," October 26, 2019, accessed January 2020, https://cannabis.anresco.com/analysis-of-illicit-vs-regulated-market-extracts/.

5. L. Lemberger et al., "Marihuana: Studies on the Disposition and Metabolism of Delta-9-Tetrahydrocannabinol in Man," *Science* 170, no. 3964 (1970): 1320–22.

6. S. Lunn et al., "Human Pharmacokinetic Parameters of Orally Administered Delta-9-Tetrahydrocannabinol Capsules Are Altered by Fed Versus Fasted Conditions and Sex Differences," *Cannabis and Cannabinoid Research* 4, no. 4 (2019): 255–64.

7. T. Nadulski et al., "Randomized, Double-Blind, Placebo-Controlled Study About the Effects of Cannabidiol (CBD) on the Pharmacokinetics of Delta-9-Tetrahydrocannabinol (THC) After Oral Application of THC Versus Standardized Cannabis Extract," *Therapeutic Drug Monitoring* 27, no. 6 (2005): 799–810.

8. C. Hess et al., "Topical Application of THC Containing Products Is Not Able to Cause Positive Cannabinoid Finding in Blood or Urine," *Forensic Science International* 272 (2017): 68–71.

9. J. D. Wilkinson et al., "Cannabinoids Inhibit Human Keratinocyte Proliferation Through a Non-CB$_1$/CB$_2$ Mechanism and Have a Potential Therapeutic Value in the Treatment of Psoriasis," *Journal of Dermatological Science* 45, no. 2 (2007): 87–92.

10. E. Gaffal et al., "Anti-inflammatory Activity of Topical THC in DNFB-Mediated Mouse Allergic Contact Dermatitis Independent of CB$_1$ and CB$_2$ Receptors," *Allergy* 68, no. 8 (2013): 994–1000.

11. A. L. Stinchcomb et al., "Human Skin Permeation of Delta-8-Tetrahydrocannabinol, Cannabidiol, and Cannabinol," *Journal of Pharmacy and Pharmacology* 56, no. 3 (2004): 291–97.

12. Gaffal et al., "Anti-inflammatory Activity of Topical THC," 994–1000; E. Gaffal et al., "Cannabinoid 1 Receptors in Keratinocytes Attenuate Fluorescein Isothiocyanate-Induced Mouse Atopic-Like Dermatitis," *Experimental Dermatology* 23, no. 6 (2014): 401–6; and H. J. Kim et al., "Topical Cannabinoid Receptor 1 Agonist Attenuates the Cutaneous Inflammatory Responses in Oxazolone-Induced Atopic Dermatitis Model," *International Journal of Dermatology* 54, no. 10 (2015): e401–8.

13. N. Q. Phan et al., "Adjuvant Topical Therapy with a Cannabinoid Receptor Agonist in Facial Postherpetic Neuralgia," *Journal der Deutschen Dermatologischen Gesellschaft* 8, no. 2 (2010): 88–91.

14. G. Appendino et al., "Antibacterial Cannabinoids from *Cannabis Sativa*: A Structure-Activity Study," *Journal of Natural Products* 71, no. 8 (2008): 1427–30.

15. D. C. Hammell et al., "Transdermal Cannabidiol Reduces Inflammation and Pain-Related Behaviours in a Rat Model of Arthritis," *European Journal of Pain* 20, no. 6 (2016): 936–48.

16. J. C. Szepietowski et al., "Efficacy and Tolerance of the Cream Containing Structured Physiological Lipids with Endocannabinoids in the Treatment of Uremic Pruritus: A Preliminary Study," *Acta Dermatovenerologica Croatica* 13, no. 2 (2005): 97–103.

Notes

17. V. Maida et al., "Topical Medical Cannabis: A New Treatment for Wound Pain—Three Cases of Pyoderma Gangrenosum," *Journal of Pain and Symptom Management* 54, no. 5 (2017): 732–36.

18. M. P. Chelliah et al., "Self-Initiated Use of Topical Cannabidiol Oil for Epidermolysis Bullosa," *Pediatric Dermatology* 35, no. 4 (2018): e224–27.

19. M. A. ElSohly et al., "Rectal Bioavailability of Delta-9-Tetrahydrocannabinol from the Hemisuccinate Ester in Monkeys," *Journal of Pharmaceutical Sciences* 80, no. 10 (1991): 942–45; and E. Perlin et al., "Disposition and Bioavailability of Various Formulations of Tetrahydrocannabinol in the Rhesus Monkey," *Journal of Pharmaceutical Sciences* 74, no. 2 (1985): 171–74.

20. ElSohly et al., "Rectal Bioavailability of Delta-9-Tetrahydrocannabinol," 942–45; and R. Brenneisen et al., "The Effect of Orally and Rectally Administered Delta-9-Tetrahydrocannabinol on Spasticity: A Pilot Study with 2 Patients," *International Journal of Clinical Pharmacology and Therapeutics* 34, no. 10 (1996): 446–52.

21. R. Schicho et al., "Topical and Systemic Cannabidiol Improves Trinitrobenzene Sulfonic Acid Colitis in Mice," *Pharmacology* 89, nos. 3–4 (2012): 149–55.

22. M. Lodzki et al., "Cannabidiol-Transdermal Delivery and Anti-inflammatory Effect in a Murine Model," *Journal of Controlled Release* 93, no. 3 (2003): 377–87.

23. A. A. Rey, "Biphasic Effects of Cannabinoids in Anxiety Responses: CB_1 and $GABA_B$ Receptors in the Balance of GABAergic and Glutamatergic Neurotransmission," *Neuropsychopharmacology* 37, no. 12 (2012): 2624–34.

24. L. Lemberger et al., "Marihuana: Studies on the Disposition and Metabolism of Delta-9-Tetrahydrocannabinol in Man," *Science* 170, no. 3964 (1970): 1320–22.

25. D. I. Abrams et al., "Cannabinoid–Opioid Interaction in Chronic Pain," *Clinical Pharmacology and Therapeutics* 90, no. 6 (2011): 844–51.

26. H. K. Borys et al., "Development of Tolerance to the Prolongation of Hexobarbitone Sleeping Time Caused by Cannabidiol," *British Journal of Pharmacology* 67, no. 1 (1979): 93–101.

27. O. Devinsky et al., "Cannabidiol in Patients with Treatment-Resistant Epilepsy: An Open-Label Interventional Trial," *Lancet Neurology* 15, no. 3 (2016): 270–78.

28. Ibid.

29. T. E. Gaston et al. and UAB CBD Program, "Interactions Between Cannabidiol and Commonly Used Antiepileptic Drugs," *Epilepsia* 58, no. 9 (2017): 1586–92.

30. L. Grayson et al., "An Interaction Between Warfarin and Cannabidiol, a Case Report," *Epilepsy and Behavior Case Reports* 9 (2018): 10–11.

31. P. Damkier et al., "Interaction Between Warfarin and Cannabis," *Basic and Clinical Pharmacology and Toxicology* 124, no. 1 (2019): 28–31.

32. Project CBD, "Project CBD Releases Primer on Cannabinoid–Drug Interactions," last modified January 14, 2019, https://www.projectcbd.org/how-to/cbd-drug-interactions.

Chapter 6: Medical Risks of Cannabis Use

1. S. Sidney, "Cardiovascular Consequences of Marijuana Use," *Journal of Clinical Pharmacology* 42, no. S1 (2002): 64–70S.

2. B. A. Fisher et al., "Cardiovascular Complications Induced by Cannabis Smoking: A Case Report and Review of the Literature," *Emergency Medicine Journal* 22, no. 9 (2005): 679–80; D. A. Kosior et al., "Paroxysmal Atrial Fibrillation Following Marijuana Intoxication: A Two-Case Report of Possible Association," *International Journal of Cardiology* 78, no. 2 (2001): 183–84; and G. K. Singh, "Atrial Fibrillation Associated with Marijuana Use," *Pediatric Cardiology* 21, no. 3 (2000): 284.

Notes

3. W. S. Aronow et al., "Effect of Marihuana and Placebo-Marihuana Smoking on Angina Pectoris," *New England Journal of Medicine* 291, no. 2 (1974): 65–67.

4. M. A. Mittleman et al., "Triggering Myocardial Infarction by Marijuana," *Circulation* 103, no. 23 (2001): 2805–9.

5. L. Frost et al., "Marijuana Use and Long-Term Mortality Among Survivors of Acute Myocardial Infarction," *American Heart Journal* 165, no. 2 (2013): 170–75.

6. D. G. Caldicott et al., "Keep Off the Grass: Marijuana Use and Acute Cardiovascular Events," *European Journal of Emergency Medicine* 12, no. 5 (2005): 236–44.

7. K. J. Mukamal et al., "An Exploratory Prospective Study of Marijuana Use and Mortality Following Acute Myocardial Infarction," *American Heart Journal* 155, no. 3 (2008): 465–70; and S. Sidney et al., "Marijuana Use and Mortality," *American Journal of Public Health* 87, no. 4 (1997): 585–90.

8. M. Axiyan et al., "Cardiovascular Disease Among US Adult Marijuana Users: National Health and Nutrition Examination Survey, 2011–2012," *Journal of the American College of Cardiology* 65, suppl. 10 (2015): A1425.

9. E. Jouanjus et al., "What Is the Current Knowledge About the Cardiovascular Risk for Users of Cannabis-Based Products? A Systematic Review," *Current Atherosclerosis Reports* 19, no. 6 (2017): 26.

10. R. Durst et al., "Cannabidiol, a Nonpsychoactive Cannabis Constituent, Protects Against Myocardial Ischemic Reperfusion Injury," *American Journal of Physiology: Heart and Circulatory Physiology* 293, no. 6 (2007): H3602–7; C. P. Stanley et al., "Is the Cardiovascular System a Therapeutic Target for Cannabidiol?," *British Journal of Clinical Pharmacology* 75, no. 2 (2013): 313–22; K. Hayakawa et al., "Cannabidiol Prevents Infarction via the Non-CB$_1$ Cannabinoid Receptor Mechanism," *Neuroreport* 15, no. 15 (2004): 2381–85; K. Mishima et al., "Cannabidiol Prevents Cerebral Infarction via a Serotonergic 5-Hydroxytryptamine1A Receptor–Dependent Mechanism," *Stroke* 36, no. 5 (2005): 1077–82; M. Ceprián et al., "Cannabidiol Reduces Brain Damage and Improves Functional Recovery in a Neonatal Rat Model of Arterial Ischemic Stroke," *Neuropharmacology* 116 (2017): 151–59; and K. Hayakawa et al., "Delayed Treatment with Cannabidiol Has a Cerebroprotective Action via a Cannabinoid Receptor-Independent Myeloperoxidase-Inhibiting Mechanism," *Journal of Neurochemistry* 102, no. 5 (2007): 1488–96.

11. D. P. Tashkin et al., "Acute Pulmonary Physiologic Effects of Smoked Marijuana and Oral Delta-9-Tetrahydrocannabinol in Healthy Young Men," *New England Journal of Medicine* 289, no. 7 (1973): 336–41; and D. P. Tashkin et al., "Acute Effects of Smoked Marijuana and Oral Delta-9-Tetrahydrocannabinol on Specific Airway Conductance in Asthmatic Subjects," *American Review of Respiratory Disease* 109, no. 4 (1974): 420–28.

12. S. J. Williams et al., "Bronchodilator Effect of Delta-1-Tetrahydrocannabinol Administered by Aerosol of Asthmatic Patients," *Thorax* 31, no. 6 (1976): 720–23; and A. A. Falk et al., "Uptake, Distribution, and Elimination of Alpha-Pinene in Man After Exposure by Inhalation," *Scandinavian Journal of Work, Environment, and Health* 16, no. 5 (1990): 372–78.

13. D. P. Tashkin et al., "Respiratory Symptoms and Lung Function in Habitual Heavy Smokers of Marijuana Alone, Smokers of Marijuana and Tobacco, Smokers of Tobacco Alone, and Nonsmokers," *American Review of Respiratory Disease* 135, no. 1 (1987): 209–16; and J. W. Bloom et al., "Respiratory Effects of Non-Tobacco Cigarettes," *BMJ (Clinical Research Edition)* 295, no. 6612 (1987): 1516–18.

14. Tashkin et al., "Respiratory Symptoms and Lung Function in Habitual Heavy Smokers," 209–16; and Bloom et al., "Respiratory Effects of Non-Tobacco Cigarettes," 1516–18.

15. D. P. Tashkin et al., "Impact of Changes in Regular Use of Marijuana and/or Tobacco on Chronic Bronchitis," *Journal of Chronic Obstructive Pulmonary Disease* 9, no. 4 (2012): 367–74.

16. Tashkin et al., "Respiratory Symptoms and Lung Function in Habitual Heavy Smokers," 209–16; S. Aldington et al., "Effects of Cannabis on Pulmonary Structure, Function, and Symptoms," *Thorax*

Notes

62, no. 12 (2007): 1058–63; and R. J. Hancox et al., "Effects of Cannabis on Lung Function: A Population-Based Cohort Study," *European Respiratory Journal* 35, no. 1 (2010): 42–47.

17. S. Sidney et al., "Marijuana Use and Cancer Incidence (California, United States)," *Cancer Causes and Control* 8, no. 5 (1997): 722–28; and G. C. Baldwin et al., "Marijuana and Cocaine Impair Alveolar Macrophage Function and Cytokine Production," *American Journal of Respiratory and Critical Care Medicine* 156, no. 5 (1997): 1606–13.

18. M. Hashibe et al., "Marijuana Use and the Risk of Lung and Upper Aerodigestive Tract Cancers: Results of a Population-Based Case-Control Study," *Cancer Epidemiology, Biomarkers, and Prevention* 15, no. 10 (2006): 1829–34.

19. W. C. Tan et al., "Marijuana and Chronic Obstructive Lung Disease: A Population-Based Study," *Canadian Medical Association Journal* 180, no. 8 (2009): 814–20.

20. D. P. Tashkin, "Effects of Marijuana Smoking on the Lung," *Annals of the American Thoracic Society* 10, no. 3 (2013): 239–47.

21. B. F. Sexton et al., *The Influence of Cannabis on Driving*, TRL Report 477 (Crowthorne, England: Transport Research Laboratory, 2000); and A. M. Smiley et al., "Driving Simulator Studies of Marijuana Alone and in Combination with Alcohol," in *Proceedings of the 25th Conference of the American Association for Automotive Medicine* (Chicago: Association for the Advancement of Automotive Medicine, 1981), 107–16.

22. M. Bédard et al., "The Impact of Cannabis on Driving," *Canadian Journal of Public Health* 98, no. 1 (2007): 6–11.

23. O. H. Drummer, "The Involvement of Drugs in Drivers of Motor Vehicles Killed in Australian Road Traffic Crashes," *Accident: Analysis and Prevention* 36, no. 2 (2004): 239–48; and F. Grotenhermen et al., *Developing Science-Based Per Se Limits for Driving Under the Influence of Cannabis (DUIC): Findings and Recommendations by an Expert Panel* (Hürth, Germany: Nova-Institut, 2005).

24. K. W. Terhune et al., *The Incidence and Role of Drugs in Fatally Injured Drivers: Final Report* (Buffalo, NY; Washington, DC: Calspan Advanced Technology Center; National Highway Traffic Safety Administration, 1992).

25. R. L. Hartman et al., "Cannabis Effects on Driving Longitudinal Control with and Without Alcohol," *Journal of Applied Toxicology* 36, no. 11 (2016): 1418–29.

26. F. Grotenhermen, "Pharmacokinetics and Pharmacodynamics of Cannabinoids," *Clinical Pharmacokinetics* 42, no. 4 (2003): 327–60.

27. K. S. Grant et al., "Cannabis Use During Pregnancy: Pharmacokinetics and Effects on Child Development," *Pharmacology and Therapeutics* 182 (2018): 133–51.

28. T. D. Warner et al., "It's Not Your Mother's Marijuana: Effects on Maternal–Fetal Health and the Developing Child," *Clinics in Perinatology* 41, no. 4 (2014): 877–94.

29. B. Zuckerman et al., "Validity of Self-Reporting of Marijuana and Cocaine Use Among Pregnant Adolescents," *Journal of Pediatrics* 115, no. 5, pt. 1 (1989): 812–15; C. R. Warshak et al., "Association Between Marijuana Use and Adverse Obstetrical and Neonatal Outcomes," *Journal of Perinatology* 35, no. 12 (2015): 991–95; and M.-J. Saurel-Cubizolles et al., "Cannabis Use During Pregnancy in France in 2010," *BJOG: An International Journal of Obstetrics and Gynaecology* 121, no. 8 (2014): 971–77.

30. H. El Marroun et al., "Intrauterine Cannabis Exposure Affects Fetal Growth Trajectories: The Generation R Study," *Journal of the American Academy of Child and Adolescent Psychiatry* 48, no. 12 (2009): 1173–81.

31. Warshak et al., "Association Between Marijuana Use and Adverse Obstetrical and Neonatal Outcomes," 991–95.

32. P. A. Fried et al., "Growth from Birth to Early Adolescence in Offspring Prenatally Exposed to Cigarettes and Marijuana," *Neurotoxicology and Teratology* 21, no. 5 (1999): 513–25; and N. L. Day et al.,

"Alcohol, Marijuana, and Tobacco: Effects of Prenatal Exposure on Offspring Growth and Morphology at Age Six," *Alcoholism: Clinical and Experimental Research* 18, no. 4 (1994): 786–94.

33. P. A. Fried et al., "Neonatal Neurological Status in a Low-Risk Population After Prenatal Exposure to Cigarettes, Marijuana, and Alcohol," *Journal of Developmental and Behavioral Pediatrics* 8, no. 6 (1987): 318–26; and M. S. Scher et al., "The Effects of Prenatal Alcohol and Marijuana Exposure: Disturbances in Neonatal Sleep Cycling and Arousal," *Pediatric Research* 24, no. 1 (1988): 101–5.

34. C. A. Torres et al., "Totality of the Evidence Suggests Prenatal Cannabis Exposure Does Not Lead to Cognitive Impairments: A Systematic and Critical Review," *Frontiers in Psychology* 11 (2020): 816.

35. T. T.-Y. Lee et al., "Timing Is Everything: Evidence for a Role of Corticolimbic Endocannabinoids in Modulating Hypothalamic–Pituitary–Adrenal Axis Activity Across Developmental Periods," *Neuroscience* 204 (2012): 17–30; and B. Chadwick et al., "Cannabis Use During Adolescent Development: Susceptibility to Psychiatric Illness," *Frontiers in Psychiatry* 4 (2013): 129.

36. J. Díaz-Alonso et al., "Endocannabinoids via CB_1 Receptors Act as Neurogenic Niche Cues During Cortical Development," *Philosophical Transactions of the Royal Society of London: Series B, Biological Sciences* 367, no. 1607 (2012): 3229–41.

37. D. T. Malone et al., "Adolescent Cannabis Use and Psychosis: Epidemiology and Neurodevelopmental Models," *British Journal of Pharmacology* 160, no. 3 (2010): 511–22.

38. T. Rubino et al., "Chronic Delta-9-Tetrahydrocannabinol During Adolescence Provokes Sex-Dependent Changes in the Emotional Profile in Adult Rats: Behavioral and Biochemical Correlates," *Neuropsychopharmacology* 33, no. 11 (2008): 2760–71; T. Rubino et al., "Long Lasting Consequences of Cannabis Exposure in Adolescence," *Molecular and Cellular Endocrinology* 286, nos. 1–2, suppl. 1 (2008): S108–13; and V. Trezza et al., "Bidirectional Cannabinoid Modulation of Social Behavior in Adolescent Rats," *Psychopharmacology* (Berlin) 197, no. 2 (2008): 217–27.

39. J. Renard et al., "Long-Term Consequences of Adolescent Cannabinoid Exposure in Adult Psychopathology," *Frontiers in Neuroscience* 8 (2014): 361; and M. H. Meier et al., "Persistent Cannabis Users Show Neuropsychological Decline from Childhood to Midlife," *PNAS* 109, no. 40 (2012): E2657–64.

40. M. H. Meier et al., "Associations Between Adolescent Cannabis Use and Neuropsychological Decline: A Longitudinal Co-Twin Control Study," *Addiction* 113, no. 2 (2018): 257–65.

41. G. Sugranyes et al., "Cannabis Use and Age of Diagnosis of Schizophrenia," *European Psychiatry* 24, no. 5 (2009): 282–86; L. Arseneault et al., "Cannabis Use in Adolescence and Risk for Adult Psychosis: Longitudinal Prospective Study," *BMJ (Clinical Research Edition)* 325, no. 7374 (2002): 1212–13; and N. C. Stefanis et al., "Early Adolescent Cannabis Exposure and Positive and Negative Dimensions of Psychosis," *Addiction* 99, no. 10 (2004): 1333–41.

Part II: Medical Symptoms and Conditions

1. "About ADAA: Facts & Statistics," Anxiety and Depression Association of America website, accessed January 2020, https://adaa.org/about-adaa/press-room/facts-statistics.

2. B. Bandelow et al., "World Federation of Societies of Biological Psychiatry (WFSBP) Guidelines for the Pharmacological Treatment of Anxiety, Obsessive-Compulsive, and Post-Traumatic Stress Disorders—First Revision," *World Journal Biology Psychiatry* 9, no. 4 (2008): 248–312.

3. M. Morena et al., "Neurobiological Interactions Between Stress and the Endocannabinoid System," *Neuropsychopharmacology* 41, no. 1 (2016): 80–102.

4. I. Katona et al., "Distribution of CB_1 Cannabinoid Receptors in the Amygdala and Their Role in the Control of GABAergic Transmission," *Journal of Neuroscience* 21, no. 23 (2001): 9506–18; and F. R. Bambico et al., "Cannabinoids Elicit Antidepressant-Like Behavior and Activate Serotonergic Neurons Through the Medial Prefrontal Cortex," *Journal of Neuroscience* 27, no. 43 (2007): 11700–11.

Notes

5. M. Martin et al., "Involvement of CB$_1$ Cannabinoid Receptors in Emotional Behaviour," *Psychopharmacology* (Berlin) 159, no. 4 (2002): 379–87; J. Haller et al., "CB$_1$ Cannabinoid Receptors Mediate Anxiolytic Effects: Convergent Genetic and Pharmacological Evidence with CB$_1$-Specific Agents," *Behavioural Pharmacology* 15, no. 4 (2004): 299–304; and L. Urigüen et al., "Impaired Action of Anxiolytic Drugs in Mice Deficient in Cannabinoid CB$_1$ Receptors," *Neuropharmacology* 46, no. 7 (2004): 966–73.

6. G. Gobbi et al., "Antidepressant-Like Activity and Modulation of Brain Monoaminergic Transmission by Blockade of Anandamide Hydrolysis," *PNAS* 102, no. 51 (2005): 18620–25.

7. I. Dincheva et al., "FAAH Genetic Variation Enhances Fronto-Amygdala Function in Mouse and Human," *Nature Communications* 6 (2015): 6395.

8. M. N. Hill et al., "Serum Endocannabinoid Content Is Altered in Females with Depressive Disorders: A Preliminary Report," *Pharmacopsychiatry* 41, no. 2 (2008): 48–53.

9. M. N. Hill et al., "Circulating Endocannabinoids and N-Acyl Ethanolamines Are Differentially Regulated in Major Depression and Following Exposure to Social Stress," *Psychoneuroendocrinology* 34, no. 8 (2009): 1257–62.

10. B. L. Hungund et al., "Upregulation of CB$_1$ Receptors and Agonist-Stimulated [35S]GTP-Gamma-S Binding in the Prefrontal Cortex of Depressed Suicide Victims," *Molecular Psychiatry* 9, no. 2 (2004): 184–90.

11. K. Y. Vinod et al., "Elevated Levels of Endocannabinoids and CB$_1$ Receptor-Mediated G-Protein Signaling in the Prefrontal Cortex of Alcoholic Suicide Victims," *Biological Psychiatry* 57, no. 5 (2005): 480–86.

12. M. N. Hill et al., "Differential Effects of the Antidepressants Tranylcypromine and Fluoxetine on Limbic Cannabinoid Receptor Binding and Endocannabinoid Contents," *Journal of Neural Transmission* (Vienna) 115, no. 12 (2008): 1673–79.

13. A. Levy, "A World Without Pain," *The New Yorker*, January 13, 2020.

14. Z. Walsh et al., "Medical Cannabis and Mental Health: A Guided Systematic Review," *Clinical Psychology Review* 51 (2017): 15–29.

15. T. Deckman et al., "Can Marijuana Reduce Social Pain?," *Social Psychological and Personality Science* 5, no. 2 (2014): 131–39; and T. F. Denson et al., "Decreased Depression in Marijuana Users," *Addictive Behaviors* 31, no. 4 (2006): 738–42.

16. J. D. Kosiba et al., "Patient-Reported Use of Medical Cannabis for Pain, Anxiety, and Depression Symptoms: Systematic Review and Meta-Analysis," *Social Science and Medicine* 233 (2019): 181–92; M. Sexton et al., "A Cross-Sectional Survey of Medical Cannabis Users: Patterns of Use and Perceived Efficacy," *Cannabis and Cannabinoid Research* 1, no. 1 (2016): 131–38; P. Lucas et al., "Medical Cannabis Access, Use, and Substitution for Prescription Opioids and Other Substances: A Survey of Authorized Medical Cannabis Patients," *International Journal on Drug Policy* 42 (2017): 30–35; and H. Nunberg et al., "An Analysis of Applicants Presenting to a Medical Marijuana Specialty Practice in California," *Journal of Drug Policy Analysis* 4, no. 1 (2011): 1.

17. S. Shannon et al., "Cannabidiol in Anxiety and Sleep: A Large Case Series," *Permanente Journal* 23, no. 18-041 (2019).

18. M. P. Viveros et al., "Endocannabinoid System and Stress and Anxiety Responses," *Pharmacology Biochemistry and Behavior* 81, no. 2 (2005): 331–42.

19. A. W. Zuardi et al., "Action of Cannabidiol on the Anxiety and Other Effects Produced by Delta-9-THC in Normal Subjects," *Psychopharmacology* (Berlin) 76, no. 3 (1982): 245–50.

20. L. E. Hollister, "Hunger and Appetite After Single Doses of Marihuana, Alcohol, and Dextroamphetamine," *Clinical Pharmacology and Therapeutics* 12, no. 1 (1971): 44–49; and R. W. Foltin et al., "Effects of Smoked Marijuana on Food Intake and Body Weight of Humans Living in a Residential Laboratory," *Appetite* 11, no. 1 (1988): 1–14.

21. J. E. Beal et al., "Dronabinol as a Treatment for Anorexia Associated with Weight Loss in Patients with AIDS," *Journal of Pain and Symptom Management* 10, no. 2 (1995): 89–97.

22. M. Herkenham et al., "Cannabinoid Receptor Localization in Brain," *PNAS* 87, no. 5 (1990): 1932–36; and C. M. Williams et al., "Hyperphagia in Pre-Fed Rats Following Oral Delta-9-THC," *Physiology and Behavior* 65, no. 2 (1998): 343–46.

23. S. Gill et al., "Hypothalamic Ghrelin Signaling in Cannabis Induced Feeding," poster, Department of Integrative Physiology and Neurosciences, Washington State University, 2019; and B. Kola et al., "The Orexigenic Effect of Ghrelin Is Mediated Through Central Activation of the Endogenous Cannabinoid System," *PLoS One* 3, no. 3 (2008): e1797.

24. C. M. Williams et al., "Anandamide Induces Overeating: Mediation by Central Cannabinoid (CB$_1$) Receptors," *Psychopharmacology* (Berlin) 143, no. 3 (1999): 315–17.

25. J. A. Farrimond et al., "A Low-Delta-9-Tetrahydrocannabinol Cannabis Extract Induces Hyperphagia in Rats," *Behavioural Pharmacology* 21, no. 8 (2010): 769–72.

26. Foltin et al., "Effects of Smoked Marijuana on Food Intake and Body Weight," 1–14.

27. L. Volicer, "Effects of Dronabinol on Anorexia and Disturbed Behavior in Patients with Alzheimer's Disease," *International Journal of Geriatric Psychiatry* 12, no. 9 (1997): 913–19.

28. S. A. Hussain et al., "Perceived Efficacy of Cannabidiol-Enriched Cannabis Extracts for Treatment of Pediatric Epilepsy: A Potential Role for Infantile Spasms and Lennox-Gastaut Syndrome," *Epilepsy and Behavior* 47 (2015): 138–41.

29. W. Elliott et al., "Cannabidiol Oral Solution (Epidiolex)," *Internal Medicine Alert* (Atlanta) 40, no. 16 (2018); and B. K. O'Connell et al., "Cannabinoids in Treatment-Resistant Epilepsy: A Review," *Epilepsy and Behavior* 70, pt. B (2017): 341–48.

30. L. Tudge et al., "Neural Effects of Cannabinoid CB$_1$ Neutral Antagonist Tetrahydrocannabivarin on Food Reward and Aversion in Healthy Volunteers," *International Journal of Neuropsychopharmacology* 18, no. 6 (2015): pyu094.

31. O. Alshaarawy et al., "Are Cannabis Users Less Likely to Gain Weight? Results from a National 3-Year Prospective Study," *International Journal of Epidemiology* 48, no. 5 (2019): 1695–1700; and B. Le Foll et al., "Cannabis and Delta-9-Tetrahydrocannabinol (THC) for Weight Loss?," *Medical Hypotheses* 80, no. 5 (2013): 564–67.

32. E. A. Penner et al., "The Impact of Marijuana Use on Glucose, Insulin, and Insulin Resistance Among US Adults," *American Journal of Medicine* 126, no. 7 (2013): 583–89; T. B. Rajavashisth et al., "Decreased Prevalence of Diabetes in Marijuana Users: Cross-Sectional Data from the National Health and Nutrition Examination Survey (NHANES) III," *BMJ Open* 2, no. 1 (2012): e000494; and E. Smit et al., "Dietary Intake and Nutritional Status of US Adult Marijuana Users: Results from the Third National Health and Nutrition Examination Survey," *Public Health Nutrition* 4, no. 3 (2001): 781–86.

33. American Society of Nephrology, "Avoid Nonsteroidal Anti-inflammatory Drugs (NSAIDS) in Individuals with Hypertension or Heart Failure or CKD of All Causes, Including Diabetes," news release, Choosing Wisely website, April 4, 2012, accessed December 2019, https://www.choosing wisely.org/clinician-lists/american-society-nephrology-nsaids-in-individuals-with-hypertension-heart -failure-or-chronic-kidney-disease/.

34. W. Swift et al., "Survey of Australians Using Cannabis for Medical Purposes," *Harm Reduction Journal* 2, no. 1 (2005): 18; and M. A. Ware et al., "The Medicinal Use of Cannabis in the UK: Results of a Nationwide Survey," *International Journal of Clinical Practice* 59, no. 3 (2005): 291–95.

35. Nunberg et al., "An Analysis of Applicants Presenting to a Medical Marijuana Specialty Practice," 1.

36. D. R. Sagar et al., "Tonic Modulation of Spinal Hyperexcitability by the Endocannabinoid Receptor System in a Rat Model of Osteoarthritis Pain," *Arthritis and Rheumatism* 62, no. 12 (2010): 3666–76.

37. B. L. Kidd et al., "Mechanisms of Inflammatory Pain," *British Journal of Anaesthesia* 87, no. 1 (2001): 3–11.

Notes

38. A. M. Malfait et al., "The Nonpsychoactive Cannabis Constituent Cannabidiol Is an Oral Antiarthritic Therapeutic in Murine Collagen-Induced Arthritis," *PNAS* 97, no. 17 (2000): 9561–66.

39. P. F. Sumariwalla et al., "A Novel Synthetic, Nonpsychoactive Cannabinoid Acid (HU-320) with Anti-inflammatory Properties in Murine Collagen-Induced Arthritis," *Arthritis and Rheumatism* 50, no. 3 (2004): 985–98.

40. D. C. Hammell et al., "Transdermal Cannabidiol Reduces Inflammation and Pain-Related Behaviours in a Rat Model of Arthritis," *European Journal of Pain* 20, no. 6 (2016): 936–48.

41. H. T. Philpott et al., "Attenuation of Early Phase Inflammation by Cannabidiol Prevents Pain and Nerve Damage in Rat Osteoarthritis," *Pain* 158, no. 12 (2017): 2442–51.

42. L.-J. Gamble et al., "Pharmacokinetics, Safety, and Clinical Efficacy of Cannabidiol Treatment in Osteoarthritic Dogs," *Frontiers in Veterinary Science* 5 (2018): 165.

43. J. L. Croxford et al., "Cannabinoids and the Immune System: Potential for the Treatment of Inflammatory Diseases?," *Journal of Neuroimmunology* 166, nos. 1–2 (2005): 3–18.

44. D. R. Blake et al., "Preliminary Assessment of the Efficacy, Tolerability, and Safety of a Cannabis-Based Medicine (Sativex) in the Treatment of Pain Caused by Rheumatoid Arthritis," *Rheumatology* (Oxford, England) 45, no. 1 (2006): 50–52.

45. D. P. Tashkin et al., "Acute Pulmonary Physiologic Effects of Smoked Marijuana and Oral Delta-9-Tetrahydrocannabinol in Healthy Young Men," *New England Journal of Medicine* 289, no. 7 (1973): 336–41.

46. D. P. Tashkin et al., "Effects of Smoked Marijuana in Experimentally Induced Asthma," *American Review of Respiratory Disease* 112, no. 3 (1975): 377–86.

47. R. T. Abboud et al., "Effect of Oral Administration of Delta-9-Tetrahydrocannabinol on Airway Mechanics in Normal and Asthmatic Subjects," *Chest* 70, no. 4 (1976): 480–85.

48. S. Grassin-Delyle et al., "Cannabinoids Inhibit Cholinergic Contraction in Human Airways Through Prejunctional CB_1 Receptors," *British Journal of Pharmacology* 171, no. 11 (2014): 2767–77.

49. L. Giannini et al., "Activation of Cannabinoid Receptors Prevents Antigen-Induced Asthma-Like Reaction in Guinea Pigs," *Journal of Cellular and Molecular Medicine* 12, no. 6A (2008): 2381–94.

50. D. P. Tashkin et al., "Respiratory and Immunologic Consequences of Marijuana Smoking," *Journal of Clinical Pharmacology* 42, no. S1 (2002): 71-81S; and D. P. Tashkin et al., "Smoked Marijuana as a Cause of Lung Injury," *Monaldi Archives for Chest Disease* 63, no. 2 (2005): 93–100.

51. S. N. Visser et al., "Trends in the Parent-Report of Health Care Provider Diagnosed and Medicated Attention Deficit/Hyperactivity Disorder: United States, 2003–2011," *Journal of the American Academy of Child and Adolescent Psychiatry* 53, no. 1 (2014): 34–46.

52. J. N. Epstein et al., "Changes in the Definition of ADHD in DSM-5: Subtle but Important," *Neuropsychiatry* (London) 3, no. 5 (2013): 455–58.

53. N. Del Campo et al., "The Roles of Dopamine and Noradrenaline in the Pathophysiology and Treatment of Attention-Deficit/Hyperactivity Disorder," *Biological Psychiatry* 69, no. 12 (2011): e145–57.

54. D. Centonze et al., "Altered Anandamide Degradation in Attention-Deficit/Hyperactivity Disorder," *Neurology* 72, no. 17 (2009): 1526–27; C. J. Hillard et al., "Contributions of Endocannabinoid Signaling to Psychiatric Disorders in Humans: Genetic and Biochemical Evidence," *Neuroscience* 204 (2012): 207–29; and A. T. Lu et al., "Association of the Cannabinoid Receptor Gene (CNR1) with ADHD and Post-Traumatic Stress Disorder," *American Journal of Medical Genetics; Part B: Neuropsychiatric Genetics* 147B, no. 8 (2008): 1488–94.

55. P. Strohbeck-Kuehner et al., "Cannabis Improves Symptoms of ADHD," *Cannabinoids* 3, no. 1 (2008): 1–3.

56. E. Milz et al., "Successful Therapy of Treatment Resistant Adult ADHD with Cannabis: Experience from a Medical Practice with 30 Patients," in *Abstract Book of the 7th Annual European Workshop on*

Notes

Cannabinoid Research and IACM 8th Conference on Cannabinoids in Medicine, 17–19 September 2015, Sestri Levante, Italy (Rüthen, Germany: International Association for Cannabinoid Medicines, 2015), 85.

57. R. E. Cooper et al., "Cannabinoids in Attention-Deficit/Hyperactivity Disorder: A Randomised-Controlled Trial," *European Neuropsychopharmacology* 27, no. 8 (2017): 795–808.

58. J. Y. Hergenrather et al., "Cannabinoid and Terpenoid Doses Are Associated with Adult ADHD Status of Medical Cannabis Patients," *Rambam Maimonides Medical Journal* 11, no. 1 (2020): e0001.

59. H. Faras et al., "Autism Spectrum Disorders," *Annals of Saudi Medicine* 30, no. 4 (2010): 295–300.

60. B. A. Adler et al., "Drug-Refractory Aggression, Self-Injurious Behavior, and Severe Tantrums in Autism Spectrum Disorders: A Chart Review Study," *Autism* 19, no. 1 (2015): 102–6.

61. K. Ballaban-Gil et al., "Epilepsy and Epileptiform EEG: Association with Autism and Language Disorders," *Mental Retardation and Developmental Disabilities Research Reviews* 6, no. 4 (2000): 300–8.

62. R. Canitano, "Epilepsy in Autism Spectrum Disorders," *European Child and Adolescent Psychiatry* 16, no. 1 (2007): 61–66; P. M. Levisohn, "The Autism-Epilepsy Connection," *Epilepsia* 48, suppl. 9 (2007): 33–35; and M. L. Lewis et al., "Comorbid Epilepsy in Autism Spectrum Disorder: Implications of Postnatal Inflammation for Brain Excitability," *Epilepsia* 59, no. 7 (2018): 1316–26.

63. M. Maccarrone et al., "Abnormal mGlu 5 Receptor/Endocannabinoid Coupling in Mice Lacking FMRP and BC1 RNA," *Neuropsychopharmacology* 35, no. 7 (2010): 1500–9.

64. S. T. Schultz, "Can Autism Be Triggered by Acetaminophen Activation of the Endocannabinoid System?," *Acta Neurobiologiae Experimentalis* 70, no. 2 (2009): 227–31.

65. D. M. Kerr et al., "Alterations in the Endocannabinoid System in the Rat Valproic Acid Model of Autism," *Behavioural Brain Research* 249 (2013): 124–32.

66. D. Siniscalco et al., "Cannabinoid Receptor Type 2, but Not Type 1, Is Up-Regulated in Peripheral Blood Mononuclear Cells of Children Affected by Autistic Disorders," *Journal of Autism and Developmental Disorders* 43, no. 11 (2013): 2686–95.

67. D. S. Karhson et al., "Plasma Anandamide Concentrations Are Lower in Children with Autism Spectrum Disorder," *Molecular Autism* 9, no. 1 (2018): 18.

68. A. Aran et al., "Lower Circulating Endocannabinoid Levels in Children with Autism Spectrum Disorder," *Molecular Autism* 10, no. 1 (2019): 2.

69. R. Kurz et al., "Use of Dronabinol (Delta-9-THC) in Autism: A Prospective Single-Case-Study with an Early Infantile Autistic Child," *Cannabinoids* 5, no. 4 (2010): 4–6.

70. A. Aran et al., "Brief Report: Cannabidiol-Rich Cannabis in Children with Autism Spectrum Disorder and Severe Behavioral Problems—a Retrospective Feasibility Study," *Journal of Autism and Developmental Disorders* 49, no. 3 (2019): 1284–88.

71. L. Bar-Lev Schleider et al., "Real Life Experience of Medical Cannabis Treatment in Autism: Analysis of Safety and Efficacy," *Scientific Reports* 9 (2019): 200.

72. P. Fleury-Teixeira et al., "Effects of CBD-Enriched *Cannabis Sativa* Extract on Autism Spectrum Disorder Symptoms: An Observational Study of 18 Participants Undergoing Compassionate Use," *Frontiers in Neurology* 10 (2019): 1145.

73. Bar-Lev Schleider et al., "Real Life Experience of Medical Cannabis Treatment in Autism," 200.

74. A. Oláh et al., "Targeting Cannabinoid Signaling in the Immune System: 'High'-ly Exciting Questions, Possibilities, and Challenges," *Frontiers in Immunology* 8 (2017): 1487.

75. K. D. Patel et al., "Cannabinoid CB_2 Receptors in Health and Disease," *Current Medicinal Chemistry* 17, no. 14 (2010): 1393–410.

76. M. Karsak et al., "Attenuation of Allergic Contact Dermatitis Through the Endocannabinoid System," *Science* 316, no. 5830 (2007): 1494–97; G. A. Cabral et al., "Turning Over a New Leaf: Cannabinoid and Endocannabinoid Modulation of Immune Function," *Journal of Neuroimmune Pharmacology* 10,

no. 2 (2015): 193–203; and V. Chiurchiù et al., "Endocannabinoid Signalling in Innate and Adaptive Immunity," *Immunology* 144, no. 3 (2015): 352–64.

77. P. Nagarkatti et al., "Cannabinoids as Novel Anti-inflammatory Drugs," *Future Medicinal Chemistry* 1, no. 7 (2009): 1333–49.

78. Croxford et al., "Cannabinoids and the Immune System," 3–18; and T. W. Klein, "Cannabinoid-Based Drugs as Anti-inflammatory Therapeutics," *Nature Reviews: Immunology* 5, no. 5 (2005): 400–11.

79. E. Shohami et al., "Cytokine Production in the Brain Following Closed Head Injury: Dexanabinol (HU-211) Is a Novel TNF-Alpha Inhibitor and an Effective Neuroprotectant," *Journal of Neuroimmunology* 72, no. 2 (1997): 169–77.

80. F. Massa et al., "The Endogenous Cannabinoid System Protects Against Colonic Inflammation," *Journal of Clinical Investigation* 113, no. 8 (2004): 1202–9.

81. Sumariwalla et al., "A Novel Synthetic, Nonpsychoactive Cannabinoid Acid (HU-320)," 985–98.

82. C. Di Filippo et al., "Cannabinoid CB_2 Receptor Activation Reduces Mouse Myocardial Ischemia-Reperfusion Injury: Involvement of Cytokine/Chemokines and PMN," *Journal of Leukocyte Biology* 75, no. 3 (2004): 453–59.

83. M. Sorosina et al., "Clinical Response to Nabiximols Correlates with the Downregulation of Immune Pathways in Multiple Sclerosis," *European Journal of Neurology* 25, no. 7 (2018): 934-e70.

84. A. M. Kemter et al., "The Cannabinoid Receptor 2 Is Involved in Acute Rejection of Cardiac Allografts," *Life Sciences* 138 (2015): 29–34; J. M. Sido et al., "Delta-9–Tetrahydrocannabinol Attenuates Allogeneic Host-Versus-Graft Response and Delays Skin Graft Rejection Through Activation of Cannabinoid Receptor 1 and Induction of Myeloid-Derived Suppressor Cells," *Journal of Leukocyte Biology* 98, no. 3 (2015): 435–47; W.-S. Lee et al., "Cannabidiol Limits T Cell–Mediated Chronic Autoimmune Myocarditis: Implications to Autoimmune Disorders and Organ Transplantation," *Molecular Medicine* (Cambridge, MA) 22, no. 1 (2016): 136–46; and R. Pandey et al., "Targeting Cannabinoid Receptors as a Novel Approach in the Treatment of Graft-Versus-Host Disease: Evidence from an Experimental Murine Model," *Journal of Pharmacology and Experimental Therapeutics* 338, no. 3 (2011): 819–28.

85. M. Yeshurun et al., "Cannabidiol for the Prevention of Graft-Versus-Host-Disease After Allogeneic Hematopoietic Cell Transplantation: Results of a Phase II Study," *Biology of Blood and Marrow Transplantation* 21, no. 10 (2015): 1770–75.

86. American Cancer Society, "Cancer A–Z: What Is Cancer?," last modified December 8, 2015, https://www.cancer.org/cancer/cancer-basics/what-is-cancer.html.

87. S. E. Sallan et al., "Antiemetic Effect of Delta-9-Tetrahydrocannabinol in Patients Receiving Cancer Chemotherapy," *New England Journal of Medicine* 293, no. 16 (1975): 795–97.

88. L. E. Broder et al., "A Randomized Blinded Clinical Trial Comparing Delta-9-Tetrahydrocannabinol (THC) and Hydroxyzine (HZ) as Antiemetics (AE) for Cancer Chemotherapy (CT)," in *Proceedings of the American Association for Cancer Research*, vol. 23 (Philadelphia: AACR, 1982), 514; A. Long et al., "A Randomized Double-Blind Cross-Over Comparison of the Antiemetic Activity of Levonantradol and Prochlorperazine," in *Proceedings of the American Society of Clinical Oncology*, vol. 1 (Alexandria, VA: ASCO, 1982), C-220; M. McCabe et al., "Efficacy of Tetrahydrocannabinol in Patients Refractory to Standard Antiemetic Therapy," *Investigational New Drugs* 6, no. 3 (1988): 243–46; H. S. Chan et al., "Nabilone Versus Prochlorperazine for Control of Cancer Chemotherapy-Induced Emesis in Children: A Double-Blind, Crossover Trial," *Pediatrics* 79, no. 6 (1987): 946–52; M. Pomeroy et al., "Prospective Randomized Double-Blind Trial of Nabilone Versus Domperidone in the Treatment of Cytotoxic-Induced Emesis," *Cancer Chemotherapy and Pharmacology* 17, no. 3 (1986): 285–88; and N. Niederle et al., "Crossover Comparison of the Antiemetic Efficacy of Nabilone and Alizapride in Patients with Nonseminomatous Testicular Cancer Receiving Cisplatin Therapy," *Klinische Wochenschrift* 64, no. 8 (1986): 362–65.

Notes

89. M. R. Tramèr et al., "Cannabinoids for Control of Chemotherapy Induced Nausea and Vomiting: Quantitative Systematic Review," *BMJ* 323, no. 7303 (2001): 16–21.

90. A. E. Chang et al., "Delta-9-Tetrahydrocannabinol as an Antiemetic in Cancer Patients Receiving High-Dose Methotrexate: A Prospective, Randomized Evaluation," *Annals of Internal Medicine* 91, no. 6 (1979): 819–24.

91. V. Vinciguerra et al., "Inhalation Marijuana as an Antiemetic for Cancer Chemotherapy," *New York State Journal of Medicine* 88, no. 10 (1988): 525–27.

92. A. Abrahamov et al., "An Efficient New Cannabinoid Antiemetic in Pediatric Oncology," *Life Sciences* 56, nos. 23–24 (1995): 2097–102.

93. E. Meiri et al., "Efficacy of Dronabinol Alone and in Combination with Ondansetron Versus Ondansetron Alone for Delayed Chemotherapy-Induced Nausea and Vomiting," *Current Medical Research and Opinion* 23, no. 3 (2007): 533–43.

94. National Academies of Sciences, Engineering, and Medicine, *The Health Effects of Cannabis and Cannabinoids: The Current State of Evidence and Recommendations for Research* (Washington, DC: National Academies Press, 2017).

95. R. Gorter, "Management of Anorexia-Cachexia Associated with Cancer and HIV Infection," *Oncology* 5, suppl. 9 (1991): 13–17.

96. T. F. Plasse et al., "Recent Clinical Experience with Dronabinol," *Pharmacology Biochemistry and Behavior* 40, no. 3 (1991): 695–700.

97. K. Nelson et al., "A Phase II Study of Delta-9-Tetrahydrocannabinol for Appetite Stimulation in Cancer-Associated Anorexia," *Journal of Palliative Care* 10, no. 1 (1994): 14–18.

98. A. Jatoi et al., "Dronabinol Versus Megestrol Acetate Versus Combination Therapy for Cancer-Associated Anorexia: A North Central Cancer Treatment Group Study," *Journal of Clinical Oncology* 20, no. 2 (2002): 567–73.

99. T. D. Brisbois et al., "Delta-9-Tetrahydrocannabinol May Palliate Altered Chemosensory Perception in Cancer Patients: Results of a Randomized, Double-Blind, Placebo-Controlled Pilot Trial," *Annals of Oncology* 22, no. 9 (2011): 2086–93.

100. F. Strasser et al., "Comparison of Orally Administered Cannabis Extract and Delta-9-Tetrahydrocannabinol in Treating Patients with Cancer-Related Anorexia-Cachexia Syndrome: A Multicenter, Phase III, Randomized, Double-Blind, Placebo-Controlled Clinical Trial from the Cannabis-in-Cachexia-Study-Group," *Journal of Clinical Oncology* 24, no. 21 (2006): 3394–400.

101. G. Bar-Sela et al., "The Effects of Dosage-Controlled Cannabis Capsules on Cancer-Related Cachexia and Anorexia Syndrome in Advanced Cancer Patients: Pilot Study," *Integrative Cancer Therapies* 18 (2019): 1–8.

102. P. J. Wiffen et al., "Opioids for Cancer Pain—an Overview of Cochrane Reviews," *Cochrane Database of Systematic Reviews* 7 (2017).

103. S. Deandrea et al., "Prevalence of Undertreatment in Cancer Pain. A Review of Published Literature," *Annals of Oncology* 19, no. 12 (2008): 1985–91.

104. I. A. Khasabova et al., "CB_1 and CB_2 Receptor Agonists Promote Analgesia Through Synergy in a Murine Model of Tumor Pain," *Behavioural Pharmacology* 22, nos. 5–6 (2011): 607–16.

105. L. J. Kehl et al., "A Cannabinoid Agonist Differentially Attenuates Deep Tissue Hyperalgesia in Animal Models of Cancer and Inflammatory Muscle Pain," *Pain* 103, nos. 1–2 (2003): 175–86.

106. R. Noyes Jr. et al., "Analgesic Effect of Delta-9-Tetrahydrocannabinol," *Journal of Clinical Pharmacology* 15, nos. 2–3 (1975): 139–43.

107. R. Noyes Jr. et al., "The Analgesic Properties of Delta-9-Tetrahydrocannabinol and Codeine," *Clinical Pharmacology and Therapeutics* 18, no. 1 (1975): 84–89.

108. J. R. Johnson et al., "An Open-Label Extension Study to Investigate the Long-Term Safety and Tolerability of THC/CBD Oromucosal Spray and Oromucosal THC Spray in Patients with Terminal

Cancer–Related Pain Refractory to Strong Opioid Analgesics," *Journal of Pain and Symptom Management* 46, no. 2 (2013): 207–18.

109. J. R. Johnson et al., "Multicenter, Double-Blind, Randomized, Placebo-Controlled, Parallel-Group Study of the Efficacy, Safety, and Tolerability of THC:CBD Extract and THC Extract in Patients with Intractable Cancer-Related Pain," *Journal of Pain and Symptom Management* 39, no. 2 (2010): 167–79.

110. S. D. McAllister et al., "The Antitumor Activity of Plant-Derived Non-Psychoactive Cannabinoids," *Journal of Neuroimmune Pharmacology* 10, no. 2 (2015): 255–67; B. Chakravarti et al., "Cannabinoids as Therapeutic Agents in Cancer: Current Status and Future Implications," *Oncotarget* 5, no. 15 (2014): 5852–72; G. Velasco et al., "The Use of Cannabinoids as Anticancer Agents," *Progress in Neuro-Psychopharmacology and Biological Psychiatry* 64 (2016): 259–66; G. Velasco et al., "Anticancer Mechanisms of Cannabinoids," *Current Oncology* (Toronto) 23, suppl. 2 (2016): S23–32; G. Velasco et al., "Towards the Use of Cannabinoids as Antitumour Agents," *Nature Reviews: Cancer* 12, no. 6 (2012): 436–44; S. Pisanti et al., "The Endocannabinoid Signaling System in Cancer," *Trends in Pharmacological Sciences* 34, no. 5 (2013): 273–82; R. Ramer et al., "New Insights into Antimetastatic and Antiangiogenic Effects of Cannabinoids," in *International Review of Cell and Molecular Biology,* vol. 314, ed. K. Jeon (Cambridge, MA: Academic Press, 2015), 43–116; I. Turgeman et al., "Cannabis for Cancer—Illusion or the Tip of an Iceberg: A Review of the Evidence for the Use of Cannabis and Synthetic Cannabinoids in Oncology," *Expert Opinion on Investigational Drugs* 28, no. 3 (2019): 285–96; S. Blasco-Benito et al., "Appraising the 'Entourage Effect': Antitumor Action of a Pure Cannabinoid Versus a Botanical Drug Preparation in Preclinical Models of Breast Cancer," *Biochemical Pharmacology* 157 (2018): 285–93; and R. Schwarz et al., "Targeting the Endocannabinoid System as a Potential Anticancer Approach," *Drug Metabolism Reviews* 50, no. 1 (2018): 26–53.

111. W. M. Liu et al., "Enhancing the In Vitro Cytotoxic Activity of Delta-9-Tetrahydrocannabinol in Leukemic Cells Through a Combinatorial Approach," *Leukemia and Lymphoma* 49, no. 9 (2008): 1800–1809; S. B. Gustafsson et al., "Cannabinoid Receptor-Independent Cytotoxic Effects of Cannabinoids in Human Colorectal Carcinoma Cells: Synergism with 5-Fluorouracil," *Cancer Chemotherapy and Pharmacology* 63, no. 4 (2009): 691–701; H. Miyato et al., "Pharmacological Synergism Between Cannabinoids and Paclitaxel in Gastric Cancer Cell Lines," *Journal of Surgical Research* 155, no. 1 (2009): 40–47; M. Donadelli et al., "Gemcitabine/Cannabinoid Combination Triggers Autophagy in Pancreatic Cancer Cells Through a ROS-Mediated Mechanism," *Cell Death and Disease* 2, no. 4 (2011): e152; S. M. Emery et al., "Combined Antiproliferative Effects of the Aminoalkylindole WIN 55,212-2 and Radiation in Breast Cancer Cells," *Journal of Pharmacology and Experimental Therapeutics* 348, no. 2 (2014): 293–302; K. A. Scott et al., "The Combination of Cannabidiol and Delta-9-Tetrahydrocannabinol Enhances the Anticancer Effects of Radiation in an Orthotopic Murine Glioma Model," *Molecular Cancer Therapeutics* 13, no. 12 (2014): 2955–67; S. Torres et al., "A Combined Preclinical Therapy of Cannabinoids and Temozolomide Against Glioma," *Molecular Cancer Therapeutics* 10, no. 1 (2011): 90–103; and S. M. Emery et al., "Abstract 1453: The Cannabinoid WIN 55,212-2 Enhances the Response of Breast Cancer Cells to Radiation," in *Proceedings of the 103rd Annual Meeting of the American Association for Cancer Research, March 31–April 4, 2012, Chicago, IL* (Philadelphia: AACR Publications, 2012), 1453.

112. S. J. Ward et al., "Cannabidiol Prevents the Development of Cold and Mechanical Allodynia in Paclitaxel-Treated Female C57Bl6 Mice," *Anesthesia and Analgesia* 113, no. 4 (2011): 947–50; S. J. Ward et al., "Cannabidiol Inhibits Paclitaxel-Induced Neuropathic Pain Through 5-HT$_{1A}$ Receptors Without Diminishing Nervous System Function or Chemotherapy Efficacy," *British Journal of Pharmacology* 171, no. 3 (2014): 636–45; and K. M. King et al., "Single and Combined Effects of Delta-9-Tetrahydrocannabinol and Cannabidiol in a Mouse Model of Chemotherapy-Induced Neuropathic Pain," *British Journal of Pharmacology* 174, no. 17 (2017): 2832–41.

Notes

113. Blasco-Benito et al., "Appraising the 'Entourage Effect,' " 285–93.

114. A. Greenhough et al., "The Cannabinoid Delta(9)-Tetrahydrocannabinol Inhibits RAS-MAPK and PI3K-AKT Survival Signalling and Induces BAD-Mediated Apoptosis in Colorectal Cancer Cells," *International Journal of Cancer* 121, no. 10 (2007): 2172–80.

115. S. D. McAllister et al., "Cannabinoids Selectively Inhibit Proliferation and Induce Death of Cultured Human Glioblastoma Multiforme Cells," *Journal of Neuro-Oncology* 74, no. 1 (2005): 31–40.

116. T. Powles et al., "Cannabis-Induced Cytotoxicity in Leukemic Cell Lines: The Role of the Cannabinoid Receptors and the MAPK Pathway," *Blood* 105, no. 3 (2005): 1214–21.

117. M. Haustein et al., "Cannabinoids Increase Lung Cancer Cell Lysis by Lymphokine-Activated Killer Cells via Upregulation of ICAM-1," *Biochemical Pharmacology* 92, no. 2 (2014): 312–25.

118. J. L. Armstrong et al., "Exploiting Cannabinoid-Induced Cytotoxic Autophagy to Drive Melanoma Cell Death," *Journal of Investigative Dermatology* 135, no. 6 (2015): 1629–37.

119. T. Fisher et al., "In Vitro and In Vivo Efficacy of Non-Psychoactive Cannabidiol in Neuroblastoma," *Current Oncology* (Toronto) 23, suppl. 2 (2016): S15–22.

120. A. Carracedo et al., "Cannabinoids Induce Apoptosis of Pancreatic Tumor Cells via Endoplasmic Reticulum Stress–Related Genes," *Cancer Research* 66, no. 13 (2006): 6748–55; and I. Dando et al., "Cannabinoids Inhibit Energetic Metabolism and Induce AMPK-Dependent Autophagy in Pancreatic Cancer Cells," *Cell Death and Disease* 4, no. 6 (2013): e664.

121. L. De Petrocellis et al., "Non-THC Cannabinoids Inhibit Prostate Carcinoma Growth In Vitro and In Vivo: Pro-Apoptotic Effects and Underlying Mechanisms," *British Journal of Pharmacology* 168, no. 1 (2013): 79–102.

122. M. L. Casanova et al., "Inhibition of Skin Tumor Growth and Angiogenesis In Vivo by Activation of Cannabinoid Receptors," *Journal of Clinical Investigation* 111, no. 1 (2003): 43–50.

123. M. Guzmán et al., "A Pilot Clinical Study of Delta-9-Tetrahydrocannabinol in Patients with Recurrent Glioblastoma Multiforme," *British Journal of Cancer* 95, no. 2 (2006): 197–203.

124. GW Pharmaceuticals, "GW Pharmaceuticals Achieves Positive Results in Phase 2 Proof of Concept Study in Glioma," news release, February 7, 2017, https://www.gwpharm.com/about/news/gw-pharmaceuticals-achieves-positive-results-phase-2-proof-concept-study-glioma.

125. S.-S. Hsu et al., "Anandamide-Induced Ca^{2+} Elevation Leading to p38 MAPK Phosphorylation and Subsequent Cell Death via Apoptosis in Human Osteosarcoma Cells," *Toxicology* 231, no. 1 (2007): 21–29; and A. Notaro et al., "Involvement of PAR-4 in Cannabinoid-Dependent Sensitization of Osteosarcoma Cells to TRAIL-Induced Apoptosis," *International Journal of Biological Sciences* 10, no. 5 (2014): 466–78.

126. Donadelli et al., "Gemcitabine/Cannabinoid Combination Triggers Autophagy in Pancreatic Cancer Cells," e152; and F. Niu et al., "Potentiation of the Antitumor Activity of Adriamycin Against Osteosarcoma by Cannabinoid WIN-55,212-2," *Oncology Letters* 10, no. 4 (2015): 2415–21.

127. Sexton et al., "A Cross-Sectional Survey of Medical Cannabis Users," 131–38; P. Lucas et al., "Medical Cannabis Access, Use, and Substitution for Prescription Opioids and Other Substances: A Survey of Authorized Medical Cannabis Patients," *International Journal of Drug Policy* 42 (2017): 30–35; Nunberg et al., "An Analysis of Applicants Presenting to a Medical Marijuana Specialty Practice," 1; Swift et al., "Survey of Australians Using Cannabis for Medical Purposes," 18; Ware et al., "The Medicinal Use of Cannabis in the UK," 291–95; A. Hazekamp et al., "The Prevalence and Incidence of Medicinal Cannabis on Prescription in the Netherlands," *European Journal of Clinical Pharmacology* 69, no. 8 (2013): 1575–80; and K. F. Boehnke et al., "Medical Cannabis Use Is Associated with Decreased Opiate Medication Use in a Retrospective Cross-Sectional Survey of Patients with Chronic Pain," *Journal of Pain* 17, no. 6 (2016): 739–44.

128. National Academies of Sciences, Engineering, and Medicine, *The Health Effects of Cannabis and Cannabinoids*.

Notes

129. P. F. Whiting et al., "Cannabinoids for Medical Use: A Systematic Review and Meta-Analysis," *JAMA* 313, no. 24 (2015): 2456–73.

130. M. Mücke et al., "Cannabis-Based Medicines for Chronic Neuropathic Pain in Adults," *Cochrane Database of Systematic Reviews* 3, art. no. CD012182 (2018).

131. Boehnke et al., "Medical Cannabis Use Is Associated with Decreased Opiate Medication Use," 739–44.

132. Sexton et al., "A Cross-Sectional Survey of Medical Cannabis Users," 131–38.

133. Lucas et al., "Medical Cannabis Access, Use, and Substitution for Prescription Opioids and Other Substances," 30–35.

134. J. M. Vigil et al., "Associations Between Medical Cannabis and Prescription Opioid Use in Chronic Pain Patients: A Preliminary Cohort Study," *PLoS One* 12, no. 11 (2017): e0187795.

135. R. Abuhasira et al., "Epidemiological Characteristics, Safety, and Efficacy of Medical Cannabis in the Elderly," *European Journal of Internal Medicine* 49 (2018): 44–50.

136. V. Bargnes et al., "Safety and Efficacy of Medical Cannabis in Elderly Patients: A Retrospective Review in a Neurological Outpatient Setting," *Neurology* 92, suppl. 15 (2019): P4.1–014.

137. K. M. Takakuwa et al., "The Impact of Medical Cannabis on Intermittent and Chronic Opioid Users with Back Pain: How Cannabis Diminished Prescription Opioid Usage," *Cannabis and Cannabinoid Research,* published ahead of print (January 9, 2020).

138. D. L. Cichewicz, "Synergistic Interactions Between Cannabinoid and Opioid Analgesics," *Life Sciences* 74, no. 11 (2004): 1317–24.

139. P. Ghosh et al., "Cannabis-Induced Potentiation of Morphine Analgesia in Rat—Role of Brain Monoamines," *Indian Journal of Medical Research* 70 (1979): 275–80; R. Mechoulam et al., "Recent Advances in the Use of Cannabinoids as Therapeutic Agents," in *The Cannabinoids: Chemical, Pharmacologic, and Therapeutic Aspects,* ed. S. Agurell (Cambridge, MA: Academic Press, 1984), 777–93; S. P. Welch et al., "Antinociceptive Activity of Intrathecally Administered Cannabinoids Alone, and in Combination with Morphine, in Mice," *Journal of Pharmacology and Experimental Therapeutics* 262, no. 1 (1992): 10–18; F. L. Smith et al., "The Enhancement of Morphine Antinociception in Mice by Delta-9-Tetrahydrocannabinol," *Pharmacology Biochemistry and Behavior* 60, no. 2 (1998): 559–66; and P. B. Smith et al., "Interactions Between Delta-9-Tetrahydrocannabinol and Kappa Opioids in Mice," *Journal of Pharmacology and Experimental Therapeutics* 268, no. 3 (1994): 1381–87.

140. D. I. Abrams et al., "Cannabinoid–Opioid Interaction in Chronic Pain," *Clinical Pharmacology and Therapeutics* 90, no. 6 (2011): 844–51.

141. J. D. Roberts et al., "Synergistic Affective Analgesic Interaction Between Delta-9-Tetrahydrocannabinol and Morphine," *European Journal of Pharmacology* 530, nos. 1–2 (2006): 54–58.

142. N. Atwal et al., "THC and Gabapentin Interactions in a Mouse Neuropathic Pain Model," *Neuropharmacology* 144 (2019): 115–21.

143. F. J. Evans, "Cannabinoids: The Separation of Central from Peripheral Effects on a Structural Basis," *Planta Medica* 57, suppl. 7 (1991): S60–67.

144. P. De Candia et al., "Type 2 Diabetes: How Much of an Autoimmune Disease?," *Frontiers in Endocrinology* (Lausanne) 10 (2019): 451.

145. X. Li et al., "Examination of the Immunosuppressive Effect of Delta-9-Tetrahydrocannabinol in Streptozotocin-Induced Autoimmune Diabetes," *International Immunopharmacology* 1, no. 4 (2001): 699–712.

146. L. Weiss et al., "Cannabidiol Lowers Incidence of Diabetes in Non-Obese Diabetic Mice," *Autoimmunity* 39, no. 2 (2006): 143–51.

147. L. Weiss et al., "Cannabidiol Arrests Onset of Autoimmune Diabetes in NOD Mice," *Neuropharmacology* 54, no. 1 (2008): 244–49.

Notes

148. M. Rajesh et al., "Cannabidiol Attenuates Cardiac Dysfunction, Oxidative Stress, Fibrosis, and Inflammatory and Cell Death Signaling Pathways in Diabetic Cardiomyopathy," *Journal of the American College of Cardiology* 56, no. 25 (2010): 2115–25.

149. O. Alshaarawy et al., "Cannabis Smoking and Diabetes Mellitus: Results from Meta-Analysis with Eight Independent Replication Samples," *Epidemiology* (Cambridge, MA) 26, no. 4 (2015): 597–600.

150. Penner et al., "The Impact of Marijuana Use on Glucose, Insulin, and Insulin Resistance," 583–89.

151. Rajavashisth et al., "Decreased Prevalence of Diabetes in Marijuana Users," e000494.

152. E. T. Wargent et al., "The Cannabinoid Delta-9-Tetrahydrocannabivarin (THCV) Ameliorates Insulin Sensitivity in Two Mouse Models of Obesity," *Nutrition and Diabetes* 3, no. 5 (2013): e68.

153. P. Kwan et al., "Early Identification of Refractory Epilepsy," *New England Journal of Medicine* 342, no. 5 (2000): 314–19.

154. Ibid.

155. M. J. Wallace et al., "The Endogenous Cannabinoid System Regulates Seizure Frequency and Duration in a Model of Temporal Lobe Epilepsy," *Journal of Pharmacology and Experimental Therapeutics* 307, no. 1 (2003): 129–37.

156. L. S. Deshpande et al., "Cannabinoid CB_1 Receptor Antagonists Cause Status Epilepticus–Like Activity in the Hippocampal Neuronal Culture Model of Acquired Epilepsy," *Neuroscience Letters* 411, no. 1 (2007): 11–16.

157. A. Ludányi et al., "Downregulation of the CB_1 Cannabinoid Receptor and Related Molecular Elements of the Endocannabinoid System in Epileptic Human Hippocampus," *Journal of Neuroscience* 28, no. 12 (2008): 2976–90.

158. A. Romigi et al., "Cerebrospinal Fluid Levels of the Endocannabinoid Anandamide Are Reduced in Patients with Untreated Newly Diagnosed Temporal Lobe Epilepsy," *Epilepsia* 51, no. 5 (2010): 768–72.

159. B. J. Whalley, "CBD & CBDV in Models of Acute Epilepsy," presented at Cannabidiols: Potential Use in Epilepsy and Other Neurological Disorders, NYU School of Medicine, October 4, 2013, http://faces.med.nyu.edu/research-education/cannabidiol-conference.

160. R. Mechoulam et al., "Toward Drugs Derived from Cannabis," *Naturwissenschaften* 65, no. 4 (1978): 174–79.

161. J. M. Cunha et al., "Chronic Administration of Cannabidiol to Healthy Volunteers and Epileptic Patients," *Pharmacology* 21, no. 3 (1980): 175–85.

162. F. R. Ames et al., "Anticonvulsant Effect of Cannabidiol," *South African Medical Journal* 69, no. 1 (1986): 14.

163. B. Trembly et al., "Double-Blind Clinical Study of Cannabidiol as a Secondary Anticonvulsant," presented at the Marijuana '90 International Conference on Cannabis and Cannabinoids, July 8–11, 1990, Kolymbari, Crete, https://www.epistemonikos.org/en/documents/d41032a66cdf9e8d72 44283c358128f2576a57a7.

164. A. Pelliccia et al., "Treatment with CBD in Oily Solutions of Drug-Resistant Pediatric Epilepsies," in *IACM 3rd Conference on Cannabinoids in Medicine, 9–10 September 2005, Leiden University* (Leiden, Netherlands: International Association for Cannabis as Medicine, 2005).

165. B. E. Porter et al., "Report of a Parent Survey of Cannabidiol-Enriched Cannabis Use in Pediatric Treatment-Resistant Epilepsy," *Epilepsy and Behavior* 29, no. 3 (2013): 574–77.

166. M. Gedde et al., "Whole Cannabis Extract of High Concentration Cannabidiol May Calm Seizures in Highly Refractory Pediatric Epilepsies," abstract, American Epilepsy Society, 67th Annual Meeting, December 6–10, 2013.

167. Hussain et al., "Perceived Efficacy of Cannabidiol-Enriched Cannabis Extracts," 138–41.

168. M. Tzadok et al., "CBD-Enriched Medical Cannabis for Intractable Pediatric Epilepsy: The Current Israeli Experience," *Seizure* 35 (2016): 41–44.

169. D. Sulak et al., "The Current Status of Artisanal Cannabis for the Treatment of Epilepsy in the United States," *Epilepsy and Behavior* 70, pt. B (2017): 328–33.

170. G. S. Porcari et al., "Efficacy of Artisanal Preparations of Cannabidiol for the Treatment of Epilepsy: Practical Experiences in a Tertiary Medical Center," *Epilepsy and Behavior* 80 (2018): 240–46.

171. O. Devinsky et al., "Effect of Cannabidiol on Drop Seizures in the Lennox-Gastaut Syndrome," *New England Journal of Medicine* 378, no. 20 (2018): 1888–97.

172. O. Devinsky et al., "Trial of Cannabidiol for Drug-Resistant Seizures in the Dravet Syndrome," *New England Journal of Medicine* 376, no. 21 (2017): 2011–20.

173. A. Vezzani et al., "The Role of Inflammation in Epilepsy," *Nature Reviews Neurology* 7, no. 1 (2011): 31–40; and A. Vezzani et al., "New Roles for Interleukin-1 Beta in the Mechanisms of Epilepsy," *Epilepsy Currents* 7, no. 2 (2007): 45–50.

174. E. B. Russo, "Taming THC: Potential Cannabis Synergy and Phytocannabinoid-Terpenoid Entourage Effects," *British Journal of Pharmacology* 163, no. 7 (2011): 1344–64.

175. A. C. Campos et al., "Cannabidiol, Neuroprotection, and Neuropsychiatric Disorders," *Pharmacological Research* 112 (2016): 119–27; A. C. Campos et al., "Plastic and Neuroprotective Mechanisms Involved in the Therapeutic Effects of Cannabidiol in Psychiatric Disorders," *Frontiers in Pharmacology* 8 (2017): 269; and R. A. Do Val-da Silva et al., "Protective Effects of Cannabidiol Against Seizures and Neuronal Death in a Rat Model of Mesial Temporal Lobe Epilepsy," *Frontiers in Pharmacology* 8 (2017): 131.

176. D. Ryan et al., "Cannabidiol Targets Mitochondria to Regulate Intracellular Ca^{2+} Levels," *Journal of Neuroscience* 29, no. 7 (2009): 2053–63.

177. A. Drab et al., "Endocannabinoid System and Cannabinoids in Neurogenesis—New Opportunities for Neurological Treatment? Reports from Experimental Studies," *Journal of Pre-Clinical and Clinical Research* 11, no. 1 (2017): 76–80; G. Esposito et al., "Cannabidiol Reduces Aβ-Induced Neuroinflammation and Promotes Hippocampal Neurogenesis Through PPARγ Involvement," *PLoS One* 6, no. 12 (2011); A. C. Campos et al., "The Anxiolytic Effect of Cannabidiol on Chronically Stressed Mice Depends on Hippocampal Neurogenesis: Involvement of the Endocannabinoid System," *International Journal of Neuropsychopharmacology* 16, no. 6 (2013): 1407–19; A. C. Campos et al., "Cannabinoids as Regulators of Neural Development and Adult Neurogenesis," in *Lipidomics of Stem Cells* (New York: Humana Press, 2017), 117–36; and M. V. Fogaça et al., "The Anxiolytic Effects of Cannabidiol in Chronically Stressed Mice Are Mediated by the Endocannabinoid System: Role of Neurogenesis and Dendritic Remodeling," *Neuropharmacology* 135 (2018): 22–33.

178. O. Devinsky et al., "Randomized, Dose-Ranging Safety Trial of Cannabidiol in Dravet Syndrome," *Neurology* 90, no. 14 (2018): e1204–11.

179. T. E. Gaston et al., "Interactions Between Cannabidiol and Commonly Used Antiepileptic Drugs," *Epilepsia* 58, no. 9 (2017): 1586–92.

180. I. Kaufmann et al., "Anandamide and Neutrophil Function in Patients with Fibromyalgia," *Psychoneuroendocrinology* 33, no. 5 (2008): 676–85.

181. R. E. Harris et al., "Dynamic Levels of Glutamate Within the Insula Are Associated with Improvements in Multiple Pain Domains in Fibromyalgia," *Arthritis and Rheumatism* 58, no. 3 (2008): 903–7.

182. H. Wang et al., "Circulating Cytokine Levels Compared to Pain in Patients with Fibromyalgia—a Prospective Longitudinal Study over 6 Months," *Journal of Rheumatology* 35, no. 7 (2008): 1366–70.

183. M. Schley et al., "Delta-9-THC Based Monotherapy in Fibromyalgia Patients on Experimentally Induced Pain, Axon Reflex Flare, and Pain Relief," *Current Medical Research and Opinion* 22, no. 7 (2006): 1269–76.

184. R. Q. Skrabek et al., "Nabilone for the Treatment of Pain in Fibromyalgia," *Journal of Pain* 9, no. 2 (2008): 164–73.

Notes

185. J. Fiz et al., "Cannabis Use in Patients with Fibromyalgia: Effect on Symptoms Relief and Health-Related Quality of Life," *PLoS One* 6, no. 4 (2011): e18440.

186. A. A. Izzo et al., "Cannabinoids and the Gut: New Developments and Emerging Concepts," *Pharmacology and Therapeutics* 126, no. 1 (2010): 21–38.

187. Ibid.

188. M. Camilleri et al., "Genetic Variation in Endocannabinoid Metabolism, Gastrointestinal Motility, and Sensation," *American Journal of Physiology: Gastrointestinal and Liver Physiology* 294, no. 1 (2008): G13–19.

189. O. M. E. Abdel-Salam et al., "Effect of *Cannabis Sativa* Extract on Gastric Acid Secretion, Oxidative Stress, and Gastric Mucosal Integrity in Rats," *Comparative Clinical Pathology* 24, no. 6 (2015): 1417–34; and F. Borrelli, "Cannabinoid CB_1 Receptor and Gastric Acid Secretion," *Digestive Diseases and Sciences* 52, no. 11 (2007): 3102–3.

190. A. Lehmann et al., "Cannabinoid Receptor Agonism Inhibits Transient Lower Esophageal Sphincter Relaxations and Reflux in Dogs," *Gastroenterology* 123, no. 4 (2002): 1129–34.

191. H. Beaumont et al., "Effect of Delta-9-Tetrahydrocannabinol, a Cannabinoid Receptor Agonist, on the Triggering of Transient Lower Oesophageal Sphincter Relaxations in Dogs and Humans," *British Journal of Pharmacology* 156, no. 1 (2009): 153–62.

192. M. F. Neurath, "Targeting Immune Cell Circuits and Trafficking in Inflammatory Bowel Disease," *Nature Immunology* 20, no. 8 (2019): 970–79.

193. M. Grill et al., "Members of the Endocannabinoid System Are Distinctly Regulated in Inflammatory Bowel Disease and Colorectal Cancer," *Scientific Reports* 9, no. 2358 (2019).

194. E. S. Kimball et al., "Agonists of Cannabinoid Receptor 1 and 2 Inhibit Experimental Colitis Induced by Oil of Mustard and by Dextran Sulfate Sodium," *American Journal of Physiology: Gastrointestinal and Liver Physiology* 291, no. 2 (2006): G364–71; A. Di Sabatino et al., "The Endogenous Cannabinoid System in the Gut of Patients with Inflammatory Bowel Disease," *Mucosal Immunology* 4, no. 5 (2011): 574–83; and G. D'Argenio et al., "Up-Regulation of Anandamide Levels as an Endogenous Mechanism and a Pharmacological Strategy to Limit Colon Inflammation," *FASEB Journal* 20, no. 3 (2006): 568–70.

195. D. G. Couch et al., "The Use of Cannabinoids in Colitis: A Systematic Review and Meta-Analysis," *Inflammatory Bowel Diseases* 24, no. 4 (2018): 680–97.

196. A. Swaminath et al., "The Role of Cannabis in the Management of Inflammatory Bowel Disease: A Review of Clinical, Scientific, and Regulatory Information," *Inflammatory Bowel Diseases* 25, no. 3 (2019): 427–35.

197. T. Naftali et al., "Treatment of Crohn's Disease with Cannabis: An Observational Study," *Israel Medical Association Journal* 13, no. 8 (2011): 455–58.

198. A. Lahat et al., "Impact of Cannabis Treatment on the Quality of Life, Weight, and Clinical Disease Activity in Inflammatory Bowel Disease Patients: A Pilot Prospective Study," *Digestion* 85, no. 1 (2012): 1–8.

199. J. Ravikoff Allegretti et al., "Marijuana Use Patterns Among Patients with Inflammatory Bowel Disease," *Inflammatory Bowel Diseases* 19, no. 13 (2013): 2809–14.

200. T. Naftali et al., "Cannabis Induces a Clinical Response in Patients with Crohn's Disease: A Prospective Placebo-Controlled Study," *Clinical Gastroenterology and Hepatology* 11, no. 10 (2013): 1276–80.

201. C. Mbachi et al., "Association Between Cannabis Use and Complications Related to Crohn's Disease: A Retrospective Cohort Study," *Digestive Diseases and Sciences* 64, no. 10 (2019): 2939–44.

202. R. Desai et al., "In-Hospital Outcomes of Inflammatory Bowel Disease in Cannabis Users: A Nationwide Propensity-Matched Analysis in the United States," *Annals of Translational Medicine* 7, no. 12 (2019): 252.

Notes

203. M. A. Storr et al., "The Role of the Endocannabinoid System in the Pathophysiology and Treatment of Irritable Bowel Syndrome," *Neurogastroenterology and Motility* 20, no. 8 (2008): 857–68.

204. T. K. Klooker et al., "The Cannabinoid Receptor Agonist Delta-9-Tetrahydrocannabinol Does Not Affect Visceral Sensitivity to Rectal Distension in Healthy Volunteers and IBS Patients," *Neurogastroenterology and Motility* 23, no. 1 (2011): 30–35.

205. B. S. Wong et al., "Pharmacogenetic Trial of a Cannabinoid Agonist Shows Reduced Fasting Colonic Motility in Patients with Nonconstipated Irritable Bowel Syndrome," *Gastroenterology* 141, no. 5 (2011): 1638–47.

206. B. S. Wong et al., "Randomized Pharmacodynamic and Pharmacogenetic Trial of Dronabinol Effects on Colon Transit in Irritable Bowel Syndrome–Diarrhea," *Neurogastroenterology and Motility* 24, no. 4 (2012): 358–e169.

207. R. S. Hepler et al., "Marihuana Smoking and Intraocular Pressure," *JAMA* 217, no. 10 (1971): 1392.

208. Ibid.; A. B. Lockhart et al., "The Potential Use of *Cannabis Sativa* in Ophthalmology," *West Indian Medical Journal* 26, no. 2 (1977): 66–70; J. C. Merritt et al., "Effect of Marihuana on Intraocular and Blood Pressure in Glaucoma," *Ophthalmology* 87, no. 3 (1980): 222–28; and A. Porcella et al., "The Synthetic Cannabinoid WIN55212-2 Decreases the Intraocular Pressure in Human Glaucoma Resistant to Conventional Therapies," *European Journal of Neuroscience* 13, no. 2 (2001): 409–12.

209. I. Tomida et al., "Effect of Sublingual Application of Cannabinoids on Intraocular Pressure: A Pilot Study," *Journal of Glaucoma* 15, no. 5 (2006): 349–53.

210. A. J. Flach, "Delta-9-Tetrahydrocannabinol (THC) in the Treatment of End-Stage Open-Angle Glaucoma," *Transactions of the American Ophthalmological Society* 100 (2002): 215–22.

211. Tomida et al., "Effect of Sublingual Application of Cannabinoids on Intraocular Pressure," 349–53.

212. S. Miller et al., "Delta-9-Tetrahydrocannabinol and Cannabidiol Differentially Regulate Intraocular Pressure," *Investigative Ophthalmology and Visual Science* 59, no. 15 (2018): 5904–11.

213. K. MacMillan et al., "Cannabis and Glaucoma: A Literature Review," *Dalhousie Medical Journal* 46, no. 1 (2019): 17–21.

214. V. Di Marzo et al., "Biosynthesis of Anandamide and Related Acylethanolamides in Mouse J774 Macrophages and N18 Neuroblastoma Cells," *Biochemical Journal* 316, pt. 3 (1996): 977–84.

215. S. Oka et al., "2-Arachidonoylglycerol, an Endogenous Cannabinoid Receptor Ligand, Induces the Migration of EoL-1 Human Eosinophilic Leukemia Cells and Human Peripheral Blood Eosinophils," *Journal of Leukocyte Biology* 76, no. 5 (2004): 1002–9; and N. Rayman et al., "Distinct Expression Profiles of the Peripheral Cannabinoid Receptor in Lymphoid Tissues Depending on Receptor Activation Status," *Journal of Immunology* 172, no. 4 (2004): 2111–17.

216. T. W. Klein et al., "The Cannabinoid System and Immune Modulation," *Journal of Leukocyte Biology* 74, no. 4 (2003): 486–96.

217. R. Tanasescu et al., "Cannabinoids and the Immune System: An Overview," *Immunobiology* 215, no. 8 (2010): 588–97.

218. T. W. Klein, "Cannabinoid-Based Drugs as Anti-inflammatory Therapeutics," *Nature Reviews: Immunology* 5, no. 5 (2005): 400–11.

219. R. Rao et al., "Delta-9-Tetrahydrocannabinol Attenuates Staphylococcal Enterotoxin B-Induced Inflammatory Lung Injury and Prevents Mortality in Mice by Modulation of miR-17-92 Cluster and Induction of T-Regulatory Cells," *British Journal of Pharmacology* 172, no. 7 (2015): 1792–806.

220. G. Appendino et al., "Antibacterial Cannabinoids from *Cannabis Sativa:* A Structure-Activity Study," *Journal of Natural Products* 71, no. 8 (2008): 1427–30; M. Feldman et al., "Antimicrobial Potential of Endocannabinoid and Endocannabinoid-Like Compounds Against Methicillin-Resistant Staphylococcus Aureus," *Scientific Reports* 8, no. 17696 (2018): 1–10; and B. van Klingeren et al., "Antibacterial Activity of Delta-9-Tetrahydrocannabinol and Cannabidiol," *Antonie van Leeuwenhoek* 42, nos. 1–2 (1976): 9–12.

Notes

221. C. S. Wassmann et al., "Cannabidiol Is an Effective Helper Compound in Combination with Bacitracin to Kill Gram-Positive Bacteria," *Scientific Reports* 10, no. 1 (2020): 4112.

222. P. S. Morahan et al., "Effects of Cannabinoids on Host Resistance to Listeria Monocytogenes and Herpes Simplex Virus," *Infection and Immunity* 23, no. 3 (1979): 670–74; E. M. Mishkin et al., "Delta-9-Tetrahydrocannabinol Decreases Host Resistance to Herpes Simplex Virus Type 2 Vaginal Infection in the B6C3F1 Mouse," *Journal of General Virology* 66, pt. 12 (1985): 2539–49; G. A. Cabral et al., "Delta-9-Tetrahydrocannabinol Decreases Alpha/Beta Interferon Response to Herpes Simplex Virus Type 2 in the B6C3F1 Mouse," *Proceedings of the Society for Experimental Biology and Medicine* 181, no. 2 (1986): 305–11; M. V. Solbrig et al., "Cannabinoid Rescue of Striatal Progenitor Cells in Chronic Borna Disease Viral Encephalitis in Rats," *Journal of Neurovirology* 14, no. 3 (2008): 252–60; and J. L. Croxford et al., "Immunoregulation of a Viral Model of Multiple Sclerosis Using the Synthetic Cannabinoid R+WIN55,212," *Journal of Clinical Investigation* 111, no. 8 (2003): 1231–40.

223. D. I. Abrams et al., "Short-Term Effects of Cannabinoids in Patients with HIV-1 Infection: A Randomized, Placebo-Controlled Clinical Trial," *Annals of Internal Medicine* 139, no. 4 (2003): 258–66.

224. H. I. Lowe et al., "Potential of Cannabidiol for the Treatment of Viral Hepatitis," *Pharmacognosy Research* 9, no. 1 (2017): 116–18.

225. Ibid.

226. I. Magen et al., "Cannabidiol Ameliorates Cognitive and Motor Impairments in Bile-Duct Ligated Mice via 5-HT1A Receptor Activation," *British Journal of Pharmacology* 159, no. 4 (2010): 950–57.

227. Y. Avraham et al., "Cannabidiol Improves Brain and Liver Function in a Fulminant Hepatic Failure–Induced Model of Hepatic Encephalopathy in Mice," *British Journal of Pharmacology* 162, no. 7 (2011): 1650–58.

228. P. Mukhopadhyay et al., "Cannabidiol Protects Against Hepatic Ischemia/Reperfusion Injury by Attenuating Inflammatory Signaling and Response, Oxidative/Nitrative Stress, and Cell Death," *Free Radical Biology and Medicine* 50, no. 10 (2011): 1368–81.

229. L. Yang et al., "Cannabidiol Protects Liver from Binge Alcohol–Induced Steatosis by Mechanisms Including Inhibition of Oxidative Stress and Increase in Autophagy," *Free Radical Biology and Medicine* 68 (2014): 260–67.

230. C. Hézode et al., "Daily Cannabis Smoking as a Risk Factor for Progression of Fibrosis in Chronic Hepatitis C," *Hepatology* 42, no. 1 (2005): 63–71; C. Hézode et al., "Daily Cannabis Use: A Novel Risk Factor of Steatosis Severity in Patients with Chronic Hepatitis C," *Gastroenterology* 134, no. 2 (2008): 432–39; and J. H. Ishida et al., "Influence of Cannabis Use on Severity of Hepatitis C Disease," *Clinical Gastroenterology and Hepatology* 6, no. 1 (2008): 69–75.

231. L. Brunet et al., "Marijuana Smoking Does Not Accelerate Progression of Liver Disease in HIV–Hepatitis C Coinfection: A Longitudinal Cohort Analysis," *Clinical Infectious Diseases* 57, no. 5 (2013): 663–70.

232. D. L. Sylvestre et al., "Cannabis Use Improves Retention and Virological Outcomes in Patients Treated for Hepatitis C," *European Journal of Gastroenterology and Hepatology* 18, no. 10 (2006): 1057–63.

233. E. M. Kelly et al., "Marijuana Use Is Not Associated with Progression to Advanced Liver Fibrosis in HIV/Hepatitis C Virus–Coinfected Women," *Clinical Infectious Diseases* 63, no. 4 (2016): 512–18.

234. A. C. Adejumo et al., "Cannabis Use Is Associated with Reduced Prevalence of Non-Alcoholic Fatty Liver Disease: A Cross-Sectional Study," *PLoS One* 12, no. 4 (2017): e0176416.

235. A. C. Adejumo et al., "Cannabis Use Is Associated with Reduced Prevalence of Progressive Stages of Alcoholic Liver Disease," *Liver International* 38, no. 8 (2018): 1475–86.

Notes

236. A. C. Adejumo et al., "Reduced Incidence and Better Liver Disease Outcomes Among Chronic HCV Infected Patients Who Consume Cannabis," *Canadian Journal of Gastroenterology and Hepatology* 2018 (2018): 9430953.

237. R. S. El-Mallakh, "Marijuana and Migraine," *Headache* 27, no. 8 (1987): 442–43.

238. R. Burstein et al., "EHMTI-0354. Abnormal Expression of Gene Transcripts Linked to Inflammatory Response in the Periosteum of Chronic Migraine Patients: Implications to Extracranial Origin of Headache," *Journal of Headache and Pain* 15, suppl. 1 (2014): K2.

239. P. Sarchielli et al., "Endocannabinoids in Chronic Migraine: CSF Findings Suggest a System Failure," *Neuropsychopharmacology* 32, no. 6 (2007): 1384–90.

240. C. Rossi et al., "Endocannabinoids in Platelets of Chronic Migraine Patients and Medication-Overuse Headache Patients: Relation with Serotonin Levels," *European Journal of Clinical Pharmacology* 64, no. 1 (2008): 1–8.

241. D. N. Rhyne et al., "Effects of Medical Marijuana on Migraine Headache Frequency in an Adult Population," *Pharmacotherapy* 36, no. 5 (2016): 505–10.

242. M. Nicolodi et al., "Therapeutic Use of Cannabinoids—Dose Finding, Effects, and Pilot Data of Effects in Chronic Migraine and Cluster Headache," *European Journal of Neurology* 24, suppl. 1 (2017): 287.

243. E. P. Baron et al., "Patterns of Medicinal Cannabis Use, Strain Analysis, and Substitution Effect Among Patients with Migraine, Headache, Arthritis, and Chronic Pain in a Medicinal Cannabis Cohort," *Journal of Headache and Pain* 19, no. 1 (2018): 37.

244. A. Hazekamp et al., "The Medicinal Use of Cannabis and Cannabinoids: An International Cross-Sectional Survey on Administration Forms," *Journal of Psychoactive Drugs* 45, no. 3 (2013): 199–210.

245. J. H. Kindred et al., "Cannabis Use in People with Parkinson's Disease and Multiple Sclerosis: A Web-Based Investigation," *Complementary Therapies in Medicine* 33 (2017): 99–104.

246. L. Mestre et al., "Gut Microbiota, Cannabinoid System, and Neuroimmune Interactions: New Perspectives in Multiple Sclerosis," *Biochemical Pharmacology* 157 (2018): 51–66; M. Mecha et al., "The Endocannabinoid 2-AG Enhances Spontaneous Remyelination by Targeting Microglia," *Brain, Behavior, and Immunity* 77 (2019): 110–26; and R. Kaur et al., "Endocannabinoid System: A Multi-Facet Therapeutic Target," *Current Clinical Pharmacology* 11, no. 2 (2016): 110–17.

247. J. Corey-Bloom, "Short-Term Effects of Cannabis Therapy on Spasticity in Multiple-Sclerosis," synopsis of CMCR published clinical study results, in *Center for Medicinal Cannabis Research, Report to the Legislature and Governor of the State of California,* University of California, San Diego, February 11, 2010, p. 12, https://www.cmcr.ucsd.edu/images/PDFs/CMCR_REPORT_FEB17.pdf.

248. National Academies of Sciences, Engineering, and Medicine, *The Health Effects of Cannabis and Cannabinoids*, 128.

249. F. Patti et al., "Efficacy and Safety of Cannabinoid Oromucosal Spray for Multiple Sclerosis Spasticity," *Journal of Neurology, Neurosurgery, and Psychiatry* 87, no. 9 (2016): 944–51.

250. N. Abo Youssef et al., "Cannabinoids for Treating Neurogenic Lower Urinary Tract Dysfunction in Patients with Multiple Sclerosis: A Systematic Review and Meta-Analysis," *BJU International* 119, no. 4 (2017): 515–21.

251. Sorosina et al., "Clinical Response to Nabiximols Correlates with the Downregulation of Immune Pathways," 934-e70.

252. L. Ferrè et al., "Efficacy and Safety of Nabiximols (Sativex[*]) on Multiple Sclerosis Spasticity in a Real-Life Italian Monocentric Study," *Neurological Sciences* 37, no. 2 (2016): 235–42.

253. C. Raman et al., "Amyotrophic Lateral Sclerosis: Delayed Disease Progression in Mice by Treatment with a Cannabinoid," *Amyotrophic Lateral Sclerosis and Other Motor Neuron Disorders* 5, no. 1 (2004): 33–39.

Notes

254. L. G. Bilsland et al., "Increasing Cannabinoid Levels by Pharmacological and Genetic Manipulation Delays Disease Progression in SOD1 Mice," *FASEB Journal* 20, no. 7 (2006): 1003–5.

255. K. Kim et al., "AM1241, a Cannabinoid CB_2 Receptor Selective Compound, Delays Disease Progression in a Mouse Model of Amyotrophic Lateral Sclerosis," *European Journal of Pharmacology* 542, nos. 1–3 (2006): 100–5.

256. J. L. Shoemaker, "The CB_2 Cannabinoid Agonist AM-1241 Prolongs Survival in a Transgenic Mouse Model of Amyotrophic Lateral Sclerosis when Initiated at Symptom Onset," *Journal of Neurochemistry* 101, no. 1 (2007): 87–98.

257. D. Amtmann et al., "Survey of Cannabis Use in Patients with Amyotrophic Lateral Sclerosis," *American Journal of Hospice and Palliative Care* 21, no. 2 (2004): 95–104.

258. G. T. Carter et al., "Marijuana in the Management of Amyotrophic Lateral Sclerosis," *American Journal of Hospice and Palliative Care* 18, no. 4 (2001): 264–70.

259. N. Riva et al., "Safety and Efficacy of Nabiximols on Spasticity Symptoms in Patients with Motor Neuron Disease (CANALS): A Multicentre, Double-Blind, Randomised, Placebo-Controlled, Phase 2 Trial," *Lancet: Neurology* 18, no. 2 (2019): 155–64.

260. G. Watt et al., "In Vivo Evidence for Therapeutic Properties of Cannabidiol (CBD) for Alzheimer's Disease," *Frontiers in Pharmacology* 8 (2017): 20.

261. G. Esposito et al., "The Marijuana Component Cannabidiol Inhibits Beta-Amyloid-Induced Tau Protein Hyperphosphorylation Through Wnt/Beta-Catenin Pathway Rescue in PC12 Cells," *Journal of Molecular Medicine* (Berlin) 84, no. 3 (2006): 253–58.

262. C. Cao et al., "The Potential Therapeutic Effects of THC on Alzheimer's Disease," *Journal of Alzheimer's Disease* 42, no. 3 (2014): 973–84.

263. R. M. Tolón et al., "The Activation of Cannabinoid CB_2 Receptors Stimulates In Situ and In Vitro Beta-Amyloid Removal by Human Macrophages," *Brain Research* 1283 (2009): 148–54.

264. G. Esposito et al., "CB_1 Receptor Selective Activation Inhibits Beta-Amyloid-Induced iNOS Protein Expression in C6 Cells and Subsequently Blunts Tau Protein Hyperphosphorylation in Co-cultured Neurons," *Neuroscience Letters* 404, no. 3 (2006): 342–46.

265. E. Aso et al., "CB_2 Cannabinoid Receptor Agonist Ameliorates Alzheimer-Like Phenotype in AβPP/PS1 Mice," *Journal of Alzheimer's Disease* 35, no. 4 (2013): 847–58.

266. E. Aso et al., "CB_1 Agonist ACEA Protects Neurons and Reduces the Cognitive Impairment of AβPP/PS1 Mice," *Journal of Alzheimer's Disease* 30, no. 2 (2012): 439–59.

267. E. Aso et al., "Cannabis-Based Medicine Reduces Multiple Pathological Processes in AβPP/PS1 Mice," *Journal of Alzheimer's Disease* 43, no. 3 (2015): 977–91.

268. Ibid.

269. J. Fernández-Ruiz, "The Endocannabinoid System as a Target for the Treatment of Motor Dysfunction," *British Journal of Pharmacology* 156, no. 7 (2009): 1029–40.

270. C. Blázquez et al., "Loss of Striatal Type 1 Cannabinoid Receptors Is a Key Pathogenic Factor in Huntington's Disease," *Brain* 134, pt. 1 (2011): 119–36.

271. J. Bouchard et al., "Cannabinoid Receptor 2 Signaling in Peripheral Immune Cells Modulates Disease Onset and Severity in Mouse Models of Huntington's Disease," *Journal of Neuroscience* 32, no. 50 (2012): 18259–68.

272. S. Valdeolivas et al., "Neuroprotective Properties of Cannabigerol in Huntington's Disease: Studies in R6/2 Mice and 3-Nitropropionate-Lesioned Mice," *Neurotherapeutics* 12, no. 1 (2015): 185–99.

273. O. Sagredo et al., "Cannabidiol Reduced the Striatal Atrophy Caused 3-Nitropropionic Acid In Vivo by Mechanisms Independent of the Activation of Cannabinoid, Vanilloid TRPV1, and Adenosine A2A Receptors," *European Journal of Neuroscience* 26, no. 4 (2007): 843–51; J. Palazuelos et al., "Microglial CB_2 Cannabinoid Receptors Are Neuroprotective in Huntington's Disease Excitotoxicity," *Brain* 132, pt. 11 (2009): 3152–64; O. Sagredo et al., "Cannabinoid CB_2 Receptor Agonists Protect the Striatum

Notes

Against Malonate Toxicity: Relevance for Huntington's Disease," *Glia* 57, no. 11 (2009): 1154–67; and A. Pintor et al., "The Cannabinoid Receptor Agonist WIN 55,212-2 Attenuates the Effects Induced by Quinolinic Acid in the Rat Striatum," *Neuropharmacology* 51, no. 5 (2006): 1004–12.

274. S. Valdeolivas et al., "Effects of a Sativex-Like Combination of Phytocannabinoids on Disease Progression in R6/2 Mice, an Experimental Model of Huntington's Disease," *International Journal of Molecular Sciences* 18, no. 4 (2017): E684.

275. A. Curtis et al., "Nabilone Could Treat Chorea and Irritability in Huntington's Disease," *Journal of Neuropsychiatry and Clinical Neurosciences* 18, no. 4 (2006): 553–54; A. Curtis et al., "A Pilot Study Using Nabilone for Symptomatic Treatment in Huntington's Disease," *Movement Disorders* 24, no. 15 (2009): 2254–59; and K. R. Müller-Vahl et al., "Nabilone Increases Choreatic Movements in Huntington's Disease," *Movement Disorders* 14, no. 6 (1999): 1038–40.

276. P. Consroe et al., "Controlled Clinical Trial of Cannabidiol in Huntington's Disease," *Pharmacology Biochemistry and Behavior* 40, no. 3 (1991): 701–8.

277. J. García-Caldentey et al., "Q23: A Double-Blind, Cross-Over, Placebo-Controlled, Phase II Trial of Sativex in Huntington's Disease," *Journal of Neurology, Neurosurgery, and Psychiatry* 83, suppl. 1 (2012): A62.

278. J. Fernández-Ruiz et al., "Cannabidiol for Neurodegenerative Disorders: Important New Clinical Applications for This Phytocannabinoid?," *British Journal of Clinical Pharmacology* 75, no. 2 (2013): 323–33.

279. P. J. Blanchet et al., "Chronic Pain and Pain Processing in Parkinson's Disease," *Progress in Neuro-Psychopharmacology and Biological Psychiatry* 87, pt. B (2018): 200–6.

280. C. García et al., "Cannabinoid–Dopamine Interactions in the Physiology and Physiopathology of the Basal Ganglia," *British Journal of Pharmacology* 173, no. 13 (2016): 2069–79.

281. Fernández-Ruiz, "The Endocannabinoid System as a Target for the Treatment of Motor Dysfunction," 1029–40.

282. K. A. Sieradzan et al., "Cannabinoids Reduce Levodopa-Induced Dyskinesia in Parkinson's Disease: A Pilot Study," *Neurology* 57, no. 11 (2001): 2108–11.

283. C. B. Carroll et al., "Cannabis for Dyskinesia in Parkinson Disease: A Randomized Double-Blind Crossover Study," *Neurology* 63, no. 7 (2004): 1245–50.

284. K. Venderová et al., "Survey on Cannabis Use in Parkinson's Disease: Subjective Improvement of Motor Symptoms," *Movement Disorders* 19, no. 9 (2004): 1102–6.

285. A. W. Zuardi et al., "Cannabidiol for the Treatment of Psychosis in Parkinson's Disease," *Journal of Psychopharmacology* 23, no. 8 (2009): 979–83.

286. I. Lotan et al., "Cannabis (Medical Marijuana) Treatment for Motor and Non-Motor Symptoms of Parkinson Disease: An Open-Label Observational Study," *Clinical Neuropharmacology* 37, no. 2 (2014): 41–44.

287. M. H. Chagas et al., "Effects of Cannabidiol in the Treatment of Patients with Parkinson's Disease: An Exploratory Double-Blind Trial," *Journal of Psychopharmacology* 28, no. 11 (2014): 1088–98.

288. M. H. Chagas et al., "Cannabidiol Can Improve Complex Sleep-Related Behaviours Associated with Rapid Eye Movement Sleep Behaviour Disorder in Parkinson's Disease Patients: A Case Series," *Journal of Clinical Pharmacy and Therapeutics* 39, no. 5 (2014): 564–66.

289. Y. Balash et al., "Medical Cannabis in Parkinson Disease: Real-Life Patients' Experience," *Clinical Neuropharmacology* 40, no. 6 (2017): 268–72.

290. S. M. De Faria et al., "Effects of Acute Cannabidiol Administration on Anxiety and Tremors Induced by a Simulated Public Speaking Test in Patients with Parkinson's Disease," *Journal of Psychopharmacology* 34, no. 2 (2020): 189–96.

291. C. García et al., "Symptom-Relieving and Neuroprotective Effects of the Phytocannabinoid Delta-9-THCV in Animal Models of Parkinson's Disease," *British Journal of Pharmacology* 163, no. 7 (2011): 1495–506.

Notes

292. I. Lastres-Becker et al., "Cannabinoids Provide Neuroprotection Against 6-Hydroxydopamine Toxicity In Vivo and In Vitro: Relevance to Parkinson's Disease," *Neurobiology of Disease* 19, nos. 1–2 (2005): 96–107.

293. C. M. Nievergelt et al., "International Meta-Analysis of PTSD Genome-Wide Association Studies Identifies Sex- and Ancestry-Specific Genetic Risk Loci," *Nature Communications* 10, no. 1 (2019): 4558.

294. M. Hoskins et al., "Pharmacotherapy for Post-Traumatic Stress Disorder: Systematic Review and Meta-Analysis," *British Journal of Psychiatry* 206, no. 2 (2015): 93–100.

295. Katona et al., "Distribution of CB_1 Cannabinoid Receptors in the Amygdala," 9506–18.

296. G. A. Fraser, "The Use of a Synthetic Cannabinoid in the Management of Treatment-Resistant Nightmares in Posttraumatic Stress Disorder (PTSD)," *CNS Neuroscience and Therapeutics* 15, no. 1 (2009): 84–88.

297. C. Cameron et al., "Use of a Synthetic Cannabinoid in a Correctional Population for Posttraumatic Stress Disorder—Related Insomnia and Nightmares, Chronic Pain, Harm Reduction, and Other Indications: A Retrospective Evaluation," *Journal of Clinical Psychopharmacology* 34, no. 5 (2014): 559–64.

298. A. Neumeister et al., "Elevated Brain Cannabinoid CB_1 Receptor Availability in Post-Traumatic Stress Disorder: A Positron Emission Tomography Study," *Molecular Psychiatry* 18, no. 9 (2013): 1034–40.

299. G. R. Greer et al., "PTSD Symptom Reports of Patients Evaluated for the New Mexico Medical Cannabis Program," *Journal of Psychoactive Drugs* 46, no. 1 (2014): 73–77.

300. P. Roitman et al., "Preliminary, Open-Label, Pilot Study of Add-On Oral Delta-9-Tetrahydrocannabinol in Chronic Post-Traumatic Stress Disorder," *Clinical Drug Investigation* 34, no. 8 (2014): 587–91.

301. R. Jetly et al., "The Efficacy of Nabilone, a Synthetic Cannabinoid, in the Treatment of PTSD-Associated Nightmares: A Preliminary Randomized, Double-Blind, Placebo-Controlled Cross-Over Design Study," *Psychoneuroendocrinology* 51 (2015): 585–88.

302. L. Elms et al., "Cannabidiol in the Treatment of Post-Traumatic Stress Disorder: A Case Series," *Journal of Alternative and Complementary Medicine* (New York) 25, no. 4 (2019): 392–97.

303. F.-M. Werner et al., "Classical Neurotransmitters and Neuropeptides Involved in Schizophrenia: How to Choose the Appropriate Antipsychotic Drug?," *Current Drug Therapy* 8, no. 2 (2013): 132–43.

304. M. Glass et al., "Cannabinoid Receptors in the Human Brain: A Detailed Anatomical and Quantitative Autoradiographic Study in the Fetal, Neonatal, and Adult Human Brain," *Neuroscience* 77, no. 2 (1997): 299–318.

305. A. F. Giuffrida et al., "Cerebrospinal Anandamide Levels Are Elevated in Acute Schizophrenia and Are Inversely Correlated with Psychotic Symptoms," *Neuropsychopharmacology* 29, no. 11 (2004): 2108–14.

306. H. Segal-Gavish et al., "BDNF Overexpression Prevents Cognitive Deficit Elicited by Adolescent Cannabis Exposure and Host Susceptibility Interaction," *Human Molecular Genetics* 26, no. 13 (2017): 2462–71.

307. A. W. Zuardi, "Antipsychotic Effect of Cannabidiol," *Journal of Clinical Psychiatry* 56, no. 10 (1995): 485–86.

308. F. M. Leweke et al., "Cannabidiol as an Antipsychotic: A Double-Blind, Controlled Clinical Trial of Cannabidiol vs. Amisulpiride in Acute Schizophrenia," presented at 15th Annual Symposium on Cannabinoids, International Cannabinoid Research Society, Clearwater Beach, FL, 2005.

309. F. M. Leweke et al., "Cannabidiol Enhances Anandamide Signaling and Alleviates Psychotic Symptoms of Schizophrenia," *Translational Psychiatry* 2, no. 3 (2012): e94.

310. P. McGuire et al., "Cannabidiol (CBD) as an Adjunctive Therapy in Schizophrenia: A Multicenter Randomized Controlled Trial," *American Journal of Psychiatry* 175, no. 3 (2018): 225–31.

311. C. Makiol et al., "Remission of Severe, Treatment-Resistant Schizophrenia Following Adjunctive Cannabidiol," *Australian and New Zealand Journal of Psychiatry* 53, no. 3 (2019): 262.

Notes

312. J. E. C. Hallak et al., "Performance of Schizophrenic Patients in the Stroop Color Word Test and Electrodermal Responsiveness After Acute Administration of Cannabidiol (CBD)," *Brazilian Journal of Psychiatry* 32, no. 1 (2010): 56–61.

313. D. L. Boggs et al., "The Effects of Cannabidiol (CBD) on Cognition and Symptoms in Outpatients with Chronic Schizophrenia: A Randomized Placebo Controlled Trial," *Psychopharmacology* (Berlin) 235, no. 7 (2018): 1923–32.

314. A. Oláh et al., "Differential Effectiveness of Selected Non-Psychotropic Phytocannabinoids on Human Sebocyte Functions Implicates Their Introduction in Dry/Seborrhoeic Skin and Acne Treatment," *Experimental Dermatology* 25, no. 9 (2016): 701–7.

315. E. Gaffal et al., "Anti-inflammatory Activity of Topical THC in DNFB-Mediated Mouse Allergic Contact Dermatitis Independent of CB_1 and CB_2 Receptors," *Allergy* 68, no. 8 (2013): 994–1000.

316. Karsak et al., "Attenuation of Allergic Contact Dermatitis," 1494–97.

317. Ibid.

318. G. Nam et al., "Selective Cannabinoid Receptor-1 Agonists Regulate Mast Cell Activation in an Oxazolone-Induced Atopic Dermatitis Model," *Annals of Dermatology* 28, no. 1 (2016): 22–29.

319. B. Eberlein et al., "Adjuvant Treatment of Atopic Eczema: Assessment of an Emollient Containing N-Palmitoylethanolamine (ATOPA Study)," *Journal of the European Academy of Dermatology and Venereology* 22, no. 1 (2008): 73–82.

320. J. E. Schlosburg et al., "Endocannabinoid Modulation of Scratching Response in an Acute Allergenic Model: A New Prospective Neural Therapeutic Target for Pruritus," *Journal of Pharmacology and Experimental Therapeutics* 329, no. 1 (2009): 314–23.

321. J. C. Szepietowski et al., "Efficacy and Tolerance of the Cream Containing Structured Physiological Lipids with Endocannabinoids in the Treatment of Uremic Pruritus: A Preliminary Study," *Acta Dermatovenerologica Croatica* 13, no. 2 (2005): 97–103.

322. Eberlein et al., "Adjuvant Treatment of Atopic Eczema," 73–82.

323. Szepietowski et al., "Efficacy and Tolerance of the Cream Containing Structured Physiological Lipids," 97–103; J. C. Szepietowski et al., "Emollients with Endocannabinoids in the Treatment of Uremic Pruritus: Discussion of the Therapeutic Options," *Therapeutic Apheresis and Dialysis* 9, no. 3 (2005): 277–79; and S. Ständer et al., "Topical Cannabinoid Agonists: An Effective New Possibility for Treating Chronic Pruritus" [in German], *Hautarzt* 57, no. 9 (2006): 801–7.

324. E. Ambrożewicz et al., "Pathophysiological Alterations of Redox Signaling and Endocannabinoid System in Granulocytes and Plasma of Psoriatic Patients," *Cells* 7, no. 10 (2018): E159.

325. J. D. Wilkinson et al., "Cannabinoids Inhibit Human Keratinocyte Proliferation Through a Non-CB_1/CB_2 Mechanism and Have a Potential Therapeutic Value in the Treatment of Psoriasis," *Journal of Dermatological Science* 45, no. 2 (2007): 87–92.

326. Casanova et al., "Inhibition of Skin Tumor Growth and Angiogenesis In Vivo," 43–50.

327. C. Blázquez et al., "Cannabinoid Receptors as Novel Targets for the Treatment of Melanoma," *FASEB Journal* 20, no. 14 (2006): 2633–35; Armstrong et al., "Exploiting Cannabinoid-Induced Cytotoxic Autophagy," 1629–37; M. R. Scuderi et al., "The Antimitogenic Effect of the Cannabinoid Receptor Agonist WIN55212-2 on Human Melanoma Cells Is Mediated by the Membrane Lipid Raft," *Cancer Letters* 310, no. 2 (2011): 240–49; B. Adinolfi et al., "Anticancer Activity of Anandamide in Human Cutaneous Melanoma Cells," *European Journal of Pharmacology* 718, nos. 1–3 (2013): 154–59; E. Simmerman et al., "Cannabinoids as a Potential New and Novel Treatment for Melanoma: A Pilot Study in a Murine Model," *Journal of Surgical Research* 235 (2019): 210–15; and I. Kenessey et al., "Revisiting CB_1 Receptor as Drug Target in Human Melanoma," *Pathology and Oncology Research* 18, no. 4 (2012): 857–66.

328. M. A. Dew et al., "Healthy Older Adults' Sleep Predicts All-Cause Mortality at 4 to 19 Years of Follow-Up," *Psychosomatic Medicine* 65, no. 1 (2003): 63–73.

Notes

329. Centers for Disease Control and Prevention, "1 in 3 Adults Don't Get Enough Sleep," news release, last modified February 16, 2016, accessed January 2020, https://www.cdc.gov/media/releases/2016/p0215-enough-sleep.html.

330. D. F. Kripke et al., "Hypnotics' Association with Mortality or Cancer: A Matched Cohort Study," *BMJ Open* 2, no. 1 (2012): e000850; S. Weich et al., "Effect of Anxiolytic and Hypnotic Drug Prescriptions on Mortality Hazards: Retrospective Cohort Study," *BMJ* 348 (2014): g1996; and L. Mallon et al., "Is Usage of Hypnotics Associated with Mortality?," *Sleep Medicine* 10, no. 3 (2009): 279–86.

331. P. J. Gates et al., "The Effects of Cannabinoid Administration on Sleep: A Systematic Review of Human Studies," *Sleep Medicine Reviews* 18, no. 6 (2014): 477–87.

332. Fraser, "The Use of a Synthetic Cannabinoid in the Management of Treatment-Resistant Nightmares," 84–88; Cameron et al., "Use of a Synthetic Cannabinoid in a Correctional Population," 559–64; Roitman et al., "Preliminary, Open-Label, Pilot Study of Add-On Oral Delta-9-Tetrahydrocannabinol," 587–91; and Jetly et al., "The Efficacy of Nabilone, a Synthetic Cannabinoid," 585–88.

333. H. Yang et al., "Alpha-Pinene, a Major Constituent of Pine Tree Oils, Enhances Non–Rapid Eye Movement Sleep in Mice Through $GABA_A$-Benzodiazepine Receptors," *Molecular Pharmacology* 90, no. 5 (2016): 530–39.

334. D. W. Carley et al., "Functional Role for Cannabinoids in Respiratory Stability During Sleep," *Sleep* 25, no. 4 (2002): 391–98.

335. B. Prasad et al., "Proof of Concept Trial of Dronabinol in Obstructive Sleep Apnea," *Frontiers in Psychiatry* 4 (2013): 1; D. W. Carley et al., "0558 Dronabinol Reduces AHI and Daytime Sleepiness in Patients with Moderate to Severe Obstructive Sleep Apnea Syndrome," *Sleep* 40, suppl. 1 (2017): A207–8; and D. W. Carley et al., "Pharmacotherapy of Apnea by Cannabimimetic Enhancement, the PACE Clinical Trial: Effects of Dronabinol in Obstructive Sleep Apnea," *Sleep* 41, no. 1 (2018): zsx184.

336. S. Adhikary et al., "Modulation of Inflammatory Responses by a Cannabinoid-2–Selective Agonist After Spinal Cord Injury," *Journal of Neurotrauma* 28, no. 12 (2011): 2417–27.

337. A. Hama et al., "Antinociceptive Effect of Cannabinoid Agonist WIN 55,212-2 in Rats with a Spinal Cord Injury," *Experimental Neurology* 204, no. 1 (2007): 454–57.

338. J. Malec et al., "Cannabis Effect on Spasticity in Spinal Cord Injury," *Archives of Physical Medicine and Rehabilitation* 63, no. 3 (1982): 116–18.

339. Ibid.

340. U. Hagenbach et al., "The Treatment of Spasticity with Delta-9-Tetrahydrocannabinol in Persons with Spinal Cord Injury," *Spinal Cord* 45, no. 8 (2007): 551–62.

341. S. Pooyania et al., "A Randomized, Double-Blinded, Crossover Pilot Study Assessing the Effect of Nabilone on Spasticity in Persons with Spinal Cord Injury," *Archives of Physical Medicine and Rehabilitation* 91, no. 5 (2010): 703–7.

342. B. Wilsey et al., "An Exploratory Human Laboratory Experiment Evaluating Vaporized Cannabis in the Treatment of Neuropathic Pain from Spinal Cord Injury and Disease," *Journal of Pain* 17, no. 9 (2016): 982–1000.

343. K. R. Müller-Vahl et al., "Cannabinoids: Possible Role in Patho-Physiology and Therapy of Gilles de la Tourette Syndrome," *Acta Psychiatrica Scandinavica* 98, no. 6 (1998): 502–6.

344. K. R. Müller-Vahl et al., "Treatment of Tourette's Syndrome with Delta-9-Tetrahydrocannabinol," *American Journal of Psychiatry* 156, no. 3 (1999): 495.

345. K. R. Müller-Vahl et al., "Combined Treatment of Tourette Syndrome with Delta-9-THC and Dopamine Receptor Antagonists," *Journal of Cannabis Therapeutics* 2, nos. 3–4 (2002): 145–54.

346. K. R. Müller-Vahl et al., "Treatment of Tourette's Syndrome with Delta-9-Tetrahydrocannabinol (THC): A Randomized Crossover Trial," *Pharmacopsychiatry* 35, no. 2 (2002): 57–61.

347. K. R. Müller-Vahl et al., "Delta-9-Tetrahydrocannabinol (THC) Is Effective in the Treatment of Tics in Tourette Syndrome: A 6-Week Randomized Trial," *Journal of Clinical Psychiatry* 64, no. 4 (2003): 459–65.

348. K. R. Müller-Vahl, "Cannabinoids Reduce Symptoms of Tourette's Syndrome," *Expert Opinion on Pharmacotherapy* 4, no. 10 (2003): 1717–25.

349. A. Brunnauer et al., "Cannabinoids Improve Driving Ability in a Tourette's Patient," *Psychiatry Research* 190, nos. 2–3 (2011): 382.

350. E. Jakubovski et al., "Speechlessness in Gilles de la Tourette Syndrome: Cannabis-Based Medicines Improve Severe Vocal Blocking Tics in Two Patients," *International Journal of Molecular Sciences* 18, no. 8 (2017): E1739.

351. A. Thaler et al., "Single Center Experience with Medical Cannabis in Gilles de la Tourette Syndrome," *Parkinsonism and Related Disorders* 61 (2019): 211–13.

352. N. Szejko et al., "Delta-9-Tetrahydrocannabinol for the Treatment of a Child with Tourette Syndrome: Case Report," *European Journal of Medical Case Reports* 2, no. 2 (2018): 39–41.

353. N. Szejko et al., "Vaporized Cannabis Is Effective and Well-Tolerated in an Adolescent with Tourette Syndrome," *Medical Cannabis and Cannabinoids* 2, no. 1 (2019): 60–64.

354. L. M. Milosev et al., "Treatment of Gilles de la Tourette Syndrome with Cannabis-Based Medicine: Results from a Retrospective Analysis and Online Survey," *Cannabis and Cannabinoid Research* 4, no. 4 (2019): 265–74.

355. E.-M. Pichler et al., "Pure Delta-9-Tetrahydrocannabinol and Its Combination with Cannabidiol in Treatment-Resistant Tourette Syndrome: A Case Report," *International Journal of Psychiatry in Medicine* 54, no. 2 (2019): 150–56.

356. D. J. Loane et al., "Neuroprotection for Traumatic Brain Injury: Translational Challenges and Emerging Therapeutic Strategies," *Trends in Pharmacological Sciences* 31, no. 12 (2010): 596–604.

357. C. Berger et al., "Massive Accumulation of N-Acylethanolamines After Stroke. Cell Signalling in Acute Cerebral Ischemia?," *Journal of Neurochemistry* 88, no. 5 (2004): 1159–67; H. H. Hansen et al., "Accumulation of the Anandamide Precursor and Other N-Acylethanolamine Phospholipids in Infant Rat Models of In Vivo Necrotic and Apoptotic Neuronal Death," *Journal of Neurochemistry* 76, no. 1 (2001): 39–46; and D. Panikashvili et al., "An Endogenous Cannabinoid (2-AG) Is Neuroprotective After Brain Injury," *Nature* 413, no. 6855 (2001): 527–31.

358. S. H. Kim et al., "Molecular Mechanisms of Cannabinoid Protection from Neuronal Excitotoxicity," *Molecular Pharmacology* 69, no. 3 (2006): 691–96; G. Marsicano et al., "CB_1 Cannabinoid Receptors and On-Demand Defense Against Excitotoxicity," *Science* 302, no. 5642 (2003): 84–88; and M. van der Stelt et al., "Acute Neuronal Injury, Excitotoxicity, and the Endocannabinoid System," *Molecular Neurobiology* 26, nos. 2–3 (2002): 317–46.

359. T. W. Klein, "Cannabinoid-Based Drugs as Anti-inflammatory Therapeutics," *Nature Reviews: Immunology* 5, no. 5 (2005): 400–11; S. Murikinati et al., "Activation of Cannabinoid 2 Receptors Protects Against Cerebral Ischemia by Inhibiting Neutrophil Recruitment," *FASEB Journal* 24, no. 3 (2010): 788–98; L. Walter et al., "Cannabinoids and Neuroinflammation," *British Journal of Pharmacology* 141, no. 5 (2004): 775–85; M. Guzmán et al., "Control of the Cell Survival/Death Decision by Cannabinoids," *Journal of Molecular Medicine* (Berlin) 78, no. 11 (2001): 613–25; I. Galve-Roperh et al., "Mechanisms of Control of Neuron Survival by the Endocannabinoid System," *Current Pharmaceutical Design* 14, no. 23 (2008): 2279–88; S. H. Ramirez et al., "Activation of Cannabinoid Receptor 2 Attenuates Leukocyte–Endothelial Cell Interactions and Blood–Brain Barrier Dysfunction Under Inflammatory Conditions," *Journal of Neuroscience* 32, no. 12 (2012): 4004–16; and M. T. Viscomi et al., "Selective CB_2 Receptor Agonism Protects Central Neurons from Remote Axotomy-Induced Apoptosis Through the PI3K/Akt Pathway," *Journal of Neuroscience* 29, no. 14 (2009): 4564–70.

360. D. Alonso-Alconada et al., "The Cannabinoid WIN 55,212-2 Mitigates Apoptosis and Mitochondrial Dysfunction After Hypoxia Ischemia," *Neurochemical Research* 37, no. 1 (2012): 161–70; D. Alonso-Alconada et al., "The Cannabinoid Receptor Agonist WIN 55,212-2 Reduces the Initial Cerebral Damage After Hypoxic-Ischemic Injury in Fetal Lambs," *Brain Research* 1362 (2010): 150–59; D. Fernández-López et al., "The Cannabinoid Agonist WIN 55,212 Reduces Brain Damage in an In Vivo Model of Hypoxic-Ischemic Encephalopathy in Newborn Rats," *Pediatric Research* 62, no. 3 (2007): 255–60; and D. Fernández-López et al., "The Cannabinoid WIN 55,212-2 Promotes Neural Repair After Neonatal Hypoxia-Ischemia," *Stroke* 41, no. 12 (2010): 2956–64.

361. H. Lafuente et al., "Cannabidiol Reduces Brain Damage and Improves Functional Recovery After Acute Hypoxia-Ischemia in Newborn Pigs," *Pediatric Research* 70, no. 3 (2011): 272–77.

362. M. Braun et al., "Selective Activation of Cannabinoid Receptor-2 Reduces Neuroinflammation After Traumatic Brain Injury via Alternative Macrophage Polarization," *Brain, Behavior, and Immunity* 68 (2018): 224–37.

363. C. Belardo et al., "Oral Cannabidiol Prevents Allodynia and Neurological Dysfunctions in a Mouse Model of Mild Traumatic Brain Injury," *Frontiers in Pharmacology* 10 (2019): 352.

364. B. M. Nguyen et al., "Effect of Marijuana Use on Outcomes in Traumatic Brain Injury," *American Surgeon* 80, no. 10 (2014): 979–83.

365. D. W. Lawrence et al., "Cannabis, Alcohol, and Cigarette Use During the Acute Post-Concussion Period," *Brain Injury* 34, no. 1 (2020): 42–51.

Appendix A: The History of Cannabis

1. T. H. Mikuriya, "Physical, Mental, and Moral Effects of Marijuana: The Indian Hemp Drugs Commission Report," Schaffer Library of Drug Policy website, accessed May 14, 2020, http://www.druglibrary.org/schaffer/library/effects.htm.

Appendix B: The Pharmacokinetics of Phytocannabinoids

1. F. Grotenhermen, "Pharmacokinetics and Pharmacodynamics of Cannabinoids," *Clinical Pharmacokinetics* 42, no. 4 (2003): 327–60.

2. M. N. Newmeyer et al., "Free and Glucuronide Whole Blood Cannabinoids' Pharmacokinetics After Controlled Smoked, Vaporized, and Oral Cannabis Administration in Frequent and Occasional Cannabis Users: Identification of Recent Cannabis Intake," *Clinical Chemistry* 62, no. 12 (2016): 1579–92.

3. Grotenhermen, "Pharmacokinetics and Pharmacodynamics of Cannabinoids," 327–60.

4. Ibid.

5. S. W. Toennes et al., "Comparison of Cannabinoid Pharmacokinetic Properties in Occasional and Heavy Users Smoking a Marijuana or Placebo Joint," *Journal of Analytical Toxicology* 32, no. 7 (2008): 470–77.

6. T. E. Gaston et al., "Interactions Between Cannabidiol and Commonly Used Antiepileptic Drugs," *Epilepsia* 58, no. 9 (2017): 1586–92; and S. Agurell et al., "Interactions of Delta 1-Tetrahydrocannabinol with Cannabinol and Cannabidiol Following Oral Administration in Man. Assay of Cannabinol and Cannabidiol by Mass Fragmentography with Cannabinol and Cannabidiol Following Oral Administration in Man. Assay of Cannabinol and Cannabidiol by Mass Fragmentography," *Experientia* 37, no. 10 (1981): 1090–92.

7. M. A. Huestis, "Human Cannabinoid Pharmacokinetics," *Chemistry and Biodiversity* 4, no. 8 (2007): 1770–804.

8. R. J. Dinis-Oliveira, "Metabolomics of Delta-9-Tetrahydrocannabinol: Implications in Toxicity," *Drug Metabolism Reviews* 48, no. 1 (2016): 80–87.

9. A. Ohlsson et al., "Plasma Delta-9-Tetrahydrocannabinol Concentrations and Clinical Effects After Oral and Intravenous Administration and Smoking," *Clinical Pharmacology and Therapeutics* 28, no. 3 (1980): 409–16.

10. E. L. Karschner et al., "Plasma Cannabinoid Pharmacokinetics Following Controlled Oral Delta-9-Tetrahydrocannabinol and Oromucosal Cannabis Extract Administration," *Clinical Chemistry* 57, no. 1 (2011): 66–75.

11. S. Lunn et al., "Human Pharmacokinetic Parameters of Orally Administered Delta-9-Tetrahydrocannabinol Capsules Are Altered by Fed Versus Fasted Conditions and Sex Differences," *Cannabis and Cannabinoid Research* 4, no. 4 (2019): 255–64.

12. Karschner et al., "Plasma Cannabinoid Pharmacokinetics," 66–75.

13. G. W. Guy et al., "A Phase I, Double Blind, Three-Way Crossover Study to Assess the Pharmacokinetic Profile of Cannabis Based Medicine Extract (CBME) Administered Sublingually in Variant Cannabinoid Ratios in Normal Healthy Male Volunteers (GWPK0215)," in *Cannabis: From Pariah to Prescription,* ed. E. B. Russo (New York: Routledge, 2014), 129–60.

14. A. L. Stinchcomb et al., "Human Skin Permeation of Delta-8-Tetrahydrocannabinol, Cannabidiol, and Cannabinol," *Journal of Pharmacy and Pharmacology* 56, no. 3 (2004): 291–97.

15. E. Perlin et al., "Disposition and Bioavailability of Various Formulations of Tetrahydrocannabinol in the Rhesus Monkey," *Journal of Pharmaceutical Sciences* 74, no. 2 (1985): 171–74.

16. R. Schicho et al., "Topical and Systemic Cannabidiol Improves Trinitrobenzene Sulfonic Acid Colitis in Mice," *Pharmacology* 89, nos. 3–4 (2012): 149–55.

17. S. Valiveti et al., "In Vitro/In Vivo Correlation Studies for Transdermal Delta-8-THC Development," *Journal of Pharmaceutical Sciences* 93, no. 5 (2004): 1154–64.

18. Dinis-Oliveira, "Metabolomics of Delta-9-Tetrahydrocannabinol," 80–87; C. A. Hunt et al., "Tolerance and Disposition of Tetrahydrocannabinol in Man," *Journal of Pharmacology and Experimental Therapeutics* 215, no. 1 (1980): 35–44; and N. Gunasekaran et al., "Reintoxication: The Release of Fat-Stored Delta-9-Tetrahydrocannabinol (THC) into Blood Is Enhanced by Food Deprivation or ACTH Exposure," *British Journal of Pharmacology* 158, no. 5 (2009): 1330–37.

19. L. Lemberger et al., "11-Hydroxy-Delta-9-Tetrahydrocannabinol: Pharmacology, Disposition, and Metabolism of a Major Metabolite of Marihuana in Man," *Science* 177, no. 4043 (1972): 62–64.

20. M. Eichler et al., "Heat Exposure of *Cannabis Sativa* Extracts Affects the Pharmacokinetic and Metabolic Profile in Healthy Male Subjects," *Planta Medica* 78, no. 7 (2012): 686–91.

21. W. Holubek, "Medical Risks and Toxicology," in *The Pot Book,* ed. J. Holland (Rochester, VT; Toronto: Park Street Press, 2010), 141–52.

22. Ohlsson et al., "Plasma Delta-9-Tetrahydrocannabinol Concentrations," 409–16.

23. P. Consroe et al., "Controlled Clinical Trial of Cannabidiol in Huntington's Disease," *Pharmacology Biochemistry and Behavior* 40, no. 3 (1991): 701–8.

Appendix D: Terpenoids and Their Effects

1. E. P. Baron, "Medicinal Properties of Cannabinoids, Terpenes, and Flavonoids in Cannabis, and Benefits in Migraine, Headache, and Pain: An Update on Current Evidence and Cannabis Science," *Headache* 58, no. 7 (2018): 1139–86.

Index

Note: Italic page numbers refer to illustrations and charts.

acetylcholine, 88, 168
acne, 90, 256–57
acupuncture, 182, 194, 234, 274
adolescence, 144–46
Agricultural Act of 2014, 282
AIDS, 162, 280
alcohol use, 50, 128, 131, 141, 142, 156
allergic contact dermatitis, 110, 257
alpha-pinene, *16*, 139
ALS (amyotrophic lateral sclerosis), 74, 81, 238–40
Alzheimer's disease (AD), 68, 72, 88, 99, 162, 238, 240–42
anandamide: appetite and, 162; autism spectrum disorder and, 175; CBC and, 90, 157; CBDA and, 77; CBG and, 80, 157; as endocannabinoid, 27; FAAH enzyme breaking down, 155–56, 179, 257; fibromyalgia and, 213; migraine headaches and, 232; schizophrenia and, 254; studies on levels of, 30, 156, 175
Anslinger, Harry, 278
anticonvulsants, 71, 129, 147, 149
antidepressants, 157, 159
anxiety and depression: ADHD and, 170, 172; ALS and, 240; Alzheimer's disease and, 242; appetite affected by, 162; autoimmune conditions and, 181–82; cannabis withdrawal and, 57; case study on, 159–61; CBDA for, 78; CBD reducing, 67, 69–70, 77, 157, 160; CBG for, 81, 82, 83, 157; chronic illness and, 43; chronic pain and, 194; delivery methods and, 102; delta-8-THC for, 88–89, 123; dosing and,

118; endocannabinoid system dysfunction and, 38, 155–57, 161; fibromyalgia and, 212, 215; irritable bowel syndrome and, 221; limonene and, 15, 20; management of symptoms, 154, 197, 202; migraine headaches and, 233; multiple sclerosis and, 156, 238; Parkinson's disease and, 244, 245, 246, 247, 248; phytocannabinoids improving, 157–58, 184; PTSD and, 249, 251–53; rimonabant and, 40; schizophrenia and, 256; sleep apnea and, 263; sleep disorders and, 260, 262; spinal cord injury and, 264–66; synergies between phytocannabinoids and terpenoids, 17; THC associated with anxiety, 34, 50, 53, 56, 66, 70, 106, 125–27, 145, 156–57; THC dosing and, 125, 126, 156, 157, 158; THC medicinal effects and, 63, 64, 76, 77, 125, 157, 158; THCV for, 84; Tourette syndrome and, 268, 270; traumatic brain injury and, 270, 273–74
appetite: ADHD and, 170; ALS and, 240; Alzheimer's disease and, 242; anorexia and weight loss, 185–87, 223; cannabis use for stimulation of, 53, 63, 161–63, 185, 188, 192, 207, 211; cannabis withdrawal and, 57; CB₁ receptors and, 34, 162; CBD affecting, 54, 69; CBG for, 81–82; CBN for, 72; delta-8-THC for, 89; endocannabinoid dysfunction and, 39, 202; gastrointestinal disorders and, 219, 221, 223; hepatitis C and, 229; Parkinson's disease and, 248; THC and, 34, 63, 161–63; THCV for, 84–85

arthritis: antiarthritic effect of cannabis, 164–68, 202; anti-inflammatory treatment for, 164–66, 180; case studies of, 167–68; chronic pain and, 194; collagen-induced arthritis, 165; osteoarthritis, 165, 167; rheumatoid arthritis, 3–4, 71, 131–35, 164–67, 179, 195; topical application for, 108, 109–10, 166

asthma, 168–69, 179

atopic dermatitis/eczema, 108–10, 257–58

attention deficit hyperactivity disorder (ADHD): case study on, 172–73; CB_1 receptors related to, 33; imbalance in neurotransmitters, 31–32, 170; as neurodevelopmental disorder, 169–72; pesticide side effects and, 99; research on, 171; sleep apnea and, 263; synergies between phytocannabinoids and terpenoids, 17; Tourette syndrome and, 268–69

autism spectrum disorder (ASD): CB_2 receptors and, 41, 175; CBD:THC ratios for, 114, 176–78; CBD for, 24–25, 71, 177; CBDV for, 87, 123; CBG for, 81–82; core symptoms of, 174; THCA for, 76

autoimmune and inflammatory conditions: blood-brain barrier and, 74; cannabinoid-induced anti-inflammatory effects, 179–81; case study on, 181–82; CBD for, 69, 138; endocannabinoid system dysfunction and, 30, 38, 167, 178–79, 182; pain relief for, 164–65, 167, 198–99; synergies between phytocannabinoids and terpenoids, 17. See also arthritis; diabetes; fibromyalgia; gastrointestinal disorders; multiple sclerosis (MS); psoriasis

bacteria, testing for, 98, 99

benzodiazepines, 44, 127, 157, 196

beta-caryophyllene, 16, 17, 166, 181, 209, 222, 234, 238

bioaccumlators, 21, 101

bioavailability, 106, 112

blood–brain barrier (BBB), 74, 157–58

blood pressure, 81, 137, 164, 263

brain: CB_1 receptors located in areas of, 32–34, 155; developmental risks, 136, 144–46; inflammation of, 180, 208, 209; surgery for seizures, 203–4

Bush, George H. W., 280

California: cannabis testing requirements of, 93, 95, 97–98; dispensaries of, 13, 178, 195; medical cannabis clinics of, 164, 197; medical marijuana law in, 281

Canada, 196, 250

cancer: anorexia and weight loss, 185–87, 192; anticancer properties of phytocannabinoids, 56, 69, 183; cannabis as cure for, 183, 188–91; cannabis smoke risk, 140; cannabis used for combating symptoms, 55, 126, 162, 183–88, 192–93; case study on, 191–94; CBC for, 90; CBDA for, 78, 123; CBD for, 59, 67, 68, 69; CBG for, 80, 81, 122; CBN for, 72; CDBV for, 86; chemotherapy-induced nausea and vomiting, 63, 89, 183–85, 192; colorectal cancer, 218; in Crohn's patients using cannabis, 220; delta-8-THC for, 88–89; dosage of phytocannabinoids for, 117, 190–91; endocannabinoid system and, 30; flavonoids and, 18; gastroesophageal reflux and, 217; hepatitis C and, 229, 231; inflammatory components of, 179; limonene and, 15; multiple sclerosis and, 236; pain with, 187–88, 192, 195; pesticides linked to, 99; rectal suppositories for, 111; skin cancer, 189, 190, 259–60; sleep disorders and, 261; THCA for, 75, 76; THC for, 62, 63; THCV for, 84; topical application for, 110

cannabinoid receptors: in adolescence, 144; appetite and, 162, 185; CBDV interaction with, 86; CBG interaction with, 80; delta-8-THC interaction with, 88; discovery of, 27–28; endocannabinoids binding to, 29–30, 60; in gastrointestinal disorders, 216; in immune system, 179; keys for, 28–29; location of, 32–36, 33, 60; negative allosteric modulation of, 67; THCV and, 83–84; upregulation and downregulation of, 40–42, 56, 251. See also CB_1 receptors; CB_2 receptors; endocannabinoid system

cannabinoids: acute overdose symptoms, 50; for Alzheimer's disease, 241–42; anticancer effects of, 189–90; anti-inflammatory effects of, 165; antiviral effects of, 228; in cannabis varieties, 9, 19–20, 23; chronic toxicity of, 51–53; entourage effect of, 14;

Index

for Huntington's disease, 243–44; ingestion of raw cannabinoids, 107; metabolization of, 126; for migraine headaches, 232–33; for multiple sclerosis, 49, 236–38; pain relief effects of, 194, 195; for Parkinson's disease, 245–48; profiles of, 93–95, *94*; for pruritis/itching, 258; research on, 27–28; for skin cancer, 260; for sleep disorders, 261–62; synthetic cannabinoids, 11, 48–49, 145, 153, 161, 165, 168, 180, 183, 187, 193, 213, 219, 222, 241, 257, 261, 271; for traumatic brain injury, 271. *See also* phytocannabinoids

cannabis: acute toxicity of, 49–50; addiction to, 57; adverse side effects of, 53–55; chronic toxicity of, 51–53; false claims about, xii, 161; as fat soluble, 112, 124; history of, 5, 277–83; organic certification of, 100–101; recreational use of, 49, 57, 99–100, 127, 137, 157, 220; safety of, 46–49; as Schedule I controlled substance, xi, 47–48, 59, 153, 188, 207, 279. *See also* medical cannabis

cannabis oils, 115, *115*, 116–17

cannabis plants: chemotypes, 12; chemovars of, 9, 13, 17, 19–21, 76, 92, 136, 171, 209, 233–34, 235, 242, 252; endocannabinoid system and, 31, 66; growing conditions of, 20–21, 100–101; medicinal compounds of, 5, 9; sativa or indica, 19–20; synthesis of phytocannabinoids, 11–14, *13*; trichomes of female cannabis flower, 11, *12*, 22. *See also* flavonoids; phytocannabinoids; terpenoids

cannabis research, restriction of, xi–xii, 6, 153, 166, 184, 188, 191

Cannabis Therapeutic Research Program, 224–25

cannabis use: driving under the influence with THC use, 136, 141–42; medical risks and safety of, 5, 136–38; in pediatric population, 136, 144–46; pregnancy and breastfeeding with THC use, 136, 142–44; pulmonary risks of smoking cannabis, 136, 139–41; stigma of, 216

cardiovascular disease, 39, 51, 136–38, 179–80, 260, 263

cardiovascular system, 35, 136, 137

CB_1 receptors: Alzheimer's disease and, 241; appetite and, 162, 202; asthma-like reactions and, 168–69; atopic dermatitis and, 257–58; biphasic effects of THC interacting with, 125; in brain, 32–34, 155; CBG and, 80; CBN and, 72; depression associated with increase in, 156; epilepsy and, 204; gastrointestinal system and, 35–36, 216–19; Huntington's disease and, 243; immune cells and, 179; intraocular pressure and, 224, 225; location of, *33*; multiple sclerosis and, 237; neurodegenerative disorders and, 239; pain relief and, 187; Parkinson's disease and, 246; psoriasis and, 259; PTSD and, 250; rimonabant and, 40, 202; skin and, 36, 109; skin cancer and, 260; skin disorders and, 256; THC activating, 137; THCV as neutral antagonist at, 83–84; topical application activating, 109

CB_2 receptors: ALS and, 239, 240; Alzheimer's disease and, 241; asthma-like reactions and, 168–69; autism spectrum disorders and, 41, 175; CBG and, 80; CBN and, 72; gastrointestinal system and, 35–36, 216–19; Huntington's disease and, 243; immune cells and, 179, 217; location of, 32, *33*, 35; multiple sclerosis and, 237; pain relief and, 187; Parkinson's disease and, 245; psoriasis and, 259; skin and, 36; skin cancer and, 260; skin disorders and, 256; THCA and, 75; THC activating, 137; THCV and, 84

CBC (cannabichromene), 10, 50, 73, 89–90, 157, 227, 228

CBCA (cannabichromenic acid), 11, 89

CBD (cannabidiol): for acne, 257; adverse side effects of, 54, 69; AEDs and, 209–11; for Alzheimer's disease, 241; antianxiety effects of, 157; antibacterial properties of, 227; anticancer properties of, 188, 190, 193; antiemetic properties of, 185; as antiepileptic, 205–8; anti-inflammatory effects of, 165, 166, 167, 209; antiseizure mechanisms of, 208–9, 211–12; appetite and, 163; for autism spectrum disorders, 177, 178; availability of, 58–59; binding to sites on cannabinoid receptors, 60, 67; biphasic effects of, 125; buffering effects of intoxication of THC, 70, 127; for cancer, 59, 67, 68, 69; CBD+THC, 113, 118, 119, 195, 202, 218, 223, 225, 233, 235, 236,

Index

CBD (cannabidiol) *(cont.)*
242, 259, 265, 269, 270, 274;
CBD+THC+CBDA, 77; CBD isolates, 95,
153; CBG interaction with, 81;
composition of phytocannabinoids, 12,
13–14; for diabetes, 201; distribution and
metabolism of, 288; dosing of, 122,
128–29, 177, 262–63; drug–drug
interactions, 128–30; effect on liver, 54,
69, 210, 229, 231; entourage effect, 70;
extraction process for, 21; for fibromyalgia,
214; of hemp products, 14, 19, 21–23;
inhalation of, 102; intraocular pressure
and, 225; for irritable bowel syndrome,
222; medicinal effects of, 66, 69–71, 209;
for migraine headaches, 233; molecular
structure of, *10*; for multiple sclerosis, 238;
as neuroprotectant, 209; non-cannabinoid
targets and, 66–67; as nonintoxicating,
136; overdose symptoms, 50; for
Parkinson's disease, 245, 246, 247; potency
testing, 107; pregnancy use, 143; for
psoriasis, 259; psychoactive effects of, 59,
69, 157; for PTSD, 251, 253; ratio of CBD
to THC, 20, 22–23, 56–57, 70–71, 79,
114, 119, *120*, 121–22, 124, 158, 166–67,
172, 176–77, 181–82, 196, 198–200, 202,
215, 218, 221, 236, 238, 242, 244, 251;
rectal suppositories of, 111; research on,
10, 14, 66–68; reverse tolerance with, 70,
177; Schedule I status of, 59; for
schizophrenia, 255; as single compound,
11; for sleep disorders, 262–63; synergistic
enhancement with THC, 14; topical
application of, 109, 110; transdermal
patches of, 113, 165; for traumatic brain
injury, 271–72, 274; for ulcerative colitis,
219
CBDA (cannabidiolic acid): antianxiety
benefits of, 157–58, 159; antiemetic
properties of, 185; anti-inflammation
benefits of, 166, 167, 168, 181; availability
of, 59; in cannabis tea, 107; categories of
products and effects, *120*; CBDA+THC,
79; conversion to CBD, 78, 80; for Crohn's
disease, 221; dosing of, 119, 123; for
fibromyalgia, 214; for irritable bowel
syndrome, 222; medicinal effects of,
78–80; migraine headaches and, 182, 233;
for multiple sclerosis, 238; for pain relief,

199; as precursor to CBD, 11–12; for
psoriasis, 259; research on, 77–78; side
effects of, 55; for spinal cord injury, 265; as
tinctures, 125; for traumatic brain injury,
273
CBDV (cannabidivarin), 10, 86–87, *121*,
123, 257
CBG (cannabigerol): acute overdose
symptoms, 50; for ADHD, 172;
anandamide interaction with, 80, 157;
antibacterial properties of, 227; antifungal
effects of, 228; anti-inflammation benefits
of, 166–67, 181; for anxiety, 159, 182; for
autism spectrum disorders, 178;
availability of, 59, 82–83; categories of
products and effects, *120*; CBG+CBD, 82;
dosing of, 119, 122; for fibromyalgia, 214;
medicinal effects of, 81–83; for psoriasis,
259; research on, 80–81; as secondary
phytocannabinoid, 10; side effects of, 55;
for spinal cord injury, 265; topical
application of, 109; for Tourette syndrome,
270; for traumatic brain injury, 272–73; in
Type IV, 12; for ulcerative colitis, 219
CBGA (cannabigerolic acid), 11, 80, 89
CBL (cannabicyclol), 10
CBN (cannabinol): ADHD symptoms
affected by, 171; antibacterial properties of,
227; discovery of, 71–72; inhibition of
uptake of anandamide, 157; lack of side
effects, 55; medicinal effects of, 72–73; as
phytocannabinoid, 10; for psoriasis, 259;
topical application of, 109
CBV (cannabivarin), 10
Centers for Disease Control (CDC), 50, 104,
174, 218, 260
Certificate of Analysis (COA): bacteria,
fungi, and mycotoxins testing, 98, *99*;
cannabinoid profiles, 93–95, *94*; dosing
with, 119, 122, 125; heavy metals testing,
101–2; information included in, 22–23,
93; measurement for sublingual tinctures,
107; pesticide testing, 83, 99–101, *100*; as
report of cannabis testing laboratory,
93–94; residual solvents testing, 83,
96–98, *97*; reviewing of, 113; state testing
requirements, 93, 95, 97–98; terpenoid
profiles, 20, 95–96, *96*
Charlotte's Web CBD oil, 43–45
chemotherapy, 63, 89, 111, 183–85, 192

child development, 142–46
chronic pain and neuropathy: case study on, 199–200; CBD for, 69; CBN for, 73; depression from, 156; dosing for, 124; gastrointestinal disorders and, 217, 219, 221, 223; head trauma and, 71; hepatitis C and, 229, 231; management of symptoms, 154, 194–99, 202; multiple sclerosis and, 195, 236; sleep disorders and, 261, 262; spinal cord injury and, 264, 266–67; THC medicinal effects for, 63; THCV for, 84; traumatic brain injury and, 272; types of, 194–95, 212. *See also* fibromyalgia
CHS (Cannabinoid Hyperemesis Syndrome), 55–56
cineole, 181, 238
citronellol, 181, 238
clobazam (Onfi), 129, 207, 210
Cole Memorandum (DOJ), 281, 282
Colorado, 98, 195
Controlled Substances Act, xi–xii, 47, 279
COVID-19, 227
COX enzymes, 68, 75, 78
Crohn's disease, 41, 71, 216, 218, 219–21
cyclical vomiting syndrome (CVS), 24, 25, 55
CYP2C9, 129
CYP2C19, 129
CYP3A4, 129
cytochrome P450 system, 68, 128, 129, 210
cytokines, 68, 165, 226–27

DEA (Drug Enforcement Administration), 46, 47–48, 279, 280
delivery methods: comparison of, *113*; drug–drug interactions, 129; edibles, 105–6, 126, 167, 169, 178, 222, 240; effect on dosing, 117, 118, 178, 185; effects depending on, 102–3, 105–6, 118, 237; experimentation with, 102, 118, 136, 140, 166; first pass effect, 105, 107, 108, 112, 286; ingestion, 105–7, 286; inhalation, 102–5, 138, 140–41, 184–87, 233, 237, 285–86; rectal suppositories, 111, 287; smoking, 102–3, 136, 139–41, 169; sublingual tinctures, 102, 107–8, *117*, 125, 169, 178, 233, 237, 240, 286; topical application, 102, 108–10, 166–67, 258–59, 286–87; transdermal patches,

112–13, 165, 287; vaporization, 102, 103–5, 128, 140–41, 167, 169, 185, 195, 198, 235, 237, 240
delta-8-THC (delta-8-tetrahydrocannabinol): antiemetic properties of, 184–85; availability of, 59; categories of products and effects, *121*; delta-9-THC compared to, 87–89; dosing of, 123; medicinal effects of, 88–89; side effects of, 55; topical application of, 109
depression. *See* anxiety and depression
diabetes, 18, 39, 40, 85, 164, 179, 200–203
Di Marzo, Vincenzo, 30, 39
DOJ (US Department of Justice), 280, 281, 282
dopamine, 27, 170, 245, 254
dosing: adult guidelines, 121–25; avoidance of errors in, 95; biphasic effects, 125, 168, 177; categories of products and effects, *120–21*; concentration amounts, 115, *115*, 116; drug–drug interactions, 128–29, 210; of edibles, 106, 126, 178; with needleless syringes, 115, 125; as patient-determined, self-titrating, 118, 154, 178, 190–91, 211; research methods, 153, 154; "rule it in or rule it out" method, 118–19, 159, 166, 178, 199, 213–14; for sleep disorders, 118, 262; start low and go slow method, 53, 65, 106, 117–21, 125, 242, 247; of sublingual tinctures, 108, 178; THC overdose, 126–27; therapeutic range for, 117; timing of, 123–24, 129, 136, 166, 238; with/without meals, 106, 124
Dravet syndrome, 58, 79, 207–8, 210
dronabinol (Marinol): for ALS, 240; for appetite, 161, 186; for autism, 175–76; for chemotherapy-induced nausea and vomiting, 183–84; for chronic pain, 195; for irritable bowel syndrome, 222; for sleep apnea, 263; for spinal cord injury, 266; as synthetic THC, 83; for viral infections, 228

eczema. *See* atopic dermatitis/eczema
edibles: as delivery method, 105–6, 126, 167, 169, 178, 222, 240; precautions with, 131, 205; product label example, *116*; ratio for, 115–16; for sleep disorders, 262
11-hydroxy-THC, 105, 106, 112, 126
endocannabinoid deficiency syndrome, 38–39, 61, 156

endocannabinoids, 11, 29, 30, 39, 60
endocannabinoid system: in adolescence, 144, 145; in autism spectrum disorders, 174–75; case study on, 43–45; CBD enhancing function of, 68, 70, 208; components of, 28–29, 28; discovery of, xi, xii, 26–28, 153; dysfunction of, 5, 26, 29–30, 32, 37–40, 43–45, 61, 63–64, 153, 155–57, 161, 170, 178–79, 182, 202, 204, 212–13, 215, 249–50, 254, 259; endocannabinoid deficiency syndrome, 38–39, 61, 156; in gastrointestinal system, 216–17; genetic deficiency in, 64; homeostasis of cells maintained by, 29–32, 37–38, 61, 179, 204, 209, 216, 232, 256; in Huntington's disease, 242–43, 245; individual differences in, 31–32; in joint tissues, 164; in mental health, 155; overactivity of, 39–40; in Parkinson's disease, 245; physiologic pathways regulated by, 30–31, 37, 91; receptor locations, 32–36, 33; in skin, 108; tone of, 163; upregulation and downregulation of receptors, 40–41, 42, 56, 251
enteric nervous system, 216
entourage effect, 41, 70, 89, 95, 153, 208
enzymes, 39, 60, 68, 75, 78, 80, 155–56, 179
Epidiolex, 54, 129–30, 207–8, 210
epilepsy: antiseizure mechanisms of CBD, 208–9; appetite and, 163; autism spectrum disorder related to, 174, 176; blood-brain barrier and, 74; case study on, 211–12; CBDA and, 79; CBD and, 67, 68, 205–11; CBD-rich cannabis and, 58–59, 70, 79; CBDV for, 87; diagnosis and treatment of, x–xii; endocannabinoid system dysfunction and, 39, 44–45, 204; Epidiolex for, 129; THC as antiepileptic, 204–5; types of, 203–7. See also seizures and seizure disorders
EVALI, 104
executive function, 145, 146
extracts, 107–8

FAAH (fatty acid amide hydrolase) enzyme, 68, 155, 156, 179
Farm Bill of 2014, 21
FDA (Food and Drug Administration): ALS medications approved by, 239; approval of CBD products, 54; cannabis for cancer treatment and, 190; Epidiolex approved by, 207, 210; on EVALI, 104; heavy metals testing recommended by, 101–2; Investigational New Drug (IND) program, 280; on medical claims of hemp-based CBD products, 282; migraine medications approved by, 232; terpenoids recognized as safe by, 15; testing of products containing CBD, 21
FECO (full-extract cannabis oil), 116, 117
fibromyalgia: case study on, 214–16; dosing for, 213–15; endocannabinoid system dysfunction and, 38, 39, 212–13, 215; irritable bowel syndrome and, 212, 221; pain and, 73, 181, 195, 212–15
$5HT_{1A}$, 77, 81, 84
flavonoids, 9, 18–19, 22
Fuchs, Leonhart, 278
fungi, 98, 99

GABA, 67, 262, 272
GABA receptors, 67, 81, 86, 157
Gaoni, Yehiel, 89
gastroesophageal reflux (GERD), 15, 216–18, 221
gastrointestinal disorders: appetite and, 162; case study on, 223–24; chronic abdominal pain, 217, 219, 221, 223; Crohn's disease, 41, 71, 216, 218–21; endocannabinoid dysfunction and, 217–18, 221, 223; gastroesophageal reflux, 15, 216–18, 221; hepatitis C and, 229; inflammatory bowel disease, 216, 218–21; irritable bowel syndrome, 38, 39, 76, 181, 212, 216, 217, 221–22; THCV for, 84; ulcerative colitis, 216, 218–21, 223–24
gastrointestinal system, 30, 35–36
glaucoma, 224–26
glutamate, 213, 239
glycine receptors, 62, 67
GPR3 receptors, 68
GPR6 receptors, 68
GPR12 receptors, 68
GPR18 receptors, 62, 67, 225
GPR55 (G protein-coupled receptor 55), 37, 62, 67, 75, 84, 86, 208, 216
graft-versus-host disease (GVHD), 180–81
Gruber, Staci, 52

H1N1 "swine flu," 227

H5N1 "bird flu," 227
Hashimoto's thyroiditis, 181–82
hashish, 13, 15
Health Effects of Cannabis and Cannabinoids: The Current State of Evidence and Recommendations for Research, The (National Academies of Sciences, Engineering, and Medicine), 48–49, 184, 194
heavy metals, 101–2, 104
hemp products, 14, 19, 21–23, 95, 124
hepatitis B, 228
hepatitis C (HCV), 228–31
HIV, 195, 228, 230
Howlett, Allyn, 26–27
HU-580 (cannabidiolic acid methyl ester), 78
humulene, 181, 238
Huntington's disease (HD), 39, 75, 238, 242–44

immune system: cytokines and, 165, 226–27; endocannabinoid system and, 27, 35, 178–80, 216–18, 226. *See also* autoimmune and inflammatory conditions
infectious diseases, 226–28
inflammatory bowel disease (IBD), 216, 218–21
inflammatory conditions. *See* autoimmune and inflammatory conditions
ingestion, as delivery method, 105–7, 286
inhalation, as delivery method, 102–5, 138, 140–41, 184–87, 233, 237, 285–86
insulin sensitivity, 84, 85, 202
intestines, 128, 180. *See also* gastrointestinal disorders
intraocular pressure, 63, 67, 69, 224
irritable bowel syndrome (IBS), 38, 39, 76, 181, 212, 216, 217, 221–22

journal, for dosing, 119, 159

Keppra (levetiracetam), 24, 210
keratinocytes, 258–59
ketogenic diet, 44, 203

La Guardia, Fiorello, 47, 279
Lawn, John, 48
LD50, 49–50
Lee, Martin, 22
Lennox-Gastaut syndrome (LGS), 207–8

limonene, 15, *16*, 17, 20, 169, 218, 222, 252
linalool, *16*, 17, 20, 252, 262
liver: cannabinoids metabolized by, 126; CB_1 and CB_2 receptors and, 35; drug–drug interactions affecting, 130, 210; effect of CBD on, 54, 69, 210, 229, 231; effect of THC on, 105–6; first pass effect, 105, 107–8, 112, 286; pharmaceuticals metabolized in, 54, 128
liver disease and hepatitis C, 41, 179, 228–31
lock-and-key receptor systems, 27, 28–29, 59
LOD (limit of detection), 98
LOQ (limit of quantitation), 98
LOX enzymes, 68

MAGL (monoacylglycerol lipase) enzyme, 80
Marihuana Tax Act of 1937, 47, 278
Marijuana: A Signal of Misunderstanding (National Commission on Marijuana and Drug Abuse), 47
Marijuana and Medicine: Assessing the Science Base (Institute of Medicine of the National Academies), 48
maternal cannabis use studies, 142–43
Mechoulam, Raphael, 14, 26, 89
medical cannabis: avoidance of dosing errors, 95; Certificate of Analysis (COA), 20, 22–23, 83, 92–102; chronic toxicity of, 52; drug–drug interactions, 128–30; legitimacy of, 32, 58; media attention on, 205; medicinal use vs. recreational use, 127, 157, 220; multiple cannabinoids used in regimens, 49, 53; patient precautions, 131–35; pharmacokinetics of, 5–6; ratio and concentration, 114–17; research on, 26, 47–49, 55, 59, 153–54; side effects of, 55, 119, 154, 235; treatment with, xi, xii, 5, 6, 9, 154, 155; as Type I plants, 12, 13, 14; as Type II plants, 14; as Type III plants, 21; unlicensed distributors, 98. *See also* delivery methods; dosing; endocannabinoid system
melanoma, 259–60
metabolism, 106, 117
microbial contaminants, 98, *99*
migraine headaches: autoimmune conditions and, 181–82; case study on, 234–35; endocannabinoid system dysfunction and, 38, 39, 232–35; irritable bowel syndrome

migraine headaches *(cont.)*
and, 221; pharmaceutical medications for, 231–32; symptoms of, 231, 233; THC-rich cannabis used for, 64, 118, 233
MIND, 52–53
Moreno-Sanz, Guillermo, 74
Müller-Vahl, Kirsten, 268
multiple sclerosis (MS): as autoimmune disease, 179, 180, 235–36; blood-brain barrier and, 74; cannabinoids for, 49, 236–38; chronic pain from, 195, 236, 237; depression from, 156, 238; endocannabinoid system dysfunction and, 30, 39; symptoms of, 42, 49, 236, 237, 261
Murthy, Vivek, 48
mycotoxins, 98, *99*
myrcene, 17, *17*, 20, 181, 234, 238, 242, 252, 262

nabilone, 183, 195, 213, 243, 245, 250, 264
nabiximols (Sativex): for ADHD, 171; for ALS, 240; for chronic pain, 195; for Huntington's disease, 243, 244; for multiple sclerosis, 180, 236–38; for rheumatoid arthritis, 166; for sleep disorders, 261; tolerance to, 70
National Academies of Sciences, Engineering, and Medicine (NASEM), 48, 184, 194, 237
National Commission on Marijuana and Drug Abuse, 47
National Inpatient Sample database, 220
National Institute on Drug Abuse (NID), 279
National Organization for the Reform of Marijuana Laws (NORML), 47–48, 279, 280
nausea, 34, 39, 63, 89, 183–85, 192
N-desmethylclobazam, 129, 210
neurodegenerative disorders: Alzheimer's disease, 68, 72, 88, 99, 162, 238, 240–42; amyotrophic lateral sclerosis (ALS), 74, 81, 238–40; case study on, 247–49; Huntington's disease, 39, 75, 238, 242–44; Parkinson's disease, 30, 39, 68, 85, 238–39, 244–47
neuropathy, 110, 189, 194–200, 236
neurotransmitter receptors, 15
neurotransmitters: in adolescence, 144; CBD changing flow of, 69, 70, 208; in

endocannabinoid system, 29, 170, 204, 254; fibromyalgia and, 213; imbalances in, 31–32, 161, 170; schizophrenia and, 254
New Mexico, 196–97, 250
New York State, 196, 197
Nixon, Richard, 47, 279
non-cannabinoid receptor targets, 37, 66–67
N-palmitoylethanolamide (PEA), 258
NSAIDs, 166, 194, 212

obesity, 39–40, 163, 202, 203
opioid receptors, 27, 37, 62, 68, 197–98
opioids, 50, 128, 187, 188, 197, 198
O'Shaughnessy, William, 278

pain relief, 17, 184, 186–88, 192, 195. *See also* chronic pain and neuropathy
pain sensation, 32–33
Parkinson's disease (PD), 30, 39, 68, 85, 238–39, 244–47
pediatric patients, 108, 121, 123, 172, 205–8
peripheral nervous system, 35, 136–37
permeation enhancers, 112–13
pesticides, 99–101, *100*, 104
pharmaceutical medications: for ADHD, 170–72; for ALS, 239; antiepileptic drugs (AEDs), 203–5, 209–11; for anxiety and depression, 155, 157, 159, 161; for arthritis, 164; for asthma, 169; for autism spectrum disorder, 174, 177; for autoimmune conditions, 181–82; for cancer pain, 187; for chemotherapy-induced nausea and vomiting, 183–84; for chronic pain, 194–98; drug–drug interactions, 128–30; for fibromyalgia, 212–14; for gastroesophageal reflux, 217; for glaucoma, 226; metabolization in liver, 54, 128; for migraine headaches, 231–33; for multiple sclerosis, 236; for PTSD, 249; safety of medical cannabis compared to, 49; for schizophrenia, 254; for seizure disorders, ix–x, 212; side effects of, x, xii, 132, 146–47, 159, 161, 169–72, 187, 203, 213, 217, 236, 254; single active compound of, 9; for sleep disorders, 260–62; for traumatic brain injury, 271
phytocannabinoids: as active compound of cannabis plant, 9, 10–14; antibacterial, antiviral, and antifungal effects of, 227; anticancer properties of, 188–89;

Index

availability of, 59; biphasic effects of, 125, 177; cannabis plants' profile of, 17, 19–20, 21, 22, 23; cannabis plants' synthesis of, 11–14, *13*; charts on, 6; cytokines and, 226–27; flavonoids and, 18, 19; as immune modulators, 227; medicinal effects of, 11, 14, 59, 91, *290–93*; metabolization of, 128; as neuroprotective agents, 271; nonintoxicating phytocannabinoids, 136; pharmokinetics of, 285–88; research on, xii, 10; side effects from, 54–55; terpenoids and, 15, 17. *See also specific phytocannabinoids*

pinene, 17, 169, 171, 181, 222, 238, 242, 252, 262

postsynaptic neurons, *28*, 29

post-traumatic stress disorder (PTSD), 30, 194, 249–53, 261

PPARs (peroxisome proliferator-activated receptors), 37, 62, 67, 75, 81, 216

pregnancy and breastfeeding, 136, 142–44

presynaptic neurons, 28–29, *28*

Project CBD, 22, 130

pruritis/itching, 258, 260

psoriasis, 81, 82, 108, 109, 110, 258–59

psoriatic arthritis, 164, 259

pulmonary risks, 136, 139–41

Randall, Robert, 279–80

rectal suppositories, 111, 287

Reefer Madness (film), 199, 278

Report of the Indian Hemp Drugs Commission, 46–47, 278

Research Advisory Panel of California, 224–25

rimonabant, 40, 85, 202

RSO (Rick Simpson oil), 116, 117

rufinamide (Banzel), 130, 210

Russo, Ethan, 38

Saneto, Russell, 207

SARS, 227

schizophrenia, 39, 74, 145–46, 253–56

seizures and seizure disorders: ADHD and, 172; case studies on, 23–25, 44; CBD:THC tincture for, 71; CBD and, 146–49; CBDV and, 86; definition of, 203; endocannabinoid system as physiologic regulator of, 174–75; pharmaceutical medications for, ix–x;

THCA and, 74; traumatic brain injury and, 270; types of, 203. *See also* epilepsy

serotonin, 170, 254

serotonin receptors, 62, 67, 77, 81, 84, 157

skin, 36, 109–10, 256, 259

skin cancer, 189, 190, 259–60

skin disorders: acne, 90, 256–57; allergic contact dermatitis, 110, 257; atopic dermatitis/eczema, 108–10, 257–58; endocannabinoid system and, 257–58; pruritis/itching, 258; psoriasis, 81, 82, 108, 109, 110, 258–59; skin cancer, 189, 190, 259–60

sleep apnea, 262, 263

sleep disorders: ADHD and, 172; ALS and, 240; Alzheimer's disease and, 242; anxiety and, 157, 158; appetite and, 163; arthritis and, 166, 167; autoimmune conditions and, 181–82; cannabinoid receptors and, 41; cannabis used for, 52, 184, 186, 261–62; cannabis withdrawal syndrome and, 57; case studies on, 159–60, 182, 199–200, 215, 223, 234, 235, 252, 253; CBDA and, 79; CBD for, 45, 206, 207, 211; CBD:THC ratio for, 199–200; CBG for, 82, 83; CBN for, 73; Crohn's disease and, 219; dosing and, 118, 262; drug–drug interactions and, 128; endocannabinoid system and, 38, 43; fibromyalgia and, 212–14; Huntington's disease and, 244; insomnia, 17, 82, 83, 172, 181, 250, 252, 262; management of symptoms, 154, 194, 197, 199, 202; migraine headaches and, 231, 233–35; multiple sclerosis and, 238, 261; negative impact of, 260–61; Parkinson's disease and, 246, 247; pruritis/itching and, 258, 260; psoriasis and, 259; PTSD and, 249–53, 261; research on, 261; sleep apnea, 262, 263; spinal cord injury and, 264, 265; THC+CBD extract for, 188; THC causing sleepiness, 66, 106, 126, 127; THC for, 45, 63, 64–65, 105, 262; Tourette syndrome and, 269; traumatic brain injury and, 270, 271, 272; ulcerative colitis and, 223–24

smoking, 102–3, 136, 139–41, 169

solvents, 96–98, *97*, 104

spinal cord injury, 264–67

state cannabis laws, 59, 281–83

state-regulated dispensaries, 14, 22–23, 93, 190

Index

status epilepticus, 147, 204
steroids, 44, 132, 219, 236, 257, 258
stress, 155, 202, 221–22, 231, 233–34, 249, 259
sublingual tinctures, as delivery method, 102, 107–8, *117*, 125, 169, 178, 233, 237, 240, 286
Sulak, Dustin, 207

Tashkin, Donald, 140, 168, 279
temporomandibular joint disorders, 73, 221
terpenoids: as active compound of cannabis plant, 9, 15, 158; anti-inflammation benefits of, 166, 181, 209; antiseizure effects of, 74; bronchodilatory effects of, 169; cannabis plants' profile of, 17, 19–20, 21, 23; in cannabis varieties, 9, 92; charts on, 6; as essential oils in cannabis plant, 14–15, 17, 95; flavonoids and, 18, 19; gastroesophageal reflux and, 218; geranyl diphosphate as precursor to, 11; for irritable bowel syndrome, 222; medicinal effects of, 15, *16–17*, 73, 95, 171, *296–301*; phytocannabinoids and, 15, 17; profiles of, 95–96, *96*; PTSD and, 252; schizophrenia and, 256
terpinolene, 218, 222
THC (delta-9-tetrahydrocannabinol): acute overdose symptoms, 50, 106, 107, 126–27, 205; ADHD improved with THC-rich cannabis, 171, 173; adolescent use of, 145–46; adverse side effects of, 53–54, 56, 65–66, 125–27; for allergic contact dermatitis, 257; for ALS, 239; for Alzheimer's disease, 241–42; antianxiety effects of, 158; anticancer properties of, 188–90, 193; antiemetic properties of, 183–85; as antiepileptic, 204–5; anxiety associated with use, 53, 66, 70, 127, 156–57; appetite and, 34, 63, 161–63; for asthma, 169; augmenting action of anandamide, 157; autism spectrum disorders symptoms improved with, 175–76; availability of, 59; binding to cannabinoid receptors, 60, 61, 67, 70; biphasic effects of, 125, 168; for cancer pain, 187–88, 195; Cannabinoid Hyperemesis Syndrome, 55–56; cannabis variety *indica* containing, 19; cardiovascular risks with use of, 136–38;

categories of products and effects, *120*; CBC interaction with, 90; CBD preventing anxiety and paranoia caused by, 70, 127; CBN combined with, 72–73; chronic toxicity of, 51, 52; clinical indications of, 63–66; composition of phytocannabinoids, 12, 13, 19–20; for Crohn's disease, 219, 221; for diabetes, 201; discovery of, 72; distribution and metabolism of, 287–88; dosing of, 34, 53, 65, 119, 122, 125–27, 157–58, 205; driving under the influence of, 136, 141–42; drug–drug interactions, 128–30; endocannabinoid dysfunction corrected with, 61, 63–64; for fibromyalgia, 213–14; first-time use of THC-rich cannabis, 125–26; for gastroesophageal reflux, 217–18; for glaucoma, 63, 224–25, 226; for hepatitis C, 230–31; for HIV, 228, 230; for Huntington's disease, 243; for infectious diseases, 227; ingestion of THC-rich cannabis, 105–6, 126; inhalation of THC-rich cannabis, 102; intoxicating effects of, 59, 60, 70, 76, 102, 105, 114, 127, 158, 205, 218, 221; for irritable bowel syndrome, 222; medical risks of, 61; medicinal effects of, 63–66; for migraine headaches, 64, 118, 233; molecular structure of, *10*; for multiple sclerosis, 42, 238; pain relief properties of, 195, 198, 213; for Parkinson's disease, 247; potency of THC-rich cannabis, 13, 65, 106, 107; pregnancy and breastfeeding with THC use, 136, 142–44; for psoriasis, 259; psychoactive effects of, 59, 102; for PTSD, 250, 251, 253; ratio of CBD to THC, 20, 22–23, 56–57, 70–71, 79, 114, 119, *120*, 121–22, 124, 158, 166–67, 172, 176–77, 181–82, 196, 198–200, 202, 215, 218, 221, 236, 238, 242, 244, 251; recreational use of, 49, 57, 127, 137, 156; rectal suppositories of, 111; research on, 10, 14, 26–27, 61–62; risk of dependence, 57; schizophrenia and, 146, 254–55, 256; as single compound, 11; for sleep apnea, 263; for sleep disorders, 63, 64–65, 262; for spinal cord injury, 265; synergistic enhancement with CBD, 14; synthetic THC, 153, 183, 184, 185–86, 195, 213, 217, 222, 228; THC+CBDA, 77; THC+CBD extract, 188; THC-rich edibles, 106, 205; tolerance to, 41–42,

56–57, 65–66, 76, 137, 158, 163, 173, 188, 205, 251, 270; topical application of, 108–9; for Tourette syndrome, 268–70; for traumatic brain injury, 272; for ulcerative colitis, 219, 223

THCA (tetrahydrocannabinolic acid): for ADHD, 172; antianxiety benefits of, 157–58; antiemetic properties of, 75, 185; anti-inflammation benefits of, 166, 167, 181; for autism spectrum disorders, 178; availability of, 59, 76–77; avoiding conversion to THC, 76–77; in cannabis tea, 107; categories of products and effects, 120; for Crohn's disease, 221; decarboxylation process converting to THC, 73–74; dosing of, 119, 122–23; for epilepsy, 205; for fibromyalgia, 214; for irritable bowel syndrome, 222; medicinal effects of, 75–77; for migraine headaches, 182, 233; for multiple sclerosis, 238; for pain relief, 198–99; for Parkinson's disease, 248; as precursor to CBD, 11–12; as predominant phytocannabinoid compound in raw flowers, 11, 73; for psoriasis, 259; research on, 74, 75; side effects of, 55, 76; for spinal cord injury, 265; as tinctures, 125; for Tourette syndrome, 270; for traumatic brain injury, 273; for ulcerative colitis, 224

THCV (delta-9-tetrahydrocannabivarin): for acne, 257; appetite and, 163; availability of, 59, 203; categories of products and effects, 121; dosing of, 123; medicinal effects of, 84–86, 203; as neutral antagonist at CB_1 receptors, 83–84, 202; for Parkinson's disease, 246, 247; as phytocannabinoid, 10–11; for PTSD, 252; side effects of, 55; THCV+THC, 85

tobacco, 50, 139
topical application, as delivery method, 102, 108–10, 166–67, 258–59, 286–87
topiramate (Topamax, Trokendi XR, or Qudexy XR), 130, 210
Tourette syndrome (TS), 172, 267–70
transdermal patches, 112–13, 165, 235, 287
transplants, 180–81
traumatic brain injury (TBI), 30, 270–74
triptans, 231–32
TRPA1, 80
TRP channels, 61–62, 68, 75, 78, 80, 84, 86, 90
TRPM8, 80, 84
TRPV (transient receptor potential vanilloid), 37
TRPV1, 80, 84, 216, 245
TRPV2, 80, 84
TRPV3, 84
TRPV4, 84
2-AG, 27, 77–78, 80, 156

ulcerative colitis, 216, 218–21, 223–24

valproic acid (Depakote), 54, 130, 208, 210
vaporization, as delivery method, 102, 103–5, 128, 140–41, 167, 169, 185, 195, 198, 235, 237, 240

Ware, Marc, 52
Weed (CNN documentary), 24, 58, 148
Whole Plant Access for Autism, 178
whole-plant products, 95, 135, 153, 184, 205–8, 211

Young, Francis L., 48, 280

zonisamide (Zonegran), 130, 210

About the Author

Bonni Goldstein, MD, is the medical director of Canna-Centers, a Los Angeles–based medical practice that helps patients use cannabis for serious and chronic illnesses. She specialized in pediatric emergency medicine for years before witnessing the amazing benefits of this treatment in an ill loved one. Since then, she has successfully treated thousands of adult and pediatric patients with cannabis medicine and regularly speaks about the topic at conferences and to patient groups around the world. She is a board member of the International Association for Cannabis as Medicine and is medical advisor to Weedmaps.com. Dr. Goldstein was awarded 2017 Medical Professional of the Year by Americans for Safe Access.